BLOOM & FAWCETT:

CONCISE HISTOLOGY

Don W. Fawcett, M.D.

Hersey Professor of Anatomy and Cell Biology, Emeritus
Harvard Medical School

Ronald P. Jensh, Ph.D.
Contributing Editor

Professor of Pathology, Anatomy, and Cell Biology
Jefferson Medical College of Thomas Jefferson University

CHAPMAN & HALL

 INTERNATIONAL THOMSON PUBLISHING

New York • Albany • Bonn • Boston • Cincinnati • Detroit • London
Madrid • Melbourne • Mexico City • Pacific Grove • Paris • San Francisco
Singapore • Tokyo • Toronto • Washington

Join Us on the Internet
WWW: http://www.thomson.com
EMAIL: findit@kiosk.thomson.com

thomson.com is the on-line portal for the products, services and resources available from
International Thomson Publishing (ITP).
This Internet kiosk gives users immediate access to more than 34 ITP publishers and over 20,000
products. Through *thomson.com* Internet users can search catalogs, examine subject-specific
resource centers and subscribe to electronic discussion lists. You can purchase ITP products from
your local bookseller, or directly through *thomson.com*.

Visit Chapman & Hall's Internet Resource Center for information on our new publications,
links to useful sites on the World Wide Web and an opportunity to join our e-mail mailing list.
Point your browser to: **http://www.chaphall.com/chaphall.html**
or **http://www.chaphall.com/chaphall/med.html** for Medicine

Cover design: Curtis Tow Graphics

A service of I(T)P®

Printed in the United States of America

Chapman & Hall
115 Fifth Avenue
New York, NY 10003

Chapman & Hall
2-6 Boundary Row
London SE1 8HN
England

Thomas Nelson Australia
102 Dodds Street
South Melbourne, 3205
Victoria, Australia

Chapman & Hall GmbH
Postfach 100 263
D-69442 Weinheim
Germany

International Thomson Editores
Campos Eliseos 385, Piso 7
Col. Polanco
11560 Mexico D.F
Mexico

International Thomson Publishing–Japan
Hirakawacho Kyowa Building, 3F
1-2-1 Hirakawacho-cho
Chiyoda-ku, 102 Tokyo
Japan

International Thomson Publishing Asia
221 Henderson Road #05-10
Henderson Building
Singapore 0315

1 2 3 4 5 6 7 8 9 10 XXX 01 00 99 98 97

Library of Congress Cataloging-in-Publication Data

Fawcett, Don Wayne, 1917–
    Bloom and Fawcett : concise histology / Don W. Fawcett, Ronald P.
  Jensh.
       p.   cm.
    Includes index.
    ISBN 0-412-07971-2 (alk. paper)
    1. Histology.   I. Jensh, Ronald P.   II. Title.
    [DNLM: 1. Histology.   QS 504 F278c 1996]
  QM551.F337   1996
  611'.018—dc20
  DNLM/DLC
  for Library of Congress   96-19630
                                                                         CIP

British Library Cataloging in Publication Data available

To order this or any other Chapman & Hall book, please contact **International Thomson
Publishing, 7625 Empire Drive, Florence, KY 41042.** Phone: (606) 525-6600 or 1-800-842-3636.
Fax: (606) 525-7778. e-mail: order@chaphall.com.

For a complete listing of Chapman & Hall titles, send your request to **Chapman & Hall, Dept. BC,
115 Fifth Avenue, New York, NY 10003.**

Contents

Preface

With the addition of cellular biology, molecular biology and genetics to the medical school curriculum in recent years, the time allotted to histology has been greatly shortened and the **Bloom & Fawcett Textbook of Histology** became too large for students in the courses now given. We have therefore undertaken to produce a more concise version of the textbook. It is my hope that its abridged text will better meet the needs of students, while still giving them the benefit of many of the instructive illustrations, many in color, that have been acquired over the years for the larger book.

I wish to express my deep gratitude to Professor Jay Angevine for revision of his chapter on the nervous system. I am also indebted to Dr. Ronald Jensh who has contributed outlines, key words and multiple choice examination questions for each chapter. It is hoped that these will enable the student to evaluate his/her success in assimilation of the salient features of the text.

Don W. Fawcett, M.D.

1

THE CELL

CHAPTER OUTLINE

KEY WORDS

Actin
Anaphase
Apoptosis
ATP
Autophagy
Axoneme
Centrioles
Centromere
Centrosome
Chromatin
Cilia
Cleavage Furrow
Cristae
Desmin
DNA
Dynein
Endocytosis
Endosome
Equatorial Plate
Euchromatin
Flagellum
Glucose
Heterochromatin
Heterophagy
Histones
Interphase
Keratin
Kinesin
Kinetochore

Lamellipodia
Lamins: A, B
Lipochrome
  Pigment
Lipofuchsin
Metaphase
Mitotic Spindle
Myosin
Necrosis
Neurofilaments
Nuclear Lamina
Nucleosome
Pars Fibrosa
Pars Granulosa
Pericentriolar
  Bodies
Perinuclear
  Cisterna
Phagocytosis
Pinocytosis
Plasmalemma
Polysomes
Pseudopodia
RNA: mRNA,
  tRNA
Telophase
Transcription
Tubulins
Vimentin

The cell is a unit of protoplasm limited by a cell membrane (or **plasmalemma**) and partitioned into two major compartments, a spherical or ovoid nucleus, surrounded by the **cytoplasm,** that makes up the greater part of the cell volume. The nucleus contains the genetic material of the cell, **deoxyribonucleic acid (DNA)** and associated proteins that control the synthetic activities of the cell. The cytoplasm contains two categories of formed elements: **organelles** and **inclusions.** The organelles are minute organs of the cell, each specialized for carrying out specific biochemical processes essential for its metabolism. The inclusions are metabolically inert stores of nutrients, or accumulated cell products. The organelles and inclusions are distributed in a gel-like cytoplasmic matrix containing ions and various organic molecules in its aqueous phase. It also contains slender **microfilaments,** some of which serve to stabilize cell shape, whereas others are involved in cell motility. In addition, there are slender **microtubules** that serve as tracks, along which materials are moved from place to place within the cell. Together, the microfilaments and microtubules constitute the **cytoskeleton.** In routine histological preparations viewed with the light microscope, the nucleus and some cytoplasmic inclusions are visible. The organelles can be revealed only by special staining techniques. The range of visible cell components has been vastly extended by the electron microscope which has revealed the substructure of the organelles, inclusions (Fig. 1-1) and even smaller units, down to the level of macromolecules.

CELL MEMBRANE

The cell membrane, or plasmalemma, forms the boundary between the cell and its environment. Other membranes within the cell bound the organelles, and thus segregate different biochemical activities. They limit diffusion and actively control the passage of ions and small molecules between functionally distinct compartments. Although the various membranes of the cell differ slightly in thickness and protein content, they all have the same basic molecular organization. In electron micrographs, they have a trilaminar appearance, consisting of two dense lines, 2.5–3.0 nm in thickness, separated by a less dense intermediate zone (Fig. 1-2). They consist of a bimolecular layer of mixed phospholipids, with the hydrophilic heads of the lipid molecules at the outer and inner surfaces, and their hydrophobic chains projecting toward the middle of the bilayer (Fig. 1-3). Each of the two layers of phospholipid is commonly referred to as one leaflet of the membrane. The two parallel dense lines, seen in electron micrographs, result from deposition of the heavy metal, osmium, in the hydrophilic ends of the phospholipid molecules. The intervening paler zone represents their unstained hydrocarbon chains. The lipid bilayer has the

properties of a two-dimensional fluid, within which the molecules are free to move about, if not bound to filaments in the underlying cytoplasm. Glycoproteins and glycolipids are also present within the phospholipid bilayer. Their oligosaccharide chains may form a delicate nap or mat that is called the **glycocalyx** on the outer surface of the membrane.

The simple trilaminar appearance of the cell membrane gives no hint of the diversity of its functions. The lipid bilayer permits diffusion of ions and gases into, and out of, the cell but prevents passive entry of most large molecules. Some of the many proteins in the membrane have important enzymatic functions; others serve as receptors for hormones and other signaling molecules that influence the behavior of the cell; still others form transmembrane channels that control the entry of specific ions. Some membrane proteins are involved in recognition and cohesion of like cells during organogenesis, whereas others serve as binding sites for attachment to other cells or to the extracellular matrix.

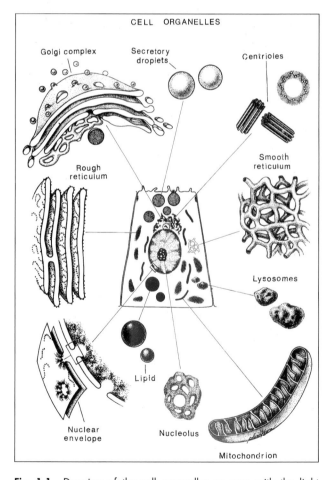

Fig. 1-1 Drawing of the cell organelles as seen with the light microscope (center). Their appearance in section and their three-dimensional forms as deduced from electron micrographs are shown around the periphery of the figure. (Drawing by Sylvia Collard/Keene.)

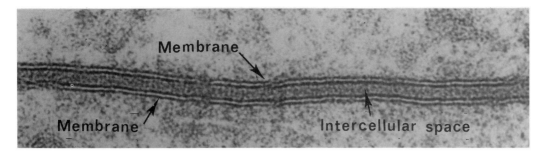

Fig. 1-2 Micrograph of the membranes of two adjoining epithelial cells and the intercellular space. Note that each membrane appears as two dense lines separated by an unstained zone representing the hydrocarbon chains of the lipid bilayer.

NUCLEUS

Nuclear Envelope

The largest of the cell organelles is its **nucleus,** a centrally located, membrane-bounded compartment that is usually round or ovoid but may be deeply infolded or lobulated in a few cell types. The nucleus is bounded by a **nuclear envelope** that is not visible with the light microscope. In electron micrographs, it is seen to consist of two parallel membranes separated by a 10–30-nm space termed the **perinuclear cisterna** (Fig. 1-4). The outer membrane is often continuous with that of tubular elements that ramify throughout the cytoplasm. At many sites around the periphery of the nucleus, the outer and inner membranes are continuous with one another small **nuclear pores** that serve as avenues of communication between the nucleoplasm and the cytoplasm (Fig. 1-4, inset). In thin sections, the pores appear to be closed by a thin pore diaphragm, but this is deceptive. In negatively stained preparations of isolated nuclear envelopes, it can be shown that there are interconnected rings of 15-nm particles attached to the inner and outer rims of the pore and projecting into it. These so-called spokes do not occlude the

pore but are evidently responsible for the specious appearance of a diaphragm in thin sections. The pore has a central channel with an effective diameter of 10 nm. Its membranous and nonmembranous components together are now referred to as the pore complex.

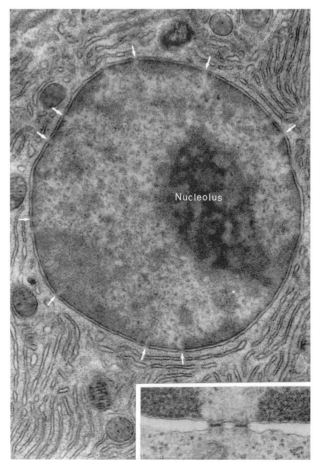

Fig. 1-4 Micrograph of a typical nucleus showing a prominent nucleolus and large aggregations of heterochromatin against the nuclear membrane, which is traversed by nuclear pores (at arrows). The inset shows two nuclear pores and their pore diaphragms at higher magnification.

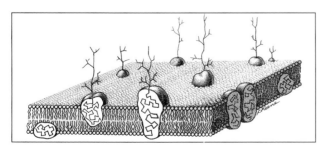

Fig. 1-3 Schematic drawing of the fluid mosaic model of the cell membrane. Globular protein molecules are positioned at different depths in the lipid bilayer depending on the distribution of their hydrophilic and hydrophobic regions. The lipid bilayer is fluid and the proteins are free to move laterally within the plane of the membrane. Terminal oligosaccharides of glycoproteins extend outward contributing to the surface coat or glycocalyx.

Nuclear Lamina

In the nucleoplasm adjacent to the nuclear envelope, there is a continuous meshwork of fine filaments, forming the **nuclear lamina.** In different cell types, this layer varies from 30 to 110 nm in thickness. Its filaments are polymers of polypeptides called lamins. **Type-A** and **type-B lamins** are distinguished on the basis their chemical properties and location. Type-A lamins are located mainly on the inner aspect of the nuclear lamina. Those of the B type predominate near its outer surface and are responsible for binding the nuclear lamina to integral proteins of the nuclear envelope. The nuclear lamina contributes to the shape and structural stability of the nucleus and there is some evidence that its lamins are involved in the organization of the nucleoplasm after cell division.

Chromatin

The nucleus is the archive of the cell, the repository of its genetic information encoded in the sequence of nucleotides in long deoxyribonucleic acid (DNA) molecules. In the period between cell divisions (interphase), most of the DNA is condensed adjacent to the nuclear envelope in clumps that stain intensely with basic dyes, and were traditionally called the **chromatin.** Some of the chromatin is not condensed but is in an extended state and is not visible with a light microscope. Its condensed, stainable portion is now designated the **heterochromatin,** and the dispersed portion is called **euchromatin.** At any given time, only the DNA of the euchromatin is actively involved in the transcription of its genetic information, and this is a very small fraction of the total.

Heterochromatin is made up of 30-nm fibrils. When isolated and subjected to high shear forces, the substructure of the fibrils is revealed. They consist of a strand of particles of basic protein, called **nucleosomes,** with a 4-nm filament of DNA wrapped helically around them. Each nucleosome is an octomer of four different **histones** (simple proteins containing numerous basic groups, **H2A, H2B, H3, and H4**). An additional type of histone (H1 or H5) is attached to the DNA filament between successive nucleosomes. The strand of nucleosomes and its associated DNA is coiled in a solenoid around a central channel to form the 30-nm fibril (Fig. 1-5). The granular appearance of heterochromatin, in section, is attributable to transverse and oblique sections of the 30-nm fibrils or higher orders of their coiling. The structure of euchromatin is largely conjectural, but it is assumed that the 30-nm fibrils are uncoiled, during transcription, to expose the appropriate nucleotide sequences of the DNA. **Transcription** is the process of synthesis of **ribonucleoprotein (RNA)** on a segment of DNA that serves as a template. In preparation for cell division, transcription ceases and all of the chromatin becomes reorganized into a number of **chromosomes,** rodlike structures of varying length in which the

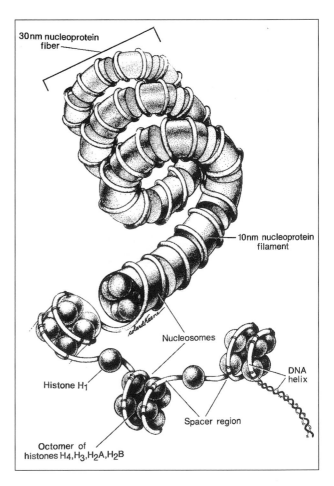

Fig. 1-5 Diagram of a 30-nm chromatin fiber showing its postulated helical structure. In the lower portion of the figure, the fiber is drawn out to maximal extension to show the core of histones in the nucleosomes with the DNA double helix wrapped around them. (Redrawn from R. Bradbury, La Recherche 9:644, 1978, and A. Worcel and C. Benyaj, Cell 12:88, 1978.)

30-nm filaments form loops radiating from a fibrillar protein core. These will be discussed later in the chapter in a section on cell division.

> *A gene is a coding sequence of nucleotides in the DNA that serves as a template for assembly of an RNA molecule that is transcribed in the synthesis of a protein. The DNA of the human haploid genome contains about 80,000 genes. Mutations of a single gene may result in a disease confined to a single organ, or one with more general effects throughout the body. Mutated genes are responsible for many inherited diseases.*

Nucleolus

An eccentrically placed, refractile body visible in the nucleus of the living cell is the **nucleolus.** In histological sections, it is stained by basic dyes but is unreactive to the

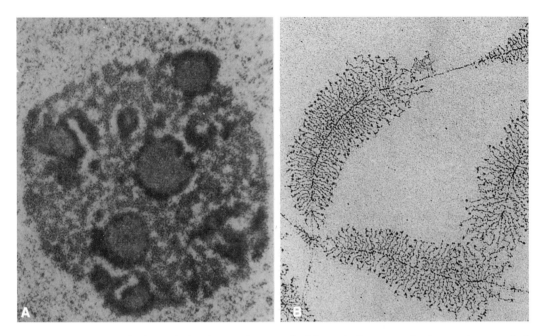

Fig. 1-6 (A) Micrograph of a nucleolus showing the network of the nucleolonema, and paler round areas called fibrillar centers. These contain the nucleolar-organizer regions of those chromosomes possessing nucleolar genes. (B) Dissociated nucleolar fibrillar centers showing rRNA-precursor molecules radiating from nucleolar genes. (Courtesy of O. Miller and C. Beatty, Science 164:164, 1969.)

Feulgen reaction for DNA. However, it is usually surrounded by a rim of nucleolus-associated chromatin (Fig. 1-4). In electron micrographs, the nucleolus appears as a network of anastomosing strands of dense granular material forming its **pars granulosa.** Within it are one or two pale, rounded areas, called fibrillar centers, surrounded by a rim of thin filaments, the **pars fibrosa** (Fig. 1-6A). The **fibrillar centers** are formed by fusion of nucleolar-organizer regions of those chromosomes possessing nucleotide sequences that code for **ribosomal ribonucleic acid (rRNA).** The pars fibrosa consists of 5–10-nm filamentous ribonucleoprotein molecules formed as transcripts of rRNA genes in the DNA. It has been possible to isolate transcriptionally active nucleolar genes of the fibrillar centers for examination with the electron microscope. In the remarkable images obtained, multiple RNA molecules can be seen radiating from a strand of DNA (ribosomal gene) in a christmas-tree-like configuration, with the transcripts quite short at one end and progressing to full-length completed molecules at the other end (Fig. 1-6B). After transcription in the fibrillar centers of the nucleolus, the RNA molecules are processed in the surrounding pars fibrosa and, there, are combined with protein imported from the cytoplasm. The resulting ribonucleoprotein accumulates in the **pars granulosa** where later steps in the formation of subunits of small granules, called **ribosomes,** are completed. These then pass into the cytoplasm, where they have an important function in protein synthesis, which will be described below. Other ribonucleic acids synthesized on the DNA of the chromatin are **messenger RNA (mRNA),** which migrate to the cytoplasm to direct the synthesis of a specific protein, and **transfer RNAs,** which transport amino acids to the site of synthesis for incorporation into a protein.

Nuclear Matrix

Little is known about the form assumed by the chromosomes in the interphase nucleus, but it has been suggested that the portions of them that constitute the heterochromatin may be deployed along a karyoskeleton, a network of fibrils, which, in the dividing cell, form the cores of the chromosomes. Such fibrils are not seen in routine preparations with the light or electron microscope. However, after digestion of nuclei with deoxyribonuclease, extraction with detergents and high-ionic-strength salt solution, a network of thin, branching 8–10-nm filaments can be seen. It is speculated that the chromatin and other nuclear components are organized around these so-called core filaments which may serve to maintain structural order within the nucleus. The possibility that these filaments are a product of the procedures required for their demonstration, and not a true reflection of the architecture of the nucleoplasm, has not been ruled out.

CYTOPLASMIC ORGANELLES

Suspended in the cytoplasmic matrix are several kinds of membrane-bounded structures that are specialized for the performance of different cell functions. A description of the form and function of the several cytoplasmic organelles follows.

Endoplasmic Reticulum

In electron micrographs, nearly all cells contain an extensive system of membrane-bounded tubules, comprising the **endoplasmic reticulum.** This organelle is not visible in the living cell, but if cell cultures are exposed to a lipophilic fluorescent dye, it is revealed as a lacelike network throughout the cytoplasm. In histological sections, continuity of the reticulum is interrupted and it appears as branching tubules of varying length. Two distinct regional differentiations of the organelle are identifiable, the **rough endoplasmic reticulum** (RER) and the **smooth endoplasmic reticulum** (SER). The RER is distinguished by the presence of 25–30-nm granules of ribonucleoprotein (ribosomes) on the surface of its membrane. These occur in groups of 8–10 uniformly spaced along a molecule of messenger RNA (Fig. 1-8, inset). The tubules are often locally expanded into broad flattened saccules, or cisternae, that may be stacked in close parallel arrays (Figs. 1-7 and 1-8). These stacks correspond to the "basophilic bodies" seen with the light microscope in protein-secreting cell types. The tubules of the SER have no adhering ribosomes and they form a close-meshed network devoid of cisternae.

The rough endoplasmic reticulum, with its associated ribosomes, is the site of synthesis of proteins for export, and of many of the proteins that are utilized within the cell. The initiation of protein synthesis begins in the cytoplasmic matrix with the attachment of a free ribosome to a signal sequence at the 5′ end of a molecule of **messenger RNA**

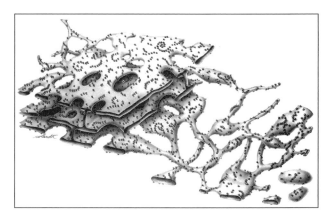

Fig. 1-7 Drawing of the three-dimensional configuration of the rough endoplasmic reticulum. It consists of branching and anastomosing tubular elements and expanded saccules, called cisternae, that are often arranged parallel. Polyribosomes occur in spirals or circles on its membrane.

(mRNA) (Figs. 1-9, 1-10). After translation of this sequence, a signal-recognition particle binds to the ribosome. This, in turn, binds to a ribosome receptor in the membrane of the endoplasmic reticulum. The ribosome moves along the mRNA molecule, reading, in each successive set of three nucleotides (codons), the instructions that determine the sequence of assembly of the amino acids that will make up the protein. Each amino acid is brought to the assembly site on the ribosome by a **transfer RNA (tRNA)** that is specific for that amino acid. The tRNA molecule rec-

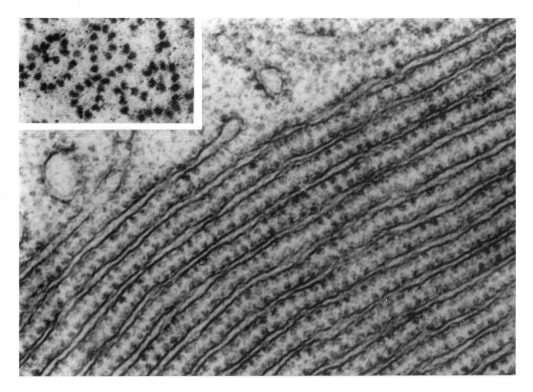

Fig. 1-8 Electron micrograph of several parallel cisternae of the rough endoplasmic reticulum, bearing numerous ribosomes on their surface. The inset shows a surface view of polyribosomes on a cisterna of the reticulum.

ognizes, and binds to, the appropriate complimentary site on the mRNA molecule. This amino acid is then inserted into the nascent polypeptide chain and the tRNA molecule is released. The ribosome then moves along to the next codon and the process is repeated, with the insertion of one amino acid after another. The mRNA molecule, the ribosomes, and the nascent polypeptide chains can be seen in a micrograph of isolated translation units (Fig. 1-9 1-10). Two integral membrane proteins of the endoplasmic reticulum (ribophorins I and II), form a transmembrane channel beneath the ribosomes, through which the lengthening polypeptide chains extend into the lumen of the reticulum. When the signal sequence reaches the lumen, it is cleaved off by a signal peptidase on the inner aspect of the membrane. As the first ribosome moves on, the second ribosome reads the same codon, and so on. This process continues, with each ribosome of the polysome assembling a molecule of the protein specified by the mRNA. When each ribosome reaches the end of the message, it separates from the membrane and from the mRNA. When the entire message has been translated, protein synthesis is terminated. The molecules that have been synthesized accumulate in the lumen of the reticulum. They are then enclosed in small transport vesicles that bud off from transitional regions of

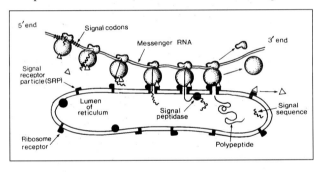

Fig. 1-9 Schematic representation of protein synthesis on ribosomes of the rough endoplasmic reticulum. When the nascent polypeptide chain emerges, its signal sequence binds to a signal-receptor protein (SRP). This, in turn, binds to a specific receptor in the membrane of the reticulum. A pore is formed through which the lengthening polypeptide chain is translocated into the lumen. The signal peptide is cleaved off, and the protein is transported in vesicles to the Golgi. (Redrawn from Walter, P. and Blobel, G. *J. Cell Biol.* 91:557, 1981.)

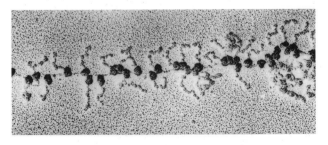

Fig. 1-10 An isolated translation unit, showing the ribosomes spaced along the thin molecule of messenger RNA with a nascent polypeptide chain emerging from each ribosome. (Micrograph courtesy of E. Kiseleva.)

the reticulum and are transported to the Golgi complex of the cell for packaging in secretory granules.

The rough and smooth endoplasmic reticulum are continuous and are regional specializations of the same organelle for different functions. As detailed above, the rough reticulum is involved in protein synthesis. The smooth reticulum varies greatly in its functions and in its extent in different cell types. It is very abundant in cells of the adrenal, ovary, and testis, where it is involved in the synthesis of steroid hormones. In the liver, it participates in reactions that are involved in the breakdown of drugs and alcohol, and detoxification of noxious chemicals that contaminate our environment. In muscle, there is a special form of smooth reticulum called the sarcoplasmic reticulum. This form of the organelle stores calcium and releases it to trigger muscle contraction.

Golgi Complex

The **Golgi complex (Golgi apparatus)** is a major organelle found in nearly all cells. It is essential in the secretory pathway and is especially conspicuous in glandular cells that produce a large volume of secretion. In such cells, it is located between the nucleus and the cell apex. It is not seen in routine histological sections but can be selectively stained by impregnation with silver or osmium in classical staining methods developed in the 1800s. It is composed of one or more stacks of smooth-surfaced cisternae that are not continuous with those of the endoplasmic reticulum (Fig. 1-11). These are often curved with their convex side toward the reticulum and the concave side toward the nucleus. In section, the lumen of a Golgi cistern is narrow throughout most of its length but is slightly expanded at either end. Numerous small vesicles are found near the ends of the cisternae. A polarity exists within the organelle. One or two cisternae at the convex, outer side of the stack are designated its cis-compartment and several at its inner side are the trans-compartment. Histochemical staining reactions reveal that the membranes of the cis and trans compartments contain different enzymes and have different functions.

In secretory cells, the small transport vesicles that bud off from the rough endoplasmic reticulum fuse with the cisterna at the cis face of the Golgi complex. The secretory product is then slowly moved through the stack by vesicles budding off from one cisterna and fusing with the next. In its transit, the product is glycosylated, sulfated, or phosphorylated, depending on the nature of the secretion. It accumulates and is concentrated in a cisterna at the trans face which rounds up, forming a membrane-bounded secretory granule. This leaves the Golgi and moves to the apical cytoplasm to join others awaiting a signal for release from the cell. Of the many proteins synthesized in the rough endoplasmic reticulum, only one may be the secretory product of the cell. The others are proteins

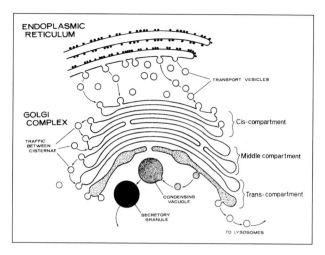

Fig. 1-11 Newly synthesized protein is transported from the endoplasmic reticulum to the Golgi complex in small vesicles that fuse with its cis compartment. The protein is transported between cisternae of the Golgi in vesicles and is modified in transit, and then concentrated in its transcompartment, where it is packaged into secretory granules for secretion.

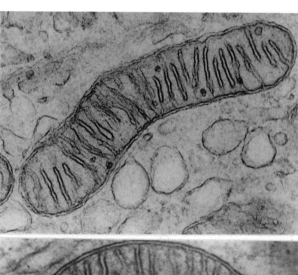

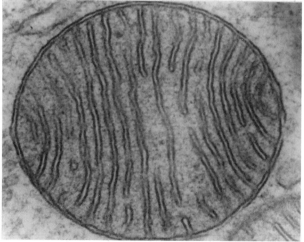

Fig. 1-12 Micrographs of mitochondria showing their limiting membranes and the cristae projecting into their interior. Mitochondria vary in shape from spherical to long flexible rods.

destined to be incorporated in other organelles or in the cell membrane. One of the several functions of the Golgi complex is to sort the proteins and add to them specific chemical groups that label them for packaging in separate vesicles for distribution to their respective destinations.

There are two secretory pathways from the Golgi complex. In most glandular cells, secretory granules accumulate in the apical cytoplasm until a neural or hormonal signal is received. The product is then released by **exocytosis,** a process in which the limiting membrane of each secretory granule fuses with the apical cell membrane, emptying its content into a system of ducts. This is called the **regulated secretory pathway.** Other cells secrete continuously in small vesicles that move from the Golgi complex to the surface and discharge their content without awaiting an external signal. This is termed the **constitutive secretory pathway.** In all cells, integral proteins for maintenance or renewal of cell components are moved in small vesicles directly from the Golgi to the appropriate intracellular site.

Mitochondria

In living cells, viewed with the phase-contrast microscope, slender rodlike **mitochondria** can be seen in the cytoplasm. They are 4–9 μm in length and 0.4–0.8 μm in diameter and are quite flexible, often changing their shape as they slowly move about in the cytoplasm. In electron micrographs, a mitochondrion is found to be limited by a smooth outer membrane and a slightly thinner inner membrane that forms varying numbers of thin folds, the **cristae mitochondriales,** that project into the interior of the organelle (Fig. 1-12). This plication is a device for increasing the surface area of the enzyme-rich inner membrane. Mitochondria are the principal site of production of the high-energy phosphate compound, **adenosine triphosphate (ATP),** that provides the energy necessary for many of the chemical reactions of the cell. In cells with high-energy requirements, the number of cristae in their mitochondria is much greater than in cells with lower energy needs.

The mitochondrial membranes bound two compartments: a large **intercristal space** in the interior of the organelle, and a smaller **membrane space,** which is the narrow interspace between the inner and outer membranes and extending between the membranes of the cristae. The membrane space has no visible content, but the intercristal space is occupied by a moderately dense mitochondrial matrix. Although the outer and inner membranes look alike, they differ in composition and physiological properties. The outer membrane contains transmembrane channels and is freely permeable to small molecules. The inner membrane is relatively impermeable and has an exceptionally high protein content. It is studded with numerous minute granules, about 10 nm in diameter that are connected to the membrane by a slender stem 3–4 nm thick and 5 nm in length. The phosphorylating system for converting ADP to ATP is located in these globular units. The intercristal space contains a few dense, more-or-less spherical **matrix granules** whose function is poorly understood. Each mitochondrion has its own DNA, consisting of a double helix in the form of a circle with a diameter of about 5.5 µm, resembling the DNA of bacteria. In evolving from symbiotic bacteria, the mitochondria have given over to the nucleus and cytoplasm of the host cell the coding and synthesis of most of their proteins. However, they still contain their own mRNA, tRNA, and rRNA. Mitochondria have a limited life span, but their numbers are maintained by a form of division that resembles the binary fission of bacteria.

> *Mutations may also occur in mitochondrial DNA, which contains genes encoding 13 proteins, all of which are part of an enzyme complex controlling oxygen consumption and its adaptation to energy needs. In Luft's disease, for example, the individual has an extremely high caloric intake, very high metabolic rate, and general weakness. Such mitochondrial diseases are inherited only through the mother.*

Lysosomes

The **lysosome** is an organelle that was not recognized by classical cytologists. Attention was first drawn to it by electron microscopic images and by histochemical reactions for acid phosphatase and 30 or more other hydrolytic enzymes. Lysosomes vary in number from a few to hundreds per cell. They are membrane-bounded, electron-dense bodies 0.2–0.8 µm in diameter, but they are so heterogeneous in size and shape that no single description encompasses all of their variations (Fig. 1-13). Their interior may appear homogeneous, or may contain dense granules of varying size in a less dense matrix. Occasionally they may contain crystals or concentric systems of lamellae. They can confidently be identified as lysosomes only by histochemical demonstration of acid phosphatase and other acid hydrolases in their interior.

Lysosomes are major agents of the waste-disposal and recycling system of the cell. Their great variety of hydrolytic enzymes are capable of digesting nearly all naturally occurring constituents of cells, as well as many foreign materials. Excess or damaged cell organelles are enclosed in a membrane to form an **autophagic vacuole**. This then fuses with a lysosome and its contents are digested. This process of controlled degradation of organelles by a healthy cell is called **autophagy** to distinguish it from **heterophagy**, which is the digestion of exogenous material taken into the cell. Undigestible residues may accumulate until the lyso-

some becomes an inactive **residual body.** A number of these may coalesce into larger masses, which are described as lipochrome pigment or **lipofuchsin pigment.** When abundant, lipochrome pigment may be visible with the light microscope as irregularly shaped yellow or brown bodies in the cytoplasm. Lysosomes also have an important role in processing substances normally taken up by cells, degrading them to split-products that can be used by the cell.

Peroxisomes

Peroxisomes are membrane-bounded bodies 0.2–1.0 µm in diameter with a content of lower density than that of lysosomes (Fig. 1-14). They are found in nearly all cell types. In metabolically active cells, such as those of the liver, they may number in the hundreds. In some animal species, the peroxisomes have a denser central region, called the **nucleoid,** which contains a crystal of urate oxidase. In primates, the nucleoid is lacking. The principal enzymes of peroxisomes are **D-amino acid oxidase, hydroxyacid oxidase, and catalase**. In the enzymatic degradation of amino acids and fatty acids, hydrogen peroxide is generated, but its potentially toxic effects are prevented by catalase of the peroxisomes, which breaks it down to water and oxygen. Several diseases have been

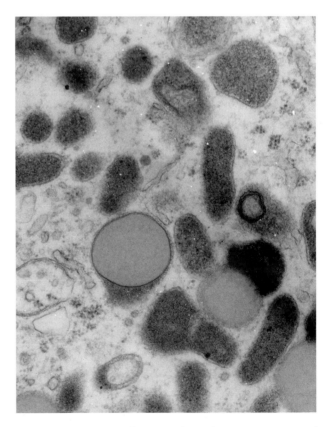

Fig. 1-13 Micrograph of an area of cytoplasm containing several lysosomes. These vary in shape and density.

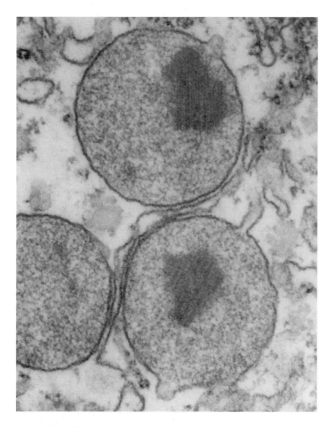

Fig. 1-14 Micrograph of two peroxisomes, each containing a dense inclusion, called the nucleoid, which is a crystal of urate oxidase. (Micrograph courtesy of D. Friend.)

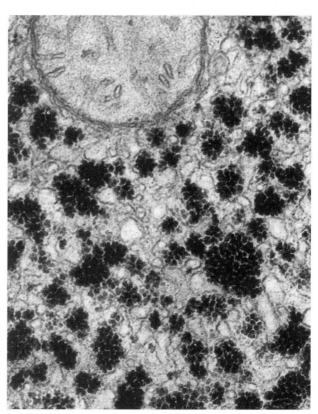

Fig. 1-15 Micrograph of an area of cytoplasm containing glycogen particles. These are aggregations of smaller subunits.

identified in which peroxisomes are not formed in normal numbers, or are deficient in one or more enzymes.

Centrosomes and Centrioles

Centrioles are self-replicating organelles, but because their structure includes a specific arrangement of microtubules, they will be described in detail following a discussion of microtubules.

CYTOPLASMIC INCLUSIONS

In addition to the organelles, which are active participants in the synthetic and metabolic activities of the cell, there are bodies in the cytoplasm that are simply stored-energy sources, or inert by-products of metabolism. These are not membrane bounded and are called cell inclusions to set them apart from cell organelles.

Glycogen

Glucose is the preferred metabolite for many cell types. When the blood glucose level is high, it is taken up and stored transiently in the cytoplasm of these cells in the form of **glycogen,** which is a polymer of glucose. When blood glucose levels are lower, glycogen is depolymerized to glucose which is metabolized to provide the energy for many cell activities. Glycogen is visible in electron micrographs in the form of 20–30-nm dense particles, widely distributed in the cytoplasm (Fig. 1-15).

Lipid

Nearly all cell types have the ability to store small quantities of lipid in their cytoplasm in the form of spherical droplets. Their lipid is extracted in the preparation of histological sections and only round, clear vacuoles remain. In electron micrographs, lipid is retained as spherical globules of varying size that stain from gray to black (Fig. 1-16). The droplets consist of **triglycerides** of fatty acids. Their metabolism yields energy and short carbon chains that can be reused in the synthesis of membranes and other lipid-containing components of the cell.

Pigment

Cell types that have a relatively long life span often contain deposits of **lipofuchsin,** a yellowish-brown pigment. These apparently represent accumulated undigestible

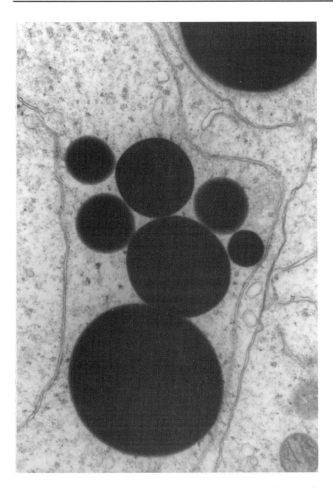

Fig. 1-16 Lipid droplets in a micrograph of an osmium-fixed cell. After gluteraldehyde fixation, they are not blackened and often appear a pale gray.

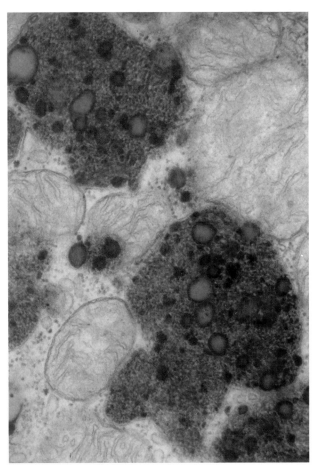

Fig. 1-17 Micrograph of lipofuchsin pigment granules. They vary in size, shape, and density of their content. The interior may appear quite heterogeneous.

residues of lysosomal activity. Unlike other inclusions, they may be bounded by a membrane. They may be dense throughout or may be aggregates of small bodies of varying density (Fig. 1-17). The storage of glycogen and lipid is transient, but lipofuchsin is enduring. It has no metabolic value, but the cell seems to have no means of clearing itself of this waste product.

There is a group of storage diseases in which a single enzyme may be lacking, resulting in accumulation of its substrate in the patient's cells. For example, in **Pompe's disease,** *the enzyme acid maltase is deficient and its substrate, glycogen, accumulates in excessive amounts in the liver, muscle, and other tissues. In other diseases of this group, there may be intracellular storage of lipid or gangliosides.*

CYTOSKELETON

The cytoplasm contains filamentous components, some of which maintain the shape of the cell, whereas others are

responsible for its motility. Others that are long slender tubules provide tracks along which particulates are moved from place to place within the cytoplasm. Collectively, these filamentous and tubular elements comprise the **cytoskeleton.** They are detectable in histological sections only where they occur in sizable bundles. The individual filaments are resolved by the electron microscope, but, because the ultrathin sections include only short segments, their three-dimensional organization is not apparent.

Microfilaments

The smallest filaments of the cytoskeleton, composed of the protein **actin,** are only about 7 nm in diameter and of varying length. Actin occurs in the cytoplasm in two forms: globular molecules of **G-actin** that are dispersed in the cytosol and are not visible with electron microscope, and **F-actin,** consisting of two identical strands coiled helically around one another to form filaments that are polymers of G-actin. Only about half of the actin in a cell is in the form of filaments. New filaments are formed, as needed, by polymerization from the pool of G-actin in the cytoplasm.

The majority of the actin filaments are in the ectoplasm, a gellike peripheral zone of the cytoplasm immediately beneath the plasmalemma. There, the filaments are crosslinked in a meshwork from which organelles are excluded. In the more fluid endoplasm, filaments are less abundant. However, under some circumstances, they may aggregate in bundles that are visible with the light or electron microscope. The contractile activity of the ectoplasm that is necessary for cell locomotion, and for the bulk uptake of substances from the environment, depends on the interaction of actin filaments with **myosin**. In muscle, both actin and myosin form filaments interdigitated in parallel array. Interaction between the heads of the molecules in the myosin filaments and the actin filaments produces a sliding of the filaments with respect to one another, resulting in shortening. In cells other than muscle, myosin does not form visible filaments and its configuration and mode of interaction with the actin filaments of the ectoplasm are still poorly understood.

Intermediate Filaments

The cytoplasm of cells also contains filaments about 10 nm in diameter that are referred to as **intermediate filaments** (Fig. 1-18). When these were first isolated from various cell types and analyzed, they proved to be not a single entity, but a family of morphologically similar, but biochemically distinct, filaments composed of subunits differing widely in molecular weight. Five categories of intermediate filaments can now be distinguished by immunocytochemical methods. All cell types contain intermediate filaments of one of these types. No one of them is common to all cells. In fibroblasts and several other cells of mesenchymal origin, the intermediate filaments consist of the 58-kDa protein **vimentin**. These may be aggregated in bundles or randomly oriented in a loose net-

work throughout the cytoplasm.

In smooth, striated, and skeletal muscle, the intermediate filaments are composed of the 53-kDa protein **desmin**. In smooth muscle, they form bundles linked together by dense bodies at sites of convergence of the actin filaments involved in contraction. They also attach to dense plaques on the inner surface of the cell membrane. They transmit the tension developed by the actin filaments and ensure a uniform distribution of force throughout the contracting cell. In striated and cardiac muscle, the desmin filaments are less abundant but form a loose network around and between the contractile components.

The intermediate filaments of many epithelial cells consist of the fibrous protein **keratin.** There are several different cytokeratins of different molecular weights. The filaments usually form a network around the nucleus with bundles radiating to the periphery to terminate in membrane specializations for cell-to-cell attachment. Such filaments are exceptionally abundant in the superficial cells of the skin, where they may occupy a large fraction of the cell volume. Keratin filaments do not undergo frequent assembly and disassembly. Their function is mechanical, stabilizing the shape of the cell and strengthening its attachment to other cells.

In the central nervous system, the intermediate filaments of the neurons, called **neurofilaments,** are made up of three polypeptides of high molecular weight (210 kDa, 160kDa, and 68 kDa). They form a typical network in the cell body, but in the axon, they are oriented parallel to its long axis. In the supporting cells of the central nervous system, the astrocytes, oligodendrocytes, and microglial cells, the intermediate filaments consist of **glial fibrillar acidic protein** (51 kDa). Their intracellular disposition is much the same as that of intermediate filaments in other cells.

Microtubules

In addition to microfilaments and intermediate filaments, the cytoplasm of nearly all cell types contains **microtubules** (Fig. 1-19). These are about 25 nm in outside diameter, with a wall 9 nm thick around a 15-nm lumen. They consist of **tubulin,** a 50-kDa protein that occurs in two forms; alpha-tubulin and beta-tubulin. Heterodimers of these two tubulins are the subunits that polymerize end-to-end to form 13 filaments that make up the wall of the microtubule (Fig. 1-20A). Microtubules are quite straight and may be several microns in length, but they can be followed in electron micrographs for only a short distance before they go out of the plane of section. Unlike the relatively stable intermediate filaments, microtubules are constantly being renewed by polymerization of subunits at one end (plus end) and depolymerization at the other end (minus end), returning subunits to the pool of subunits in the cytoplasm. Microtubules with different

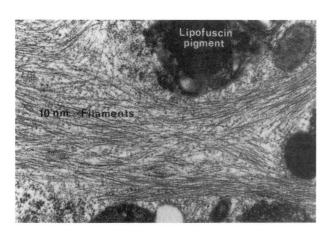

Fig. 1-18 Micrograph of an area of cytoplasm containing many intermediate filaments of the cytoskeleton. (Micrograph courtesy of W. Vogl.)

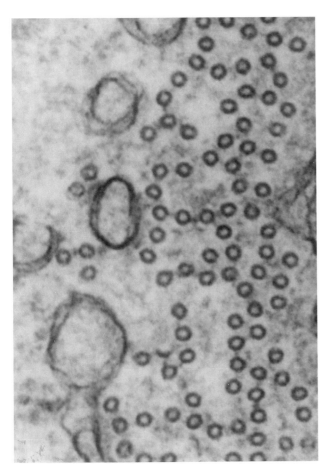

Fig. 1-19 Micrograph of an array of microtubules in cross section. A microtubule-associated protein (MAP) can be seen (at arrows) cross-linking some of the microtubules.

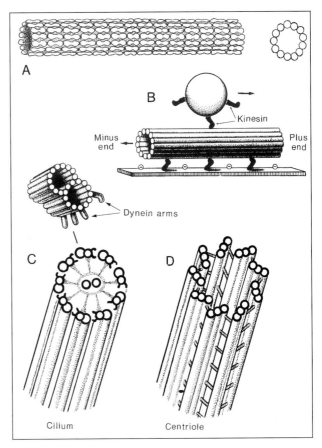

Fig. 1-20 Drawing of various forms taken by microtubules. (A) A microtubule is made up of heterodimers of two tubulins polymerized end-to-end to form 13 protofilaments that make up the wall. (B) Vesicles and organelles are moved along microtubules toward the plus end by a protein motor called kinesin. (C) Doublet microtubules with dynein arms are the motor elements of cilia. (D) Triplet microtubules form the wall of centrioles. (B redrawn from Vale, R. D., B. J. Schnapp, T. S. Reese and M. P. Sheetz, *Cell* 40:559, 1985.)

degrees of stability may coexist in the same cell, with some turning over with a half-life as short as 10 min, whereas others have a half-life of several hours.

When tubulin is extracted from cells, this fraction always contains certain other proteins that have been designated microtubule-associated proteins (MAPs). Four of these have been identified to date. Two of these, **kinesin** and **dynein,** have been found to have an important role in moving small transport vesicles along the surface of microtubules (Fig. 1-20B). One end of the kinesin molecule binds to a vesicle while the other end undergoes a cyclic interaction with successive subunits in the wall of the microtubule, moving the vesicle toward the plus end. In a similar fashion, dynein moves vesicles toward the minus end of a microtubule, thus providing for two-way traffic. A third MAP, **dynamin,** is believed to form short lateral projections at 32-nm intervals along the length of the microtubule. These may form cross-links between microtubules where they are in close proximity.

At the surface of some columnar epithelial cells, there are numerous cylindrical motile cell processes, called **cilia.** These beat to and fro, moving a blanket of mucus over the

surface of the epithelium. Spermatozoa have a longer single-cell process, the **flagellum,** that undulates to propel the cell through a fluid medium. In both cilia and flagella, the agent of their motility is the **axoneme,** a bundle of nine parallel doublet microtubules around a central pair of single microtubules (Fig. 1-20C). The doublets are made up of one complete microtubule with 13 protofilaments (subunit A), joined to an incomplete one that is C-shaped in cross section and has only 10 protofilaments (subunit B). Short lateral dynein arms project from subunit A of each doublet toward subunit B of the adjacent doublet. Although still incompletely understood, it is widely believed that ciliary and flagellar motion depend on a sliding displacement of the doublet microtubules, and this is somehow converted into a bending of the axoneme that is propagated along its length. The dynein arms generate the force moving the doublets.

In suitably stained cells, one can find a **centrosome,** a small spherical juxtanuclear area of cytoplasm having a

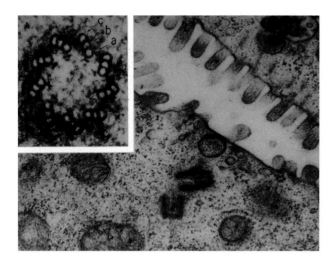

Fig. 1-21 Micrograph of a pair of centrioles near the surface of an epithelial cell. The long axes of the two centrioles are usually perpendicular to one another. The inset shows a cross section of a centriole at higher magnification. Its wall is composed of nine triplet microtubules. (Micrograph courtesy of S. Sorokin.)

slightly different texture. In its center, are the **centrioles,** two short rods with their long axes usually oriented perpendicular to one another (Fig. 1-21). There may be a few small dense bodies called **centriolar satellites** or **pericentriolar bodies** in the centrosome near them. In electron micrographs, the centrioles are hollow cylindrical structures 0.5–0.7 μm in length and about 0.2 μm in diameter with a dense wall around an electron lucent central core. The wall is made up of nine evenly spaced triplet microtubules (Figs. 1-20D and 1-21). Viewed in cross section, each triplet is set at an angle of about 40° to its respective tangent. This oblique orientation of the triplets results in a pattern resembling the vanes of a turbine. The three subunits of each triplet are designated A, B, and C, with subunit A nearest the central cavity.

The centrioles are self-replicating organelles. In preparation for cell division, a new centriole is assembled in an end-to-side relationship to each preexisting centriole. When its formation is complete, the two members of the original pair dissociate and each, with its newly formed daughter centriole and a portion of the surrounding centrosome, move to opposite poles of the cell, where they participate in the organization of the mitotic spindle, a group of microtubules along which the chromosomes move to the poles in the anaphase of cell division. Either the centrioles or the associated pericentriolar bodies are believed to initiate polymerization of the microtubules of the spindle.

CELL DIVISION

In all multicellular organisms, growth, repair, and renewal depend on the formation of new cells by the division of preexisting cells. There are two processes of division: mitosis which occurs in the somatic cells of the body, and meiosis which is confined to the germ cells that develop into ova and spermatozoa.

Mitosis

A proliferating population of cells go through a repetitive sequence of events termed the **cell cycle,** which is divided into **interphase,** the period between divisions, and **mitosis,** the events leading to the division of the cell into two daughter cells. During interphase, there is no change in the appearance of the cell, but alterations in its biochemical activity are occurring. Interphase is divided into three phases G_1, S, and G_2. In the **G_1 phase** (24 h), the cell is carrying out its normal functions without detectable change in its structure. (Cells with a long life span may remain in this phase for years.) In the **S phase** (8 h), there is a replication of its DNA and of the centrioles. In the **G_2 phase** (2.5 h), the cell synthesizes tubulin and other proteins for the generation of a mitotic spindle. This is followed by mitosis, which extends over 30–60 min. Mitosis is a continuous process, but, for descriptive purposes, it is divided into four stages: prophase, metaphase, anaphase, and telophase.

Early in the **prophase,** the chromatin is reorganized into threadlike structures which have a meandering course in the nucleoplasm. These gradually shorten to form separate rod-shaped **chromosomes,** each made up of two parallel, identical **chromatids** joined by a small body called the **centromere** or **kinetochore.** The chromosome number is constant and characteristic of each animal species. In the human, the number is 46, which is referred to as the diploid number. When nuclei of cells at this phase are smashed and spread on a slide, one can identify 22 homol-

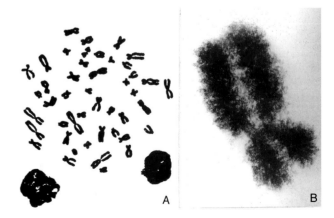

Fig. 1-22 (A) Photomicrograph of a squash preparation of metaphase chromosomes of a dividing cell. Twenty-two pairs of autosomes, and the X and Y sex chromosomes are identifiable. (Courtesy of H. Lisco and L. Lisco.) (B) Micrograph of an unsectioned metaphase chromosome showing the chromatids, primary constriction, and loops of filaments radiating from the long axis of the chromatids. (Courtesy of H. Ris.)

ogous pairs of chromosomes (Fig. 1-22A) and 2 additional **sex chromosomes** (X and Y) that differ greatly in size. In **metaphase,** the nucleolus disappears, the nucleolar envelope breaks down, and the chromosomes become aligned in a transverse plane in the middle of the cell, the **equatorial plate.** Concurrently, one pair of centrioles migrates to each pole of the cell, and there initiates polymerization of many microtubules that extend from each pole to the chromosomes on the equatorial plate, forming the **mitotic spindle.** In **anaphase,** the sister chromatids of each chromosome separate from each other and move, in opposite directions along the microtubules of the spindle, to opposite poles. No microtubule-associated protein that might serve as the motor for this movement has been identified to date. In **telophase,** a constriction, called the cleavage furrow, develops at the equator of the elongated cell and gradually deepens, cleaving it in two. The furrow is formed by contraction of subplasmalemmal actin filaments in a ringlike thickening of the ectoplasm. In the two daughter cells, a nuclear envelope is then formed around the chromosomes, which become transformed into peripheral clumps of chromatin. Upon reformation of a nucleolus, the nucleus takes on its interphase appearance.

Meiosis

Meiosis is a process of division in the germ cell line in which the number of chromosomes is reduced from the diploid number, typical of somatic cells, to the haploid number in the gametes. The diploid number is then restored by fusion of the sperm and ovum at fertilization. Reduction of chromosome number is accomplished by one replication of DNA followed by two cell divisions without an intervening S-phase. Details of meiosis will be deferred to a later chapter.

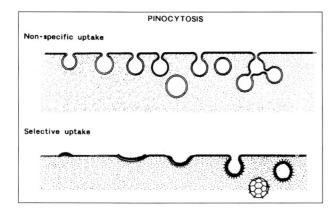

Fig. 1-23 (A) In fluid-phase pinocytosis, minute invaginations of the cell membrane detach and move into the cytoplasm as small smooth-surfaced vesicles. This process of uptake is nonselective. (B) In receptor-mediated pinocytosis, specific receptors and their ligands cluster, and this portion of the membrane invaginates to form vesicles that are enclosed in a lattice of clathrin. This form of endocytosis is selective.

ENDOCYTOSIS AND EXOCYTOSIS

Cells are bathed in extracellular fluid, from which they must obtain all materials needed for their nutrition and synthetic activities. Ions and small molecules enter by diffusion or active transport across the cell membrane. Larger molecules are taken up by **endocytosis,** a process of ingestion of fluid and solutes in invaginations of the membrane that constrict at their neck to form small vesicles (Fig. 1-23A), or larger vacuoles that move into the cytoplasm. Uptake of extracellular fluid in small vesicles is called **pinocytosis** (drinking by cells). Ingestion of solid matter by extension of cell processes that envelop and draw the particle into the cytoplasm is called **phagocytosis** (eating by cells).

Pinocytosis

Micropinocytosis, the uptake of fluid in small vesicles (80–90 nm), occurs in nearly all cell types. The volume of fluid taken up in this way is not generally appreciated because of the small number of such vesicles included in the ultrathin sections required for electron microscopy. However, scanning micrographs of isolated cell membranes reveal that they may number 50 or more per square micron of cell surface (Fig. 1-24A). A less common behavior, detectable in living cells in culture, is **macropinocytosis,** in which thin-cell processes, lamellipodia, envelop and interiorize sizable droplets of fluid (0.5–1.5 μm). Both of these mechanisms are **nonselective.**

A highly **selective** uptake of specific proteins, such as hormones, is accomplished by **receptor-mediated pinocytosis** (Fig. 1-24B). Its selectivity depends on randomly distributed specific **receptors** in the plasmalemma. After binding of extracellular protein molecules to the receptors, these cluster in a small area of membrane that invaginates to form a shallow depression. This ultimately pinches off to form a vesicle that moves into the cytoplasm (Fig. 1-23B). The membrane of these depressions has regularly spaced minute projections from its cytoplasmic surface, and they are therefore referred to as **coated pits.** Their coat is made up of molecules of a 180-kDa protein, called **clathrin,** that binds to the cytoplasmic domain of the membrane and polymerizes to form a cagelike lattice around the forming vesicle that resembles the framework of a geodesic dome (Figs. 1-23B and 1-24B). As clathrin polymerization progresses, the pits deepen and constrict at their neck to form **coated vesicles** that are easily distinguished from the smooth vesicles of the more common fluid-phase pinocytosis that is presumed to be nonselective.

After moving into the cytoplasm, the vesicles lose their clathrin coat and several of them fuse to form larger vesicles called **endosomes.** Small vesicles containing the specific receptors pinch off from these and return to the cell membrane, thus recycling the receptors. The remainder of the endosome receives enzymes from the Golgi complex

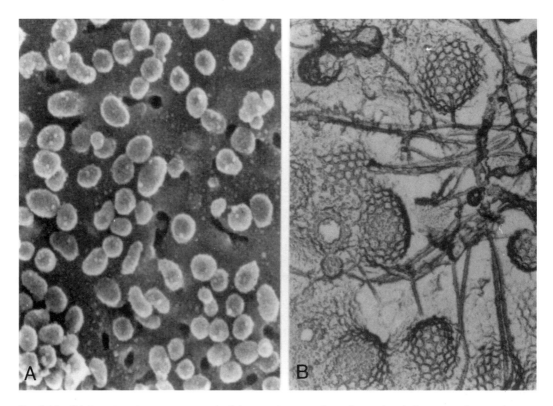

Fig. 1-24   (A) Scanning electron micrograph of the cytoplasmic surface of an isolated plasma membrane, showing a large number of forming pinocytosis vesicles. (B) A comparable preparation showing the clathrin coats of several forming coated vesicles. (A. Courtesy of T. Inoue and H. Osatako, J. Submicroscopic Cytology and Pathology 21:215, 1989. B. Courtesy of N. Hirokawa and J. Heuser.)

that processes its contents, and the endosome ultimately fuses with a lysosome.

Many other small vesicles in the cytoplasm do not arise from the cell membrane but are involved in transport from organelle to organelle. Although the majority of these appear smooth surfaced, it has recently been found that these too have a surface coat of a protein other than clathrin. It now appears that there are many kinds of vesicles, each formed with a different coating. The formation of vesicles transporting material between cisternae of the Golgi complex has been studied in some detail. Molecules of a cytoplasmic protein **adenosine diphosphate ribosylation factor (ARF)** first bind to the Golgi membrane, and this recruits protein complexes, called **coatamers,** to bind to the ARF. Their assembly, directed by ARF and energized by associated guanosine triphosphate (GTP) causes a small area of the membrane to invaginate and bud off as a coated vesicle. The coat of these vesicles does not have the geometric form of a clathrin coat and it is shed soon after formation of the vesicle, for bare membrane must contact the membrane of the target cisterna for fusion to take place. The vesicles transporting newly synthesized protein from the endoplasmic reticulum to the Golgi are formed by a similar mechanism, but they have a coat protein that differs from that involved in transport between Golgi cisternae. There is some evidence suggesting that the

composition of the coat determines which molecules will be packaged in the vesicle.

Phagocytosis

Phagocytosis is the ingestion of solid particulate matter. It is not common to all cells but occurs in certain free cells of the connective tissue (leukocytes and macrophages) that are specialized for defense against bacterial invasion. Binding of a bacterium, or other particle, to the plasmalemma is followed by extension of blunt cell processes called **pseudopodia.** These slowly elongate as their membrane advances over the surface of the bacterium in a zipperlike process of receptor binding. When the leading ends of the enveloping pseudopods meet, they fuse and the object is drawn into the cytoplasm in a vacuole bounded by a detached portion of the cell membrane. Lysosomes then fuse with the vacuole, and its content is digested.

Exocytosis

Exocytosis is the term applied to fusion of vesicles or membrane-bounded granules with the cell membrane to release their content into the extracellular space. Reference has already been made to **regulated secretion,** in which exocytosis occurs in response to a neural or hormonal stimulus, and to **constitutive secretion,** in which the product is released in small vesicles continuously transported to the cell surface. Another very common form of exocytosis is that involved in recycling of the large amount of membrane removed from the surface in pinocytosis and phagocytosis. Of the host of small vesicles visible in the cytoplasm, those coming from the plasmalemma can only be distinguished from those returning to it by exposing the cells to electron-opaque tracer molecules that are taken up with the extracellular fluid in the process of endocytosis.

CELL MOTILITY

Movement of cells is essential during embryonic development, but in the adult body, the majority of the cells are relatively fixed in their position. However, in the healing of wounds, they are capable of crawling over their substrate at a rate of 0.1–1 μm/h. The white blood cells (neutrophils, lymphocytes, and monocytes) that move out of the capillaries into the surrounding connective tissues are able to migrate through it at a rate of up to 30 μm/min. The mechanism of cell movement has been well studied. A small portion of the cell cortex changes from its normal gelated state to the fluid state, and flows outward to form a flat process called the leading lamella. The membrane on its undersurface becomes attached to the substrate by adhesion proteins. Then, the binding of myosin to actin filaments slides them past one another, drawing the cell forward. The gelated state is restored at the base of the lamella by the formation of a three-dimensional lattice of actin filaments. Repetition of this sequence of events slowly moves the cell forward. The spread of cancer cells depends on reactivation of the potential of its cells for motility.

CELL DEATH

Two processes of cell death are distinguishable, **necrosis** and **apoptosis**. Necrosis can result from anoxia, mechanical injury, or exposure to toxins. The changes observed in the dying cell include swelling, excessive clumping of the chromatin, reduced staining of the cytoplasm, and breakdown of the organelles, followed by lysis. The residues of the cell are then taken up and digested by macrophages. Apoptosis, on the other hand, is not due to injury but is a process of programmed self-destruction initiated by endogenous signals. It is important in the regulation of cell numbers in physiological conditions. The cells in the body have normal life spans ranging from a few days to 80 years or more. Programmed cell death (apoptosis) is common in those cells having a short life span. Its biochemical mechanisms are still not well understood. It is clearly an active process in which the initial event is cleavage of DNA into short segments by an endonuclease. The cytoplasm then appears to be digested by activation of one or more intrinsic proteases. What initiates this genetic program of cell death is not known, but in some instances, it may depend on environmental signals. The cell does not swell, as in necrosis, but decreases in volume, and the cytoplasm soon breaks up into small membrane-limited globules that seem to be phagocytized by neighboring cells. The scavenger cells of the body, the macrophages, seem to be less involved in the terminal events of apoptosis than they are after necrosis.

QUESTIONS*

1. Which of the organelles listed below belongs to the cytoskeleton of the cell?

   A. Golgi apparatus
   B. rough-surfaced endoplasmic reticulum
   C. smooth-surfaced endoplasmic reticulum
   D. centrioles
   E. microtubules

2. DNA is replicated during

   A. prophase
   B. G_1 of interphase
   C. S of interphase
   D. G_2 of interphase
   E. metaphase

3. Oxidative phosphorylation to adenosine triphosphate in mitochondria is associated with

   A. the matrix
   B. outer mitochondrial membrane
   C. dense granules
   D. cristae
   E. none of the above

4. The mitotic spindle is composed mostly of

   A. Golgi flattened sacs
   B. smooth-surfaced endoplasmic reticulum
   C. microtubules
   D. intermediate filaments
   E. none of the above

5. The fluid mosaic model of membrane structure

   A. contains actin filaments
   B. has hydrophobic elements directed away from the center
   C. has hydrophilic elements directed away from the center
   D. contains intermediate filaments
   E. none of the above

6. During anaphase

   A. the chromosomes uncoil becoming indistinct
   B. the chromosomes become visible and condense
   C. the chromatids separate, moving away from each other
   D. the cell contains intermediate filaments
   E. none of the above

7. In mitochondria ATP-ase activity is associated with

   A. the outer mitochondrial membrane
   B. the matrix
   C. inner mitochondrial membrane
   D. dense granules
   E. none of the above

8. All of the following are considered membranous organelles **except**

   A. lysosomes
   B. centrioles
   C. mitochondria
   D. Golgi apparatus
   E. peroxisomes

9. All of the following are considered as inclusion bodies **except**

   A. secretory granules
   B. pigment granules
   C. glycogen
   D. lipid
   E. lysosomes

10. Which of the following processes involves microtubules?

    A. movement of cilia
    B. movement of chromosomes during mitosis
    C. intracellular transport of secretory granules
    D. movement of flagella
    E. all of the above

11. The pars granulosa and pars fibrosa refer to specific portions of the

    A. nucleus
    B. nucleolus
    C. nuclear envelop
    D. RER
    E. SER

*Answers on page 307.

2

EPITHELIUM

CHAPTER OUTLINE

Classification of Epithelia
   Simple Epithelium
   Stratified Epithelium
   Pseudostratified Columnar Epithelium
   Transitional Epithelium
Epithelial Polarity
Cell Cohesion and Communication
   Zonula Occludens
   Zonula Adherens
   Macula Adherens (Desmosome)
   Gap Junction (Nexus)
Basal Lamina
Specializations of the Free Surface
   Brush Border
   Cilia
Epithelial Renewal
Transporting Epithelia
Glandular Epithelia
   Types of Exocrine Glands
   Control of Exocrine Glands
   Endocrine Glands
Histophysiology of Epithelia

KEY WORDS

Anchoring Fibers	Isochronal Rhythm
Apical Domain	Keratin, keratinized
Apocrine	Lamina Densa
Axoneme	Lamina Lucida
Basal Lamina	Laminin
Basement Membrane	Merocrine
Basolateral Domain	Mesothelium
Cell Adhesion	Metachronal Rhythm
Molecules	Microtubules
Cilia	Microvilli
Collagen	Plasmalemma
Connexons	Proteoglycans
Demilunes, serous	Pseudostratified
Dyein	Squamous
Endothelium	Stratified
Glycocalyx	Terminal Web
Goblet Cells	Transitional
Hemidesmosome	Villin
Holocrine	

Epithelium is a basic tissue consisting of closely apposed cells, forming a continuous layer covering an outside surface or lining an internal cavity. In its simplest form, it consists of polyhedral cells forming a layer one cell thick. In more complex epithelia, there may be multiple layers of cells. In all instances, the lowermost cells rest on a thin, continuous, supporting layer, the **basal lamina** or **basement membrane,** which consists of a meshwork of fine filaments. The primary function of epithelia is to form a boundary layer that can control movement of substances between the external environment and the body's internal milieu or between internal compartments of the body. The epithelia of various organs may be made up of cells specialized for absorption, secretion, or ion transport.

CLASSIFICATION OF EPITHELIA

Several categories of epithelium are assigned different names to lend precision to the description of the structure of organs. They are classified according to the number of cell layers, the shape of the cells, and the specializations of their free surface (Fig. 2-1). An epithelium made up of a single layer of cells is a **simple epithelium,** and if there are multiple layers, it is a **stratified epithelium.** The modifiers **squamous, cuboidal,** or **columnar** are added to indicate the shape of the cells of the upper layer. Thus, a single layer of flattened cells is a **simple squamous epithelium;** a single layer of tall prismatic cells is a **simple columnar**

epithelium. If the cells have, on their free surface, motile cell processes called **cilia,** it is a **ciliated columnar epithelium,** and so forth.

Simple Epithelium

In histological sections of **simple squamous epithelium,** the cells appear fusiform, or as long flat rectangles (Fig. 2-2). In surface view, after staining the cell boundaries with silver nitrate, it presents a tilelike appearance of closely adherent polygonal cells. Such an epithelium is found lining the pleural and abdominal cavities, the blood and lymph vessels, the alveoli of the lungs, and certain tubules of the kidney. The layer lining the body cavity and covering the viscera is often referred to as **mesothelium,** and that lining blood and lymph vessels as **endothelium,** but both are typical simple squamous epithelia.

Simple cuboidal epithelium appears, in section, as a row of square or rectangular profiles. In different organs, the cells vary in height from slightly taller than cuboidal, to very tall slender columns. The nuclei tend to be aligned at the same level in all of the cells. **Simple columnar epithelium** (Figs. 2-3, **2-7A** and **2-7C** [see Plate 1]) lines the gastrointestinal tract. **Ciliated columnar epithelium** is found lining the uterus and oviducts, the bronchi of the lungs, and the paranasal sinuses (Fig. 2-4).

Stratified Epithelium

In **stratified squamous epithelium** (Figs. 2-5, 2-7 [see Plate 1]), the cells vary in shape from base to free surface. Those at the base have a rounded or beveled upper end. Those above this layer are irregularly polyhedral, becoming increasingly flattened toward the surface, and in the superficial layer they are thin squamous cells. This type of epithelium is found in the epidermis of the skin, in the lining of the oral cavity, epiglottis, esophagus, and vagina. In the skin, the superficial cells are transformed into dry lifeless scales. They contain no nucleus and the cytoplasm consists largely of the fibrous scleroprotein, **keratin.** Such an epithelium is called a **keratinized stratified squamous**

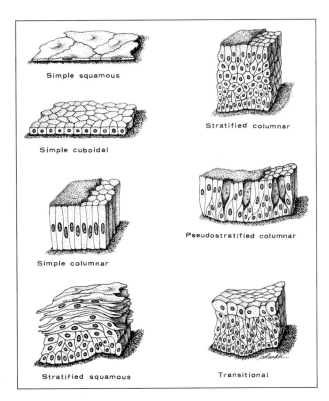

Fig. 2-1 Illustrations of the shape and arrangement of cells in the principal types of epithelium.

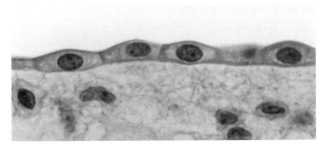

Fig. 2-2 Photomicrograph of a simple squamous epithelium. In many examples of this type of epithelium, the cells are much thinner and flatter than those illustrated here.

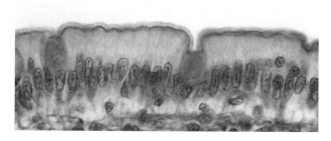

Fig. 2-3 Simple columnar epithelium with a striated border consisting of numerous, slender, parallel microvilli. This type of epithelium is found in the intestinal tract, where the cells are involved in absorption. The microvilli greatly increase the surface area exposed to the lumen.

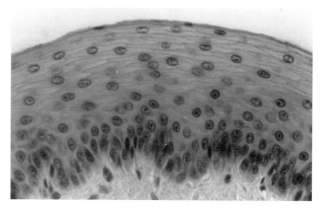

Fig. 2-5 Stratified squamous epithelium of the human esophagus. In this epithelium, the superficial cells are less heavily keratinized than in a similar type of epithelium of the skin.

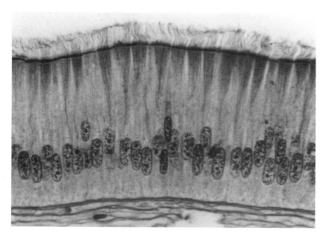

Fig. 2-4 A ciliated simple columnar epithelium. Note the relatively long cilia on the free surface, the rows of basal bodies at their base, and the stabilizing ciliary rootlets extending down into the cytoplasm.

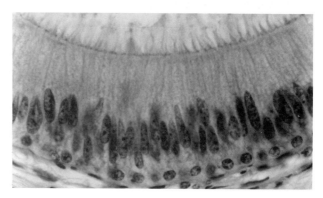

Fig. 2-6 Photomicrograph of a pseudostratified epithelium of human epididymis. Observation of two rows of nuclei is helpful in recognizing this kind of epithelium. Note, on the free surface, the long stereocilia characteristic of this epithelium.

epithelium (Fig. 2-7H [see Plate 1]).

In the uncommon **stratified columnar epithelium**, the superficial cells are columnar and the basal cells are cuboidal. One or more rows of polygonal cells may be interposed between the basal and the columnar cells. This epithelium is found only in the fornix of the conjunctiva, the cavernous urethra, and in the larger excretory ducts of some glands.

Pseudostratified Columnar Epithelium

In this epithelium, the nuclei occur at different levels, but the cells are not truly stratified. All cells are in contact with the basal lamina and some of them are typical columnar cells extending the full thickness of the epithelium, but many others resting on the basal lamina have a tapering upper end that extends only part way to the surface. Because of this arrangement, the nuclei of these two categories of cells are aligned at different levels, creating a false impression of stratification—hence the term **pseudostratified** (Figs. 2-6 and 2-7 [see Plate 1]). This epithelium is found in the male urethra and the duct of the parotid

gland, and **ciliated pseudostratified columnar epithelium** occurs in the greater part of the trachea, the primary bronchi, the auditory tube, and part of the tympanic cavity of the ear.

Transitional Epithelium

Transitional epithelium is confined to the urinary bladder, an organ that undergoes major changes in volume with its filling and emptying. The appearance of the epithelium varies greatly depending on the degree of distension of the bladder at the time of tissue fixation. In the empty bladder, it has many layers. Those at the base are cuboidal, and above these are three or four layers of polyhedral cells. In the superficial layer, the cells are very much larger than the others and have a characteristic rounded free surface. The shapes and relationships between cells change during bladder filling. When it is full, there are usually only two layers of cells: a superficial layer of large squamous cells overlying a basal layer of smaller, more-or-less cuboidal cells. Transitional epithelium is found throughout the urinary tract from the calyces of the kidney to the urethra. Some histologists prefer the term uroepithelium instead of transitional epithelium.

> *Epithelium usually maintains the structure characteristic of the organ in which it is found, but when subjected to prolonged irritation, it may become transformed to a different type better suited to resist the irritant. This is called **epithelial metaplasia**. For example, the pseudostratified ciliated epithelium of the bronchi, in very heavy smokers, may transform to stratified squamous epithelium (**squamous metaplasia**).*

EPITHELIAL POLARITY

Polarity of cells is the property of having their functions directed preferentially toward one end. Epithelial cells are polarized to carry out the vectorial functions of secretion, or transepithelial movement of ions and water. Their polarity is expressed in (1) apical specializations that amplify the area of the free surface, (2) the supranuclear position of the Golgi complex, (Fig. 2-8 [see Plate 2]), (3) the accu-

mulation of secretory products in the apical cytoplasm, and (4) in biochemical differences between the apical and basolateral regions of the membrane (Fig. 2-9). In cells other than those of epithelia, the plasmalemma is of uniform composition over their entire surface. In epithelial cells, certain membrane components are segregated in functionally distinct domains—the **apical domain** and the **basolateral domain**. The apical domain is especially rich in glycolipid, cholesterol, H^+-ATPase, ion channels, and specific transport proteins. The basolateral domain, on the other hand, contains Na^+/K^+-ATPase, anion channels, and hormone receptors. The basal component of the basolateral domain also contains binding sites for constituents of the basal lamina. Mixing of the components of the apical and basolateral domains is prevented by tight junctions that encircle the apical pole of the cell (see below).

CELL COHESION AND COMMUNICATION

The cells of epithelia maintain extensive lateral apposition. In electron micrographs, their membranes are separated by a very narrow intercellular space 15–20 nm in width, having a content of low density. This space is occu-

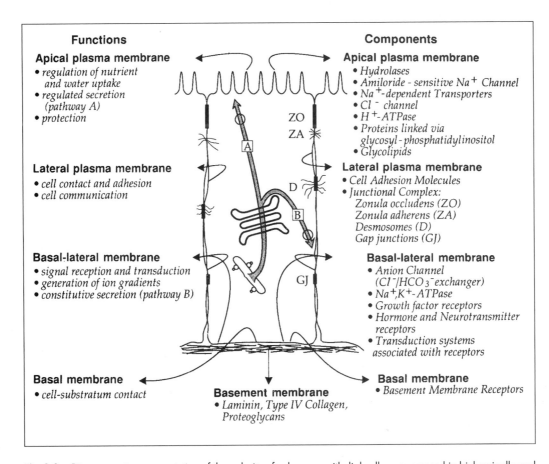

Functions

Apical plasma membrane
- regulation of nutrient and water uptake
- regulated secretion (pathway A)
- protection

Lateral plasma membrane
- cell contact and adhesion
- cell communication

Basal-lateral membrane
- signal reception and transduction
- generation of ion gradients
- constitutive secretion (pathway B)

Basal membrane
- cell-substratum contact

Basement membrane
- Laminin, Type IV Collagen, Proteoglycans

Components

Apical plasma membrane
- Hydrolases
- Amiloride-sensitive Na^+ Channel
- Na^+-dependent Transporters
- Cl^- channel
- H^+-ATPase
- Proteins linked via glycosyl-phosphatidylinositol
- Glycolipids

Lateral plasma membrane
- Cell Adhesion Molecules
- Junctional Complex:
  Zonula occludens (ZO)
  Zonula adherens (ZA)
  Desmosomes (D)
  Gap junctions (GJ)

Basal-lateral membrane
- Anion Channel (Cl^-/HCO_3^- exchanger)
- Na^+,K^+-ATPase
- Growth factor receptors
- Hormone and Neurotransmitter receptors
- Transduction systems associated with receptors

Basal membrane
- Basement Membrane Receptors

Fig. 2-9 Diagrammatic representation of the polarity of columnar epithelial cells as expressed in bichemically and functionally distinct apical, lateral, and basal domains of the plasma membrane. (From E. Rodriguez-Boulan and W. J. Nelson, Science 245:718, 1989).

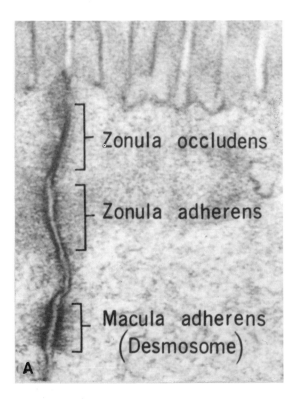

Fig. 2-10 An electron micrograph of the junctional complex between neighboring epithelial cells showing the zonula occludens, zonula adherens, and a desmosome.

pied by **proteoglycans** and a family of glycoproteins collectively called **cell adhesion molecules (CAMs)**. In addition to these macromolecules which have adhesive properties, there are local specializations of the opposing membranes that form **junctional complexes** that are the structures mainly responsible for epithelial cell cohesion (Fig. 2-10).

Zonula Occludens

In electron micrographs of a columnar epithelium, the lateral membranes of adjacent cells converge just below the free surface, obliterating the intercellular space over a distance of 0.1–0.3 μm. At high magnifications, the membranes here appear to be fused at two or more points in the junction, but they diverge slightly between these sites of fusion. Freeze-fracture preparations that cleave the lipid bilayer of membranes reveal in this region three to five slender ridges, or fibers, that run more or less parallel to the surface of the epithelium and are interconnected, forming a loose network on the inner half-membrane (**P-face**) (Fig. 2-11). A corresponding pattern of shallow grooves is found on the opposing half-membrane (**E-face**). The number of rows of these ridges corresponds to the number of sites of apparent membrane fusion, seen in thin sections. Thus, the cells are firmly attached along a series of linear membrane fusions. This beltlike junction, called the **zonula occludens**, courses around the entire circumference of each cell near its apex, closing the intercellular spaces and preventing large and small molecules from traversing the epithelium via a paracellular route. It also prevents diffusion of integral membrane proteins from the apical to the lateral domain of the plasmalemma.

Zonula Adherens

The **zonula adherens** is a beltlike specialization of the membranes and subjacent cytoplasm that encircles the cells of an epithelium immediately below the zonula occludens. The opposing membranes are 15–20 nm apart and very fine transverse striations are detectable in this narrow intercellular space. Freeze-fracture preparations reveal no

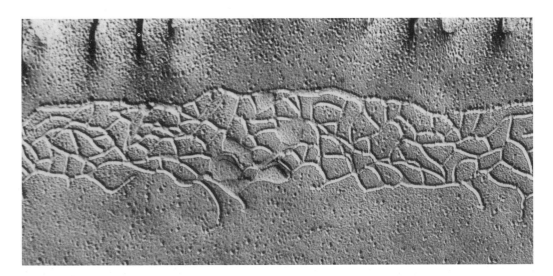

Fig. 2-11 Electron micrograph of a freeze-fracture replica of the zonula occludens in intestinal epithelium. A reticular pattern of anastomosing strands are seen on the P-face of the cleaved lateral cell membrane, just below the brush-border. (Micrograph courtesy of J. P. Revel.)

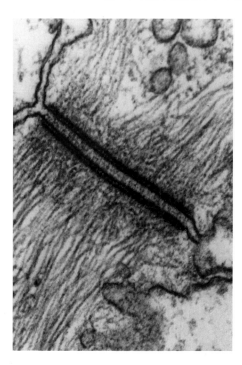

Fig. 2-12 Electron micrograph of a desmosome from epidermal epithelium showing the attachment plaque and associated filaments. (Micrograph courtesy of D. Kelly.)

intracellular components that distinguish this from other regions of the membrane. The most conspicuous feature of the zonula adherens is a dense area of the cytoplasm closely associated with the junctional membrane. At high magnifications, this dense plaque is a mat of fine filaments, some of which appear to be continuous with those of the actin-rich transverse zone of the apical cytoplasm called the **terminal web**. In addition to actin, immunocytochemical staining localizes myosin, alpha-actinin, and vinculin in the cytoplasmic density of the junction and it is thought that these are involved in cross-linking its integral filaments and binding them to the microfilaments of the terminal web and to the cell membrane. A specific, glycoprotein, **cell adhesion molecule (A-CAM)** is localized in the interspace between the membranes. In addition to being a site of cell adherence, the zonula adherens probably has an important role in stabilizing and joining the terminal web of adjoining cells.

Macula Adherens (Desmosome)

The **desmosomes** are not encircling bands like those described above, but are discrete plaques scattered over the lateral surfaces of the cells. The membranes at these junctions are 20–25 nm apart. A thin, dense line can sometimes be seen in the intercellular space midway between the membranes. The most conspicuous component of the junction is an electron-dense disk or plaque on the cytoplasmic side of the opposing membranes (Fig. 2-10 and 2-12). Very fine filaments, called **transmembrane linkers**, extend

across the intercellular space, apparently holding the membranes and their associated dense disks together at a uniform distance. Intermediate filaments of the cytoplasm of both cells converge on the desmosomes and terminate in their dense disk. Thus, the desmosomes are not only sites of cell-to-cell attachment, they also contribute to the stability of the epithelium as a whole by linking the cytoskeleton of adjoining cells.

Stratified squamous epithelium is atypical, in that zonulae occludentes and zonulae adherentes are lacking. Instead, the epithelium is rendered impervious to fluid and solutes by deposition of a complex lipid in the intercellular spaces. However, desmosomes are exceptionally abundant, and at the base of the epithelium, there are also numerous **hemidesmosomes** which bind the cells firmly to the basal lamina.

Gap Junction (Nexus)

The **gap junction,** or nexus, is a specialization of opposing cell membranes that permits passage of ions and small molecules from cell to cell. The intercellular space is narrowed to about 3 nm and, at high magnifications, minute structures, called **connexons** can be seen bridging the gap. In freeze-fracture replicas of the P-face of the membranes, the junction appears as a round area of closely spaced particles of uniform size (Fig. 2-13). When gap junctions are isolated and negatively stained with lanthanum, the particles (connexons) appear as hexagonally packed annular units with a center-to-center spacing of 9 nm. They are cylindrical and have a wall made up of six short rodlike subunits around a central pore 1.5–2.0 nm in diameter. The connexons in opposing membranes are in register and project 1.5 nm into the intercellular gap, where they are linked end-to-end. Their central pores thus form channels connecting the cytoplasm of neighboring cells. Ions, cyclic AMP, amino acids, and other small molecules can pass freely through these channels. Gap junctions thus have an important role in coordinating the activities of cells throughout the epithelium. *p. 105d – in cardiac muscle*

BASAL LAMINA

Between an epithelium and the underlying connective tissue is a thin supporting layer traditionally called the **basement membrane**. The term basal lamina is probably preferable because, since the advent of the electron microscope, we have come to think of a membrane as a lipid bilayer. Two layers are distinguishable in the basal lamina, but neither is lipid in nature. There is a zone of very low density immediately beneath the epithelium, the **lamina lucida**, and an outer zone of greater density, the **lamina densa**, facing the underlying connective tissue. The two zones are usually of similar thickness (40–50 nm), but, in

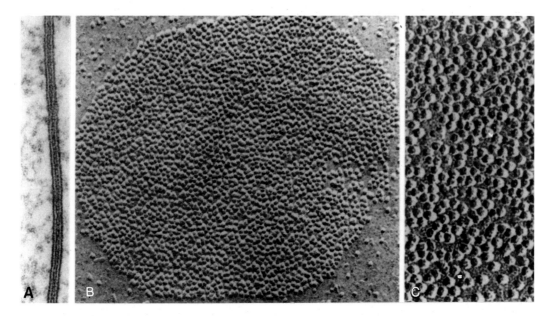

Fig. 2-13 (A) Micrograph of a gap junction as it appears in thin section. No intercellular gap is seen between the membranes. (B) Freeze-fracture replica of the P-face of a gap junction, showing the large number of intramembrane particles. (C) At higher magnification, a small pore can be resolved in the middle of each particle, through which ions and small molecules can pass from cell to cell.

rare instances, the lamina densa may be considerably thicker. It consists of a meshwork of interwoven 4-nm filaments. Little substructure is resolved in the lamina lucida, but in some preparations, it is traversed by very fine strands running from the lamina densa to the cell membranes at the base of the epithelium.

The principal chemical constituents of the basal lamina are the proteoglycans, **laminin**, and **type-IV collagen**. This type of collagen occurs exclusively in the basal lamina. Its long chains are cross-linked to form the resilient three-dimensional network comprising the lamina densa. The large glycoprotein, laminin (900 kDa), is localized mainly in the lamina lucida and its molecules are bound at one end to specific receptors in the cell membrane, and at the other end, to the collagen of the lamina densa. Slender **anchoring fibers** of **type-VII collagen** course downward from the basal lamina, looping around collagen fibers of the connective tissue and terminating in **anchoring plaques**. These are dense bodies in the extracellular matrix that have a substructure similar to that of the lamina densa and contain both type-IV and type-VII collagen. Anchoring fibers (Fig. 2-14) are abundant beneath the stratified squamous epithelium of the epidermis, especially in those areas that are subject to frictional stress. They are less common under other epithelia.

The primary function of the basal lamina is to support the epithelium, but it also serves as a passive molecular sieve or ultrafilter. This is especially evident in the kidney, where urine is formed as an ultrafiltrate of the blood passing through the glomerular capillaries. The basal lamina of the capillaries holds back molecules on the basis of their size, shape, and electrostatic charge.

SPECIALIZATIONS OF THE FREE SURFACE

Brush Border

Absorptive columnar epithelia, studied with the light microscope, have a refractile free border that exhibits fine vertical striations. With the electron microscope, this so-called **brush border** is found to consist of slender cylindrical cell processes, 1–2 μm long and 80–90 nm in diameter, called **microvilli**. They are closely packed with about 60 per square micron of epithelial surface. Delicate

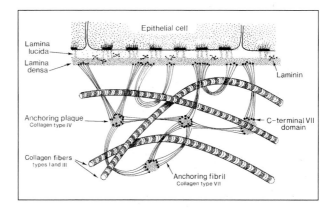

Fig. 2-14 Schematic of the anchoring fibril network beneath an epithelium. The anchoring fibrils are believed to be lateral aggregations of type-VII procollagen molecules. They originate in the basal lamina and insert into anchoring plaques consisting of type-IV collagen. (Redrawn from D. R. Keene, L. Y. Sakai, G. P. Lunstrum, N. P. Morris and R. E. Burgeson, Journal of Cell Biology 104:611, 1987).

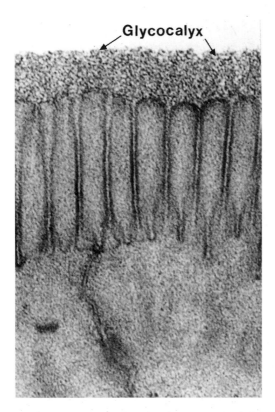

Glycocalyx

Fig. 2-15 Electron micrograph of a few microvilli of the brush border of an intestinal epithelial cell, showing the glycocalyx covering the ends of the microvilli.

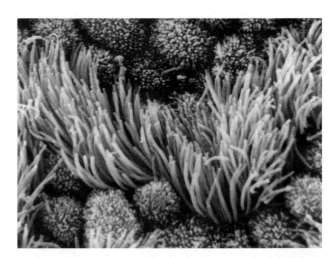

Fig. 2-16 Scanning electron micrograph of the luminal surface of the human oviduct, showing the apical ends of the ciliated and nonciliated cells. The latter bear short microvilli. (Courtesy of P. Gaddum-Rosse, R. Blandau, and R. Tiersch, American Journal of Anatomy 138:269, 1973.)

branching filaments projecting from their tips form a fuzzy coat on the surface of the epithelium, called the **glycocalyx** (Fig. 2-15). These minute filaments are terminal oligosaccharide chains of integral membrane proteins. In the epithelium lining the intestine, each microvillus contains a bundle of 25–35 actin filaments that are attached to the membrane at the tip and extend downward into the apical cytoplasm, where they intermingle with the filaments of the terminal web. The actin filaments are cross-linked by a polypeptide called **villin**. At intervals of 33 nm along its length, this core filament bundle is linked to the membrane by short filaments. The brush border is a specialization for increasing the absorptive and digestive efficiency of the epithelium. It achieves a 15–30-fold increase in the area of membrane exposed to the lumen. In epithelia not involved in absorption or transport, microvilli are few in number and usually lack core filaments.

Cilia

Cilia are motile cell processes, 7–10 μm in length and 0.3 μm in diameter, that execute rapid to-and-fro oscillations (Fig. 2-16). They are arranged in rows on the apical cell surface. When observed in living cells, cilia are seen to beat in a constant direction. If the rate of beat is slowed

down by high-speed cinematographic recordings, each cilium is seen to stiffen on the rapid forward, or effective stroke, and to bend more slowly on the recovery stroke. Cilia may have an **isochronal rhythm** in which they all beat synchronously, but, more commonly, they have a **metachronal rhythm** in which cilia in successive rows start their beat in sequence, so that each row is slightly more advanced in the cycle than the one behind it. This results in waves that can be seen sweeping over the epithelium like the waves that run before the wind in a field of wheat. The effect of this coordinated activity of the cilia is to move a blanket of mucus slowly over the surface of the epithelium, or to move fluid and particulate matter through the lumen of a tubular organ.

As described in Chapter 1, each cilium has a core complex, the **axoneme**, which consists of a central pair of **microtubules** with nine evenly spaced doublet microtubules around them (Fig. 2-17). Spaced at 24-nm intervals along each doublet, there are pairs of short **dynein** arms which project from subunit A toward subunit B of the next doublet. At the base of each cilium there is a **basal body** with an internal structure identical to that of a centriole. The nine doublets of the ciliary axoneme are continuous with the two inner subunits of the triplet microtubules of the basal body.

The exact mechanism of ciliary beat is still poorly understood, but it is generally agreed that the dynein arms are the motor elements. It is postulated that binding of ATP causes them to attach transiently to the adjacent doublet and change their conformation. Upon hydrolysis of the ATP, they detach and then reattach at a lower level on the adjacent doublet. Rapid repetition of this cycle of attachment and detachment is believed to cause a sliding of the doublets with respect to one another, resulting in bending.

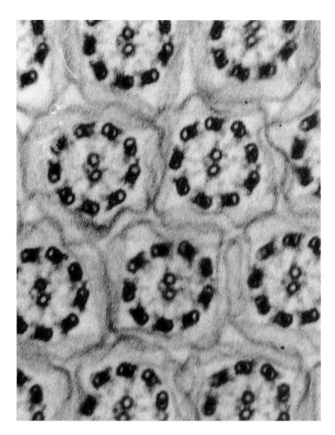

Fig. 2-17 Micrograph of cross sections of cilia on a ciliated columnar epithelium, showing the doublet microtubules with dynein arms that are the motor elements of the cilia.

To account for the change in direction of bending, it is suggested that dynein arms are active on one side of the axoneme in the effective stroke and that those on the other side are active in the recovery stroke.

> In the inherited disease **immotile cilia syndrome (Kartagener's disease)** *all cilia in the body are immotile due to the absence of the dynein arms on their axoneme. The epithelium in the respiratory tract fails to move the blanket of mucus and this leads to partial obstruction of the airway, chronic bronchitis, and ultimately to bronchiectasis (distension and disruption of the alveoli of the lungs).*

EPITHELIAL RENEWAL

The various epithelia of the body are constantly being renewed. Cells reaching the end of their limited life span are exfoliated (shed) or undergo apoptosis (programmed cell death) in situ and are replaced by division of other cells. In simple epithelia, all cells retain the ability to divide, but in stratified epithelia, the great majority lose their capacity for division in the course of their differenti-

ation, and mitosis is confined to stem cells near the basal lamina. Some of the progeny of these cells differentiate as they move upward in the epithelium, while others remain on the basal lamina as members of the population of stem cells. In the repair of mechanically damaged epithelium, cells at the margins of the defect form a thin sheet that migrates over the denuded area of the basal lamina. Somewhat later, cells at the margins of the wound begin to divide to provide the cells needed to restore the epithelium to its normal thickness.

TRANSPORTING EPITHELIA

The intestinal epithelium is able to move water, sodium ions, glucose, and amino acids from the gut lumen to the extracellular fluid beneath the basal lamina. The membrane of the microvilli is permeable to sodium ions, which are in higher concentration in the lumen than in the cytoplasm. Sodium, therefore, enters the cell down its concentration gradient. Concurrently, binding of glucose to a specific protein in the membrane of the microvilli causes a change in its conformation that permits entry of glucose. A Na^+/K^+-ATPase, confined to the basolateral membrane, pumps sodium ions out at the cell base, maintaining the concentration gradient. Glucose leaves at the cell base by **facilitated diffusion** (movement of molecules across a cell membrane using carrier molecules temporarily complexed to the molecule being transported). The efficiency of transepithelial transport is enhanced by the large surface area of the microvilli. In the transporting epithelium in the kidney tubules, the basolateral surface is also amplified by interdigitating columnar ridges on the sides of the cells and by deep infolding at the cell base.

GLANDULAR EPITHELIA

Secretory cells take up small molecules from the blood and utilize them in the synthesis of a specific product that accumulates in the apical cytoplasm in the form of secretory granules. Assemblages of secretory cells constitute **glands,** which usually form as invaginations of an epithelium. Glands are of two kinds. Those that secrete their product onto an internal or external surface through a system of ducts are called **exocrine glands**; those that release their product into the blood for transport to distant target tissues are called **endocrine glands**.

Types of Exocrine Glands

Solitary secretory cells may occur in an absorptive epithelium such as that of the intestines. These are called **goblet cells**, owing to their expanded apical region and

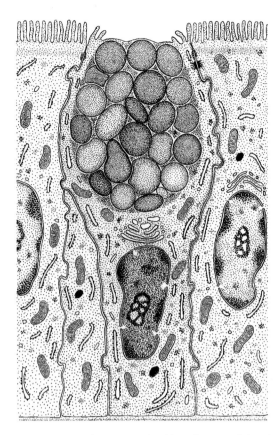

Fig. 2-18 *Drawing of an intestinal goblet cell, a unicellular gland. The nucleus is often displaced to the cell base and deformed by the accumulated mucus.*

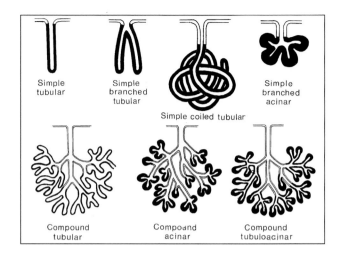

Fig. 2-19 Principal types of exocrine glands. The part of the gland consisting of secretory cells is shown in black. The glands in the lower row are depicted at lower magnification than those above. (Redrawn and modified from L. C. Junquiera, J. Carniero, and R. O. Kelley, *Basic Histology, 7th ed.* Appleton and Lange, 1992.)

more slender basal portion (Fig. 2-18). They secrete mucus which lubricates and protects the surface of the epithelium. Thus, they can be described as intramural unicellular mucus-secreting glands. Although they do not conform to the definition of a gland as an assemblage of secretory cells, goblet cells are regarded as unicellular glands. More common are the multicellular glands which range in size from small clusters of cells to tens of thousands, forming the parenchyma of whole organs such as the pancreas or the liver.

Two components are recognized in exocrine glands: the **secretory units (acini)** that synthesize the product, and the **ducts** that convey it to an inner or outer epithelial surface. The cells lining the ducts may concentrate and, in some instances, slightly alter the composition of the secretion. Glands that have a single unbranched duct are called **simple glands**. Larger glands having a highly branched duct system are **compound glands** (Fig. 2-19). The secretory portion of simple glands may be straight, coiled, or branched, and they are described accordingly as **simple tubular, simple coiled tubular,** and **simple branched tubular**. If the secretory units have a rounded or bulbar form, they are designated **simple acinar** and **simple branched acinar** glands. In a **compound acinar gland**, the bulbous acini of its terminal secretory portions are made up of pyramidal secretory cells around a very small

lumen (Fig. 2-20 [See Plate 2]). Quite commonly, however, secretory cells form the walls of short tubules with acini along their sides and at their ends. Such glands are more accurately described as **compound tubuloacinar glands** (viz. pancreas and salivary glands).

Glands may also be classified on the basis of the nature of their secretions. Thus, they may be described as **mucous glands, serous glands,** or **mixed glands**. Mucous glands secrete mucus and serous glands produce a watery secretion often rich in enzymes. Mixed glands contain both mucous and serous cells with the mucous cells making up the major portion of the gland and the serous cells forming crescentic caps, called **serous demilunes**, over the ends of the acini. The cells of the serous demilunes communicate with the lumen of the acinus via secretory canaliculi between the mucous cells.

Large compound glands like the pancreas are enclosed in a connective tissue capsule. Thinner connective tissue septa extend from the capsule into the gland passing between the masses of acini associated with the larger branches of the main duct, dividing the gland into grossly visible lobes. These, in turn, are partitioned into small lobules by thinner septa between the ramifications of smaller ducts.

Glands may also be classified according to the mode of release of their product. In **merocrine glands**, such as the pancreas, the product is released by exocytosis of secretory granules. Less common are **holocrine glands**, in which the whole cell is shed and the secretion contains residues of gland cells, as well as the secretory product. The sebaceous glands of the skin are an example. Relatively rare are **apocrine glands**, in which the apical portion of the cell, containing the product, is pinched off and released into the duct system. In the mammary gland, release of the protein component of the milk is merocrine, but the lipid component accumulates in the cell apex in large droplets that project into the lumen and are pinched off, surrounded by a portion of the plasmalemma or, sometimes, by a thin film of cytoplasm. This is one of the very few examples of apocrine secretion.

Control of Exocrine Secretion

Many exocrine glands secrete continuously, at a low rate, but are stimulated to increase their output when a greater amount of the product is required. The stimulus differs from gland to gland. Some are activated by the autonomic nervous system, whereas others respond to a blood-borne hormone. There is no microscopic clue to the involvement of a hormone, but control by the nervous system can be inferred from the finding of nerve endings in close contact with the base of some of the glandular cells. Both control mechanisms may coexist in the same gland. In the pancreas, for example, there are numerous nerve endings on acini, but physiological studies show that the gland is also responsive to the hormone gastrin, produced by the stomach, and to secretin and cholecystokinin, secreted by the duodenum.

Endocrine Glands

Endocrine glands are assemblages of secretory cells that have no duct system. Their product is a **hormone,** a chemical messenger that is released into the blood or lymph for transport to distant target cells that have specific receptors for that hormone in their plasmalemma. Endocrine glands arise in the embryo as tubular invaginations or solid outgrowths from an epithelium, but later in development, they lose their connection with the epitheli-

um from which they arose and become compact masses of epithelial cells penetrated by a rich network of fenestrated capillaries. This intimate relation between the cells and the capillaries facilitates delivery of their hormones into the blood. Some endocrine glands, such as the hypophysis and adrenal, form distinct organs. In the pancreas, however, small aggregations of endocrine cells, the islets of Langerhans, are scattered through the parenchyma of that exocrine gland. Similarly, in the testis, clusters of Leydig cells, which secrete sex hormones, are located in the interstitial tissue between the seminiferous tubules, which are the exocrine portion of that gland. Hormones are usually proteins, polypeptides, or steroids. The principal endocrine glands are the hypophysis, thyroid, adrenals, ovaries, testes, and placenta. Their microscopic structure will be considered later, in separate chapters.

HISTOPHYSIOLOGY OF EPITHELIA

As stated earlier, an epithelium is a continuous layer of cells that covers an external surface or lines in an internal cavity. Its organization and function are adapted to the local needs. On external surfaces, the epithelium is specialized for protection and prevention of dehydration. On various internal surfaces it may be specialized for absorption, secretion, or movement of fluid and particulate matter along its surface. To carry out these functions, the intercellular spaces are sealed by tight junctions to prevent passive diffusion across the epithelium, and there are gap junctions that permit the spread of signalling molecules from cell to cell to coordinate their activities and enable the entire epithelium to function as a unit. The specializations of the various epithelia will be discussed in more appropriate context in later chapters.

QUESTIONS*

1. Cellular morphologic changes or alterations in epithelia to strengthen their attachment to one another include

   A. maculae
   B. desmosomes
   C. tight junctions
   D. zonulae
   E. all of the above

2. Epithelium can be classified according to

   A. the number of cells in the layer above the basal lamina
   B. the shape of the cells lining the lumen
   C. cellular specializations
   D. all of the above
   E. none of the above

3. Goblet cells can be observed in the

   A. urinary bladder
   B. esophagus
   C. oral cavity
   D. small intestine
   E. ovary

4. Cilia

   A. are nonmotile
   B. are found in the esophagus
   C. are significantly smaller than microvilli
   D. are adapted to move luminal material
   E. increase significantly the absorptive surface of cells

5. All epithelia which comprise a simple lining rest on

   A. connective tissue
   B. elastic fibers
   C. basal lamina
   D. papillae
   E. capillaries

6. Stratified squamous epithelium would be best for lining what organ?

   A. esophagus
   B. trachea
   C. stomach
   D. small intestine
   E. urinary bladder

7. Which of the following do not contribute to the strengthening of intercellular attachments in epithelia?

   A. maculae
   B. cilia
   C. desmosomes
   D. zonulae
   E. tight junctions

8. If you were to build a urinary bladder, keeping in mind the interrelationship between structure and function, which type of epithelium would you use?

   A. simple cuboidal
   B. keratinized stratified squamous
   C. pseudostratified columnar
   D. stratified squamous nonkeratinized
   E. transitional

9. Which type of cellular structural modification would best suit the needs of the respiratory system?

   A. stereocilia
   B. brush border
   C. keratinization
   D. striated border
   E. cilia

10. Which of the following statements about epithelium and epithelial cells is **not** true?

    A. basal cells always rest on a basement membrane (lamina).
    B. epithelial cells are incapable of reproduction.
    C. may contain modified cells related to functional specificity.
    D. may be composed of more than one cell layer.
    E. separate the external and internal environments.

*Answers on page 307.

3

BLOOD

CHAPTER OUTLINE

KEY WORDS

ABO Typing
Anisocytosis
Ankyrin
Antigens A and B
Blood Plasma
Carbaminohemo-
    globin
Chemotaxis
Crenation
Cytokine
Echinocytes
Erythroblasts
Erythrocyte Ghost
Erythrocytes
Fibrinogen
Granulocytes
Granulomere Platelet
    Factors
Hemoglobin
Hemolysis
Hemophilia
Heparin
Hereditary Ellipso-
    cytosis

Hereditary
    Spherocytosis
Hyalomere
Leukocytes
Lymphocytes; T and B
Macrocytes
Microcytes
Mononuclear
Phagocyte System
Oxyhemoglobin
Phagocytins
Platelets
Polychromato-
    philic
Prothrombin
Reticulocytes
Rouleaux
Sickle Cell Anemia
Spectrin
Thrombin
Thromboplastids
Thrombospondin

Blood is a tissue composed of the **erythrocytes** (red blood cells), **leukocytes** (white blood cells), and **platelets** suspended in a liquid matrix, the **blood plasma**. It circulates in the blood vessels to maintain logistical support and communication between all of the other tissues of the body. It distributes oxygen from the lungs and nutrients from the gastrointestinal tract. It carries carbon dioxide from the tissues back to the lungs, and nitrogenous wastes to the kidneys for excretion. It also plays an essential role in the integrative function of the endocrine system by carrying hormones from their site of origin to their distant target tissues. Its volume in the human is about 5 liters.

Blood cells were once thought to carry out their principal functions in the bloodstream, but when it became possible to radiolabel cells and trace their migrations, it was found that only the erythrocytes and platelets function within the confines of the vascular system. The leukocytes are only transiently in the blood, which simply serves as a vehicle for their transport and dissemination. They are constantly migrating through the walls of capillaries and venules to become free cells wandering through the connective tissues of the body.

A knowledge of the appearance, and normal numbers, of the blood cells is important to the medical practitioner, as no tissue is examined more often for diagnostic purposes. Examination of stained blood smears not only yields information about diseases that primarily affect the blood but also provides indirect evidence of viral, bacterial, or parasitic infections that may enable the physician to identify the disease, follow its course, and evaluate the effectiveness of its treatment.

ERYTHROCYTES

Erythrocytes are the minute corpuscles that impart a red color to the blood, owing to their content of the oxygen-carrying pigment, **hemoglobin**. They number about $5,500,000/mm^3$ in the human male, and $5,000,000/mm^3$ in the female. In total, they present a surface area of 3800 m^2. This surface area, roughly the size of a football field, is available for gas exchange. The function of the erythrocytes is the transport of oxygen (O_2) and carbon dioxide (CO_2). As blood passes through the lungs, oxygen combines with the hemoglobin to form **oxyhemoglobin.** As the blood passes through the peripheral capillaries, O_2 is released and diffuses into the tissues. Concurrently, CO_2 diffuses from the tissues into the blood, combining with erythrocyte hemoglobin to form **carbaminohemoglobin.** In the lungs, the CO_2 dissociates from hemoglobin, diffuses into the alveoli, and is eliminated in exhalation.

Structure

Erythrocytes develop in the bone marrow from nucleated precursors but before entering the blood; they extrude their nucleus and other organelles and are reduced to membrane-limited corpuscles containing cytoplasm, which consists predominantly of hemoglobin in solution. In blood-smears stained with Wright's blood-stain, erythrocytes are pink (Fig. 3-1 [see Plate 2]). Their form is that of a biconcave disk with a thickness of 1.9 μm near the periphery and somewhat less in the center (Fig 3-2). This shape is well adapted to their function, for it presents, for gas exchange, a surface area 20–30% greater that a sphere of the same volume. In the blood, erythrocytes are 8.5 μm in diameter, but in the dehydrated state, in dried blood smears, they measure 7.6 μm. Their life span in the circulation is about 120 days. It follows from this datum that in excess of 2 million erythrocytes must enter the bloodstream every second, as an equal number are lost. The mechanism of their disposal is not entirely clear, but it is known that the aging erythrocytes are taken up and digested by phagocytic Kupffer cells in the liver and by macrophages in the spleen.

*Anemia is the term applied to any significant reduction in total mass of erythrocytes or in their content of hemoglobin, resulting in a reduced oxygen-carrying capacity of the blood. A deficiency in dietary intake of iron needed for hemoglobin synthesis may result in **iron-deficiency anemia**. Deficiencies of vitamin B_{12} or of folic acid may lead to **megaloblastic anemia** in which there is a retarded production of erythrocytes of larger than normal size.*

In stained blood smears, the great majority of erythrocytes stain a deep pink, but a small number that have recently entered the circulation, from the bone marrow, have a bluish or greenish tint, owing to the basophilic staining of residual ribosomes in their cytoplasm. Such polychromatophilic erythrocytes are commonly called **reticulocytes**, for when stained with Brilliant Cresyl Blue their ribonucleoprotein is precipitated by the dye as a delicate basophilic network in an otherwise acidophilic cytoplasm. Within 24 h of entering the blood, the maturing reticulocytes lose their basophilia. In the adult human, the number of reticulocytes averages about 8% of the total number of erythrocytes. The **reticulocyte count**, made on appropriately stained blood smears, is used clinically as a rough index of the rate of erythrocyte production. In patients with anemia, an elevated reticulocyte count is an encouraging sign of response to treatment.

Erythrocytes are quite pliable and may be deformed to bell-like or paraboloid shapes when flowing through small capillaries. Their shape is also influenced by the osmolarity of the surrounding medium. In moderately hypotonic solutions, they become cup-shaped and in solutions that are still more hypotonic, their swelling stretches the membrane and it becomes leaky, permitting the hemoglobin to escape, leaving behind the empty membrane called an **erythrocyte ghost**. Hypotonic disruption of erythrocytes is

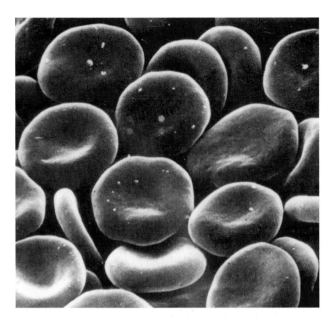

Fig. 3-2 A scanning electron micrograph of erythrocytes illustrating their discoid biconcave shape. (Micrograph courtesy of D. Phillips.)

called **hemolysis**. In fresh blood, examined in vitro, the discoid erythrocytes often form aggregates that resemble stacks of coins. These are called **rouleaux**. The basis of rouleaux formation is not understood. It does not occur in the circulation.

The maintenance of the normal biconcave shape of the erythrocytes is dependant on their content of adenosine triphosphate (ATP). When this falls below a critical level, they assume the shape of a small sphere with 10–30 radiating conical protuberances. In this form, they are called **echinocytes**, and the adoption of this shape is called *crenation*. If crenated erythrocytes are allowed time to regenerate ATP, this shape change is reversed.

Ultrastructure

The biconcave shape of erythrocytes is clearly revealed in scanning electron micrographs (Fig. 3-2). In thin sections, the membrane is unremarkable, but immediately beneath it, there is a network of filaments forming the so-called **membrane skeleton**. This is composed of **actin, spectrin,** and two associated proteins designated **band 4.1** and **band 4.9** on the basis of their electrophoretic mobility in gels. The major component of this network is spectrin, composed of two polypeptide chains that form filaments 200 nm in length. These are bound at their ends to nodal structures consisting of actin and the band 4.1 and band 4.9 proteins. Near the middle of each short strand of spectrin there is a binding site for **ankyrin**, a phosphoprotein that serves to link the network to an integral protein of the erythrocyte membrane. The actin of erythrocytes does not form filaments of the kind seen in the cytoskeleton of other cell types, but it forms short polymers only 7 nm in

length which are stabilized by **tropomyosin.** These complexes are components of the nodal structures that join the ends of the spectrin filaments together to form a network. In their 120-day life span, erythrocytes must withstand frequent deformations during thousands of passages through the vascular system. Their membrane skeleton provides them with the necessary stability and resilience to resist these stresses.

Departures from the normal size and shape of erythrocytes are encountered in a number of anemias, and a terminology has developed to describe these. Erythrocytes with a diameter greater than 9 μm are called **macrocytes** and those with diameters less than 6 μm are **microcytes**. The occurrence of large numbers of erythrocytes varying in size is termed **anisocytosis**.

> *In an hereditary disease, called **sickle-cell anemia**, a substitution of one amino acid in hemoglobin makes the molecule insoluble at low-oxygen tensions and it crystallizes within the erythrocytes, altering their shape. In **hereditary spherocytosis**, a deficiency of spectrin alters the cytoskeleton, resulting in alteration of cell shape.*

BLOOD-GROUP ANTIGENS

All cell membranes have carbohydrate chains of integral glycolipids and glycoproteins exposed on their surface. Two specific carbohydrate chains of the human erythrocyte membrane are antigenic and may result in a severe immune reaction after an incompatible blood transfusion. These are designated **antigen-A** and **antigen-B** and are the basis of the **ABO blood-group typing system**. The erythrocytes of some individuals have antigen-A on their membrane, some have antigen-B, others have both, and still others have neither. Thus, there are four major blood groups, **A, B, AB,** and **O**. For reasons that are not clear, all individuals have, in their blood plasma, antibodies against the antigens that do not occur on their own erythrocytes. Therefore, before giving a transfusion, it is necessary to determine what antigens occur on the erythrocytes of the donor and what antibodies are present in the plasma of the recipient. Failure to carry out this cross-matching may result in massive intravascular agglutination and lysis of erythrocytes in the recipient of a transfusion.

BLOOD PLATELETS

Blood platelets, or **thromboplastids**, are minute, colorless, anucleate corpuscles found in the blood of all mammals. They are thin, ovoid, biconvex disks 2–3 μm in diameter (Fig. 3-3). When viewed in section, they are fusiform. In the human, their number ranges from 150,000

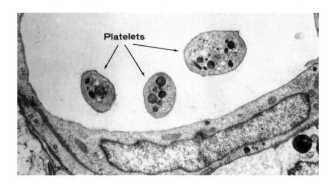

Fig. 3-3 Electron micrograph of three blood platelets in the lumen of a capillary. Note their dense azurophilic granules.

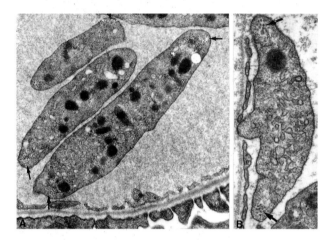

Fig. 3-4 (A) Electron micrograph of platelets. The arrows point to cross sections of a circumferential band of microtubules that maintain their shape. (Courtesy of D. Bainton.)
(B) Cross sections of the microtubules are more clearly visible in this section of a platelet adjacent to the wall of a fenestrated capillary (Courtesy of D. Friend.)

to 300,000/mm³ blood. In stained blood smears, they exhibit two concentric zones: a thin, pale, peripheral zone called the **hyalomere**, and a larger and more deeply stained central region, the **granulomere**. The latter contains small **azurophilic granules**. Platelets function in the clotting of blood at sites of injury to blood vessels and thus help to prevent excessive blood loss.

Ultrastructure

Electron micrographs of platelets reveal the structural components that maintain their flattened discoid shape. In equatorial sections, a circumferential band of 10–15 microtubules is visible in the hyalomere immediately beneath the plasmalemma. In cross section, this appears as a cluster of small circular profiles at either end of the platelet (Fig. 3-4). The hyalomere contains no other formed elements, but it is exceptionally rich in actin and myosin. These are normally present in monomeric form, but when platelets are activated

in the clotting process, actin polymerizes into the filamentous form necessary for contraction.

The granulomere contains small aggregations of glycogen particles and slender membrane-limited canaliculi that open onto the platelet surface at several sites. These are believed to serve as pathways for discharge of secretory products of activated platelets. The most conspicuous components of the granulomere are two or more categories of small dense granules. The so-called **alpha granules** correspond to the azurophil granules seen with the light microscope. They contain several substances with important functions: (1) **platelet factor IV**, which counteracts the anticoagulant heparin, (2) **von Willebrandt factor**, a glycoprotein that facilitates the adhesion of platelets to sites of injury to the blood vessel wall, (3) **platelet-derived growth factor**, which stimulates repair of damaged vessel walls, and (4) **thrombospondin**, a glycoprotein responsible for platelet aggregation in the process of blood clotting. In some species, platelets also contain **beta granules** that store **serotonin, ATP**, and **ADP**, which are potent promoters of platelet aggregation.

Function

Circulating platelets constantly patrol the vascular system for endothelial damage. The magnitude of their defensive mission is evident from the estimate that, during each minute, approximately 10^{12} platelets pass over 1000 m² of capillary surface, lined by 7×10^{11} endothelial cells. They normally exhibit no tendency to adhere to each other or to the vessel wall, but if any disruption of the endothelium is detected, they adhere to each other and to the site of injury, to initiate blood clotting, which limits blood loss and begins the process of repair. Platelets quickly adhere to the collagen exposed at a site of injury, via a collagen-binding

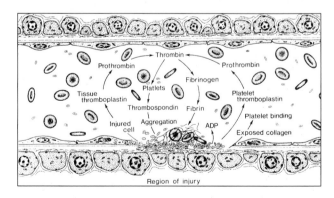

Fig. 3-5 Schematic representation of the initiating events in the formation of a blood clot in an injured vessel. Platelets adhere to the site of injury and release ADP and adhesive glycoproteins, which accelerate platelet aggregation. Tissue thromboplastin released from injured cells induces conversion of plasma prothrombin to thrombin. This catalyzes conversion of plasma fibrinogen to fibrin, which polymerizes to form fibers enmeshing platelets and impounding erythrocytes in a gelatinous clot.

protein in their membrane. Adhesion activates the platelets and causes them to release an adhesive glycoprotein and ADP, which is a potent inducer of platelet aggregation. This results in adherence of many more platelets to those already bound to the collagen. These new platelets, in turn, are activated, and their products contribute to further platelet aggregation that results in formation of a **platelet thrombus** occluding the lumen of the vessel (Fig. 3-5).

Concurrently, other complex reactions of clotting are set in motion. A substance called **tissue thromboplastin**, released by injured endothelial cells, initiates a series of reactions in the blood plasma that convert **prothrombin** to **thrombin**. Thrombin, in turn, catalyzes the conversion of a constituent of the plasma called **fibrinogen** to **fibrin**, which polymerizes to form a meshwork of fine fibrils among the aggregating platelets. These fibrils bind erythrocytes together to form a gelatinous **blood clot** (Fig. 3-6).

> *Hemophilia is an inherited defect in factor VIII, one of the clotting factors. The gene involved is located on the X chromosome so this disease usually affects males. Daughters of hemophiliacs are carriers and the sons of such carriers have a 50% chance of inheriting the disease. These patients bleed into muscles, joints, and body cavities for hours or days after an injury. Surgery and even dental extractions must be carried out with extreme care to prevent excess bleeding.*

Inherited abnormalities of platelets, or deficiencies of the accessory plasma factors, are responsible for a number of diseases. The best known is **hemophilia**, which is due to the absence of only one of the many plasma factors necessary for blood clotting.

LEUKOCYTES

The **leukocytes** are a group of cell types that are concerned with the defenses of the body against invading foreign matter. They are divided into two categories: **granular leukocytes** (**granulocytes**) and **agranular leukocytes**, depending on whether their cytoplasm contains specific granules that bind the dyes in Wright's blood stain. There are three types of granulocytes, **eosinophils, basophils**, and **neutrophils**. The agranular leukocytes include **monocytes** and **lymphocytes** (Fig. 3-7 [see Plate 3]).

A relatively small fraction of the life span of leukocytes is spent in the blood. Granulocytes spend no more than 2 days and lymphocytes less than 1 day there before migrating across the wall of capillaries into the connective tissue. They are spherical and inactive in the blood but exhibit varying degrees of amoeboid motility as they wander over the solid substrate afforded by the fibers of the connective tissue.

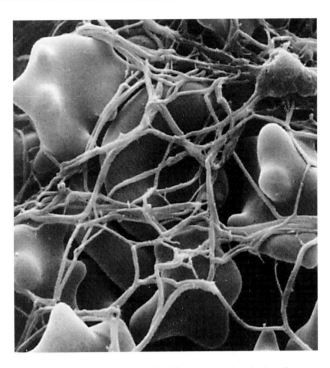

Fig. 3-6 Scanning micrograph of an early blood clot showing crenated erythrocytes in a meshwork of fibrin.

The number of leukocytes in the circulation ranges from 5000 to 9000/mm³ of blood. The number varies somewhat with the age of the individual, and even with the time of day. The large number in the tissues and organs cannot be quantitated. Minor variations in the leukocyte count are of little clinical significance, but in the presence of an infection anywhere in the body, the blood leukocyte count may rise to 20,000–40,000/mm³. The relative numbers of the several kinds of leukocytes, the **differential leukocyte count**, is normally fairly constant: neutrophils 55–60%; eosinophils 1–3%; basophils 0–0.7%; lymphocytes 25–33%; monocytes 3–7%. Different diseases affect the number of certain cell types more than others, and the differential leukocyte count is often helpful in making a diagnosis.

Neutrophilic Leukocytes

Neutrophils, also called **polymorphonuclear leukocytes**, are the most abundant of the granular leukocytes. There are 3000–6000/mm³ and about 25 billion in the entire circulation. They are 7 μm in diameter in fresh blood and 10–12 μm in diameter in dried blood smears. Mature neutrophils are easily recognized by their characteristic nucleus which has two to four lobules connected by narrow constrictions (Figs. 3-7A, and 3-7D [see Plate 3], and 3-8). Immature neutrophils which have recently entered the circulation from the bone marrow have a simple elongated nucleus and are referred to as **band forms**. The number of these in a differential leukocyte count is a useful index of the rate of entry of new neutrophils into the

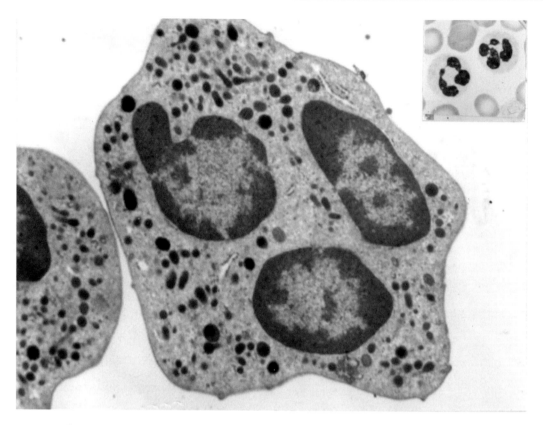

Fig. 3-8 Electron micrograph of a polymorphonuclear leukocyte. Thin sections create the false impression that the cell is multinucleate. The three lobes of the nucleus shown here are continuous with one another in other planes of section. The continuity of the lobulated single nucleus is more apparent in blood smears (inset, upper right).

circulation. In the neutrophils of the human female, the chromatin representing the condensed X chromosome may form an additional minute lobule often referred to as the **"drumstick,"** because of its characteristic shape. Thus, it is possible to determine the genetic sex of an individual by examining a large number of neutrophils in a blood smear for the presence of this minute nuclear appendage.

The cytoplasm of neutrophils is stippled with numerous small granules of two kinds: **specific granules**, which have little affinity for dyes, and a smaller number of **azurophilic granules**, which are somewhat larger and stain more intensely. In electron micrographs, a small Golgi complex is found among the lobules of the nucleus. There are a few mitochondria and a rudimentary endoplasmic reticulum. Aggregations of granules of glycogen in the cytoplasm are common. The specific and azurophilic granules are widely dispersed in the cytoplasm but are excluded from a thin ectoplasmic zone rich in actin filaments. The specific granules vary in shape from round to elongate. The slightly larger azurophil granules are more electron dense. The two types of granules are not easily identified in micrographs, but they can be distinguished by histochemical reactions. The azurophil granules give a positive reaction for the enzymes peroxidase, acid phosphatase, and glucuronidase, whereas the specific granules react positively for alkaline phosphatase, collagenase,

lysozyme, lactoferritin, and several basic proteins collectively called **phagocytins**. The latter are believed to have nonenzymatic antibacterial activity.

Functions of the Neutrophil

Neutrophils are in the front line of the body's defense against bacterial invasion. Their motility enables them to mobilize at a site of infection, where they phagocytize and digest bacteria (Fig. 3-9). A locally generated chemical

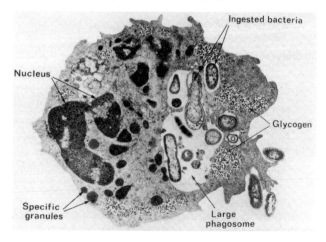

Fig. 3-9 Micrograph of a neutrophil engaged in phagocytosis of bacteria. Note several bacteria in vacuoles within the cytoplasm.

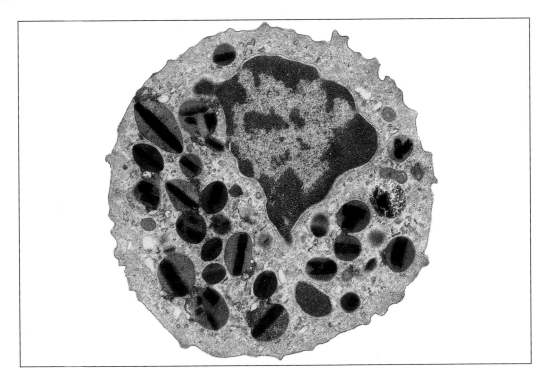

Fig. 3-10 Electron micrograph of an eosinophilic leukocyte. Note the large specific granules containing dense rhombohedral crystals.

mediator carried in the blood from the site of infection to the bone marrow stimulates increased production and release of neutrophils into the blood. These migrate through the endothelium of capillaries at the site of bacterial invasion and migrate up the concentration gradient of bacterial products to join the neutrophils already mobilized there. This migration up the gradient of a chemoattractant is called **chemotaxis**. The pus that accumulates at sites of infection consists of hundreds of thousands of dead and dying neutrophils and other leukocytes that have completed their mission and reached the end of their life span.

Eosinophilic Leukocytes

Eosinophilic leukocytes (**eosinophils**) are 9 μm in diameter in suspension and about 12 μm in diameter in blood smears. They are easily distinguished from neutrophils by their relatively large specific granules which stain pink with Wright's blood stain (Figs. 3-7B and 3-7E [see Plate 3]). Their nucleus is bilobed and its chromatin less coarse than that of neutrophils. There is a small Golgi complex and a few mitochondria. The specific granules are the most conspicuous component of the cytoplasm. These exhibit a striking interspecific variation in their ultrastructure. In the human, they are membrane limited and contain single or multiple crystals in a finely granular matrix of moderate density (Fig. 3-10). Such crystals are lacking in other mammalian species. A few relatively

small azurophilic granules are also present in the cytoplasm of eosinophils.

Functions

After entering the blood from the bone marrow, eosinophils circulate for only 6–10 h before migrating into the connective tissue, where they spend the remainder of their 8–12-day life span. Unlike neutrophils, they do not phagocytize and destroy bacteria intracellularly. One of their major functions seems to be to take up and dispose of antigen–antibody complexes formed in allergic conditions such as asthma and hay fever. They are especially abundant beneath the epithelia of the respiratory and gastrointestinal tracts, where entry of foreign proteins is most likely to occur. They are attracted to sites of **histamine** release, and the enzymes in their granules are capable of degrading this and other mediators of allergic reactions. The specific granules of eosinophils contain several hydrolases including **aryl sulfatase, ß-glucuronidase, acid phosphatase,** and **ribonuclease.** In addition, they contain three **cationic proteins** not found in lysosomes of other cell types. These are **major basophilic protein** (MBP), **eosinophil cationic protein** (ECP), and **eosinophil-derived neurotoxin.** The significance of these proteins is still under investigation, but they are believed to be important in the role of eosinophils in allergic reactions and in defense against parasitic infections. In both of these conditions, the number of eosinophils in the blood and tissues is greatly increased. MBP and ECP are both cytotoxic for

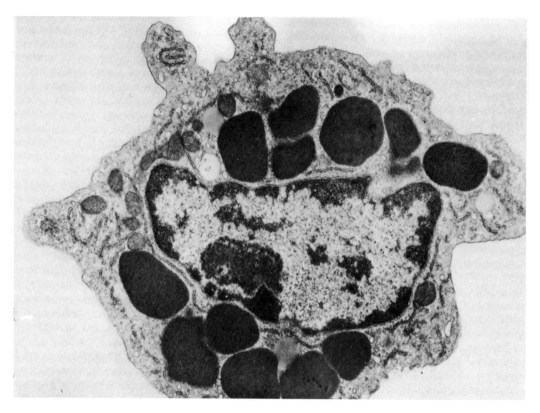

Fig. 3-11 Electron micrograph of a basophilic leukocyte. The large granules vary in shape and often in density. Note the presence of tubules and cisternae of the rough endoplasmic reticulum.

Schistosoma mansoni and *Trypanosoma cruzi*, two protozoan parasites affecting man.

Basophilic Leukocytes

The **basophilic leukocytes** are the least numerous of the granulocytes, accounting for only 0.5% of the total white blood cell count. They are about the same size as neutrophils, measuring 12 μm in diameter in stained smears. The nucleus is less heterochromatic than that of other leukocytes and is U- or J-shaped and therefore may appear bilobed in histological sections (Fig. 3-7C [see Plate 3]). The specific granules are few in number and much larger than those of eosinophils. The granules are **metachromatic**, staining purple with Toluidine Blue or alcoholic thionine.

In electron micrographs, basophils have a small Golgi complex, a few mitochondria, and somewhat more endoplasmic reticulum than other leukocytes. Particles of glycogen are not uncommon. The membrane-bounded specific granules are round or ovoid and 0.5 μm in diameter, with an interior consisting of closely packed small particles in a less-dense matrix (Fig. 3-11). They contain **heparin**, which is responsible for their metachromatic staining, and **histamine**. There is no evidence that they contain any of the lysosomal hydrolases.

Function

The basophils of the blood and the **mast cells** of the connective tissue share certain properties, but differ in others. The mast cells are larger and have many more granules. Both have large metachromatic granules containing histamine and heparin. Basophils are short-lived, and mast cells long-lived. Mast cells are relatively sessile, whereas basophils are motile, as evidenced by their assembly at sites of inflammation. Both release histamine and heparin and evidently have similar functions. It is not yet settled whether they arise from the same or different stem cells.

MONOCYTES

Monocytes account for 3–8% of the circulating leukocytes. They are spherical cells 10–12 μm in diameter in suspension, but they may measure up to 17 μm in diameter in blood smears. The eccentric nucleus is round, or more commonly kidney-shaped. Its chromatin stains less intensely than that of other agranular leukocytes (Figs. 3-7J and 3-7K [see Plate 3]). The cytoplasm has a pale blue-gray color in stained smears and contains a few small azurophilic granules.

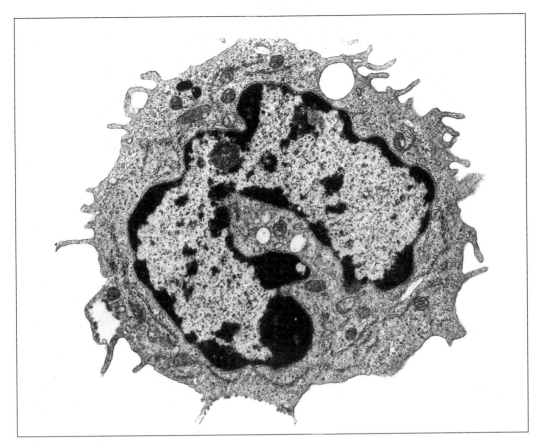

Fig. 3-12 Electron micrograph of a monocyte. It has a deeply indented nucleus, a few mitochondria, some endoplasmic reticulum and occasional lysosomes, but no specific granules.

In electron micrographs, the monocyte has a few short, slender processes. The chromatin of the nucleus is largely dispersed, but there are a few small clumps of condensed chromatin adjacent to the nuclear envelope (Fig. 3–12). One or two nucleoli are usually visible. The cytoplasm contains a small Golgi complex, a few cisternal profiles of endoplasmic reticulum, scattered glycogen particles, and a moderate number of ribosomes. There are also a few small, dense granules corresponding to the azurophilic granules seen in blood smears.

Functions

Monocytes originate in the bone marrow and circulate in the blood for 1–4 days before entering the connective tissue. There they differentiate into **tissue macrophages**, voracious phagocytic cells that take on the housekeeping chore of ingesting senescent cells, cellular debris, and any foreign matter, including invading bacteria. Together with the **alveolar macrophages** of the lung and the **Kupffer cells** of the liver, they comprise the **mononuclear phagocyte system** of the body. Monocytes and the macrophages also play an indispensible role in humoral immune responses by processing antigens and presenting them to lymphocytes to initiate the production of antibodies.

LYMPHOCYTES

Lymphocytes are the second most numerous class of leukocytes, accounting for 20–35% of the circulating white blood cells. In blood smears, they are small, round cells 7–16 μm in diameter, with a deeply staining, slightly indented nucleus, and a thin rim of clear blue cytoplasm (Figs. 3-7G and 3-7I [see Plate 3]). They contain no specific granules but may have a few small azurophil granules. In electron micrographs, a very small Golgi complex and one or two small mitochondria can be identified (Fig. 3–13). The endoplasmic reticulum is lacking but there are many free ribosomes in the cytoplasm.

The vast majority of the lymphocytes are at the low end of their size range and are referred to as **small lymphocytes.** Others with a somewhat wider rim of cytoplasm are called **large lymphocytes**. These may reach a diameter of 17 μm. The functional implications of these size differences are not entirely clear, and these descriptive terms, based on size, are no longer widely used. With advances in our understanding of immunology, more interest has centered upon two major categories of lymphocytes: **B lymphocytes** and **T lymphocytes** that differ in their developmental background, life span, and functions. They

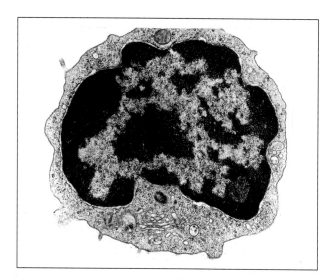

Fig. 3-13 Micrograph of a small lymphocyte. It has nucleus with large clumps of condensed chromatin, surrounded by a thin rim of cytoplasm. This section contains a very small Golgi complex, a centriole, and a single mitochondrion.

are not morphologically distinguishable, but they do have distinctive molecules in their surface membrane that serve as type-specific markers, and they can, therefore, be distinguished by immunocytochemical methods.

The lymphocytes are the principal agents of the body's humoral defense response to invasion by bacteria and viruses. The B lymphocytes produce the **antibodies** that resist infection. There are two major categories of T lymphocytes, **helper T lymphocytes**, which release signaling molecules to attract and activate B lymphocytes, and **cytotoxic T lymphocytes**, which secrete substances that kill virus-infected cells or foreign cells of tissue transplanted from another individual. The explanation of the way in which the lymphocytes carry out their important

defensive role will be deferred to Chapter 12, the Immune System.

Vast numbers of lymphocytes are found in the parenchyma of the lymph nodes and spleen. The great majority of these are B lymphocytes that have arisen from precursors in the bone marrow and have been carried to these organs in the blood. After a stay of varying duration in the these organs, they return to the blood via the lymph. B lymphocytes have a normal life span of several months, and during this time, they recirculate through the blood, lymph nodes, spleen, and lymph many times. The T lymphocytes have a very different life history. Stem cells destined to give rise to T lymphocytes originate in the bone marrow but soon enter the blood and settle in the cortex of the thymus, where they proliferate. As their progeny move through the cortex of the thymus to its medulla, they differentiate, acquiring the surface markers and receptors characteristic of T lymphocytes. After entering the blood from the thymus, they join the population of continuously recycling lymphocytes. They make up 70% or more of the small lymphocytes of the blood and have a life span, in humans, that may extend over several years.

Cytokines (Lymphokines)

Hormones are signaling molecules secreted by glandular cells and transported in the blood to distant target cells. **Cytokines** are molecules involved in intercellular communication by diffusion over short distances to target cells that have specific receptors for those molecules on their surface. The lymphocytes secrete a dozen or more signaling molecules that influence the behavior of other cells. These were formerly called **lymphokines**, but it has since been found that some of these same molecules are secreted by other cell types, and the more general term **cytokine** is now preferred.

p.49b

QUESTIONS*

1. Which of the following blood granulocytes contains very large metachromatic granules?

   A. basophil
   B. mast cell
   C. monocyte
   D. neutrophil
   E. lymphocyte

2. In prenatal life, nucleated erythrocytes are mainly or exclusively formed by which one, if any, of the following?

   A. liver
   B. spleen
   C. thymus
   D. yolk sac
   E. none of the above

3. A macrophage can originate from which of the following cells?

   A. reticular cell
   B. neutrophil
   C. plasma cell
   D. monocyte
   E. none of the above

4. A cell containing both a hyalomere and granulomere regions is a

   A. promyelocyte
   B. monocyte
   C. platelet
   D. basophil
   E. none of the above

5. Monocytes

   A. represent over 20% of the WBCs
   B. represent 1% of the WBCs
   C. represent approximately 30% of the WBCs
   D. represent approximately 5% of the WBCs
   E. none of the above

6. In the early stages of an inflammatory response, which of the following blood cells would predominate?

   A. macrophages
   B. monocytes
   C. basophils
   D. neutrophils
   E. plasma cells

7. A person suffering from an active parasitic infections would be expected to have a high count of

   A. neutrophils
   B. basophils
   C. eosinophils
   D. rubricytes
   E. myelocytes

8. Macrocytosis, microcytosis, spherocytoses, and ellipsocytosis all refer to abnormalities of the

   A. neutrophils
   B. erythrocytes
   C. monocytes
   D. basophiles
   E. lymphocytes

9. The most prominant nucleated cells in the circulation are

   A. neutrophils
   B. basophils
   C. eosinophils
   D. monocytes
   E. erythrocytes

10. Lymphocytes are

   A. the most numerous of the leukocytic cells
   B. contain large azurophilic granules
   C. give rise to tissue macrophages
   D. the principle agents in the humoral defense response
   E. typically exhibit multilobed nuclei

*Answers on page 307.

4

CONNECTIVE TISSUE

CHAPTER OUTLINE

KEY WORDS

Connective tissue consists of widely separated cells in an abundant extracellular matrix consisting of strong fibers embedded in a gellike ground substance. It is found throughout the body, supporting and binding together other structural elements. It forms the capsules of organs and thin septa that partition their epithelial functional units. It is the tissue through which the blood vessels enter and leave an organ, and the aqueous phase of its ground substance is the medium through which all nutrients and waste products diffuse in their transit between the blood and the parenchymal cells of the organs.

The relative abundance of cells, fibers, and ground substance varies from region to region and different terms are used to facilitate histological description. The term **loose connective tissue** is applied to areas in which the fibers are only moderately abundant and loosely interwoven. The term **dense connective tissue** is applied to areas in which the fibers are very abundant and closely packed. Modifiers are added to these terms to indicate the disposition of the fibers. Where they are closely interwoven, in seemingly random orientation, the tissue is described as **dense irregular connective tissue**. Where the fibers are closely packed in parallel bundles, as in tendons, or where they are interwoven in a plane to form a flat sheet, as in aponeuroses, the tissue is called **dense regular connective tissue**.

THE GROUND SUBSTANCE

The ground substance occupies all space between the cells and fibers of connective tissue. In fresh tissue, it is a colorless, translucent substance with the consistency of a highly hydrated gel. It is poorly preserved in routine histological preparations, but its residues can be detected by their staining with certain dyes or with a histochemical reaction for carbohydrates. The major polysaccharides of the ground substance are **glycosaminoglycans**. These large molecules are long linear polymers of disaccharide subunits. The major glycosaminoglycans of connective tissue are **chondroitin sulfate, keratin sulfate, heparin sulfate**, and **hyaluronic acid**. With the exception of hyaluronic acid, these occur covalently bound to a core protein to form still larger molecules called **proteoglycans** (Fig. 4-1). These very large molecules are major constituents of the ground substance. Hyaluronic acid does not bind to a core protein. It is a very large polymer of some 5000 disaccharides in a chain that would be nearly 2.5 μm in length. It is abundant in loose connective tissue. One of its important properties is its high viscosity in aqueous solution, which contributes to the gellike consistency of the ground substance. Its gelated state is no barrier to diffusion of metabolites through its aqueous phase, but it is probably a significant impediment to the spread of bacteria that may enter the tissues. It is interesting that some invasive species of bacteria have countered by acquiring the ability to synthesize the enzyme **hyaluro-**

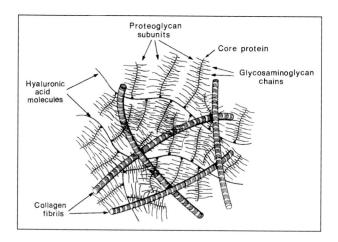

Fig. 4-1 Drawing of the extracellular matrix of cartilage, a form of connective tissue in which the matrix has a gellike consistency. The interstices between the collagen fibers are occupied by long, entwined proteogylcan molecules with hundreds of polysaccharide side chains.

nidase to depolymerize the hyaluronic acid of the ground substance.

Long, entwined proteoglycan molecules with their hundreds of glycosaminoglycan side chains are believed to occupy most of the spaces between the connective tissue fibers (Fig. 4-1). There is no satisfactory method for verification of this concept by electron microscopy, for during specimen preparation, the glycosaminoglycan chains collapse onto the core protein and the proteoglycans appear only as 10–20 nm granules in the interstices of the extracellular matrix.

In addition to these predominant components of the ground substance, there are lesser amounts of three structural or adhesion glycoproteins: **fibronectin, thrombospondin,** and **laminin**. These participate in cell binding to the connective tissue fibers or form layers supporting epithelia. The membranes of some cells have receptors that bind directly to collagen fibers, but the attachment of other cells is mediated by one of these glycoproteins. Fibronectin is a large glycoprotein (440 kDa) in the ground substance and in the basal lamina of epithelia. Along the length of this long, flexible molecule, there are binding domains for cells, collagen fibers, and glycosaminoglycans. These various binding sites are the basis for its role in connecting cells to the fibrous and amorphous components of the connective tissue. Laminin is a glycoprotein with a molecular weight of about one million. It is the major constituent of the basal lamina of epithelia. It binds to cell membranes, to **type-IV collagen**, and to heparan sulfate proteoglycan. These interactions play a major role in the assembly of the basal lamina. Thrombospondin is a 450-kDa glycoprotein that also binds to cells, collagen fibers, and fibronectin. The primary function of these adhesion glycoproteins is to maintain attachment of cells to their substrate, but evidence is accumulating that they also influence the state of differentiation of the cells and the organization of their cytoskeleton.

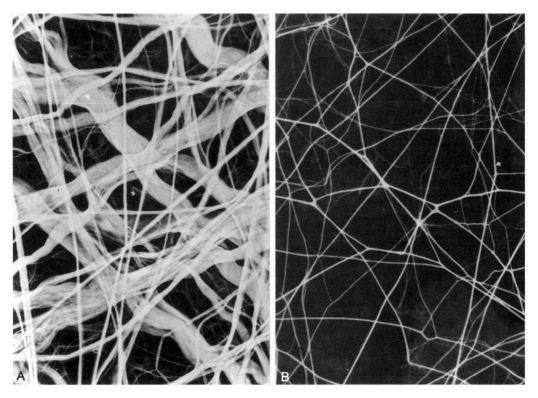

Fig. 4-2 Photomicrograph of extracellular fibers in a thin spread of mesentery. (A) Collagen fibers; (B) elastic fibers. Preparation stained with a silver method and printed as a negative to more closely simulate their fresh appearance.

EXTRACELLULAR FIBERS

Collagen Fibers

Collagen fibers are the predominant fibrous component of connective tissues. In histological sections, they are acidophilic, staining pink with hematoxylin and eosin, blue with Mallory's trichrome stain, and green with Masson's stain. In unstained spreads of loose connective tissue, they appear as randomly oriented, colorless strands ranging from 0.5 to 10 μm in diameter and of indefinite length (Fig. 4-2A). A faint longitudinal striation is evident in the larger fibers, suggesting that they are made up of smaller subunits. This is borne out in electron micrographs, where collagen fibers are seen to be bundles of unit fibrils 50–90 nm in diameter (Fig. 4-3). When stained with lead, collagen fibers are cross-striated, with denser staining transverse bands repeating every 64 nm along their length. This cross-banding is also evident in shadowed preparations of the isolated unit fibrils (Fig. 4-4). The fibrils are polymers of **tropocollagen** molecules, 280 nm in length and 1.4 nm in diameter. Each tropocollagen molecule is made up of three intertwined polypeptide chains. Two of the amino acids in these chains, **hydroxyproline** and **hydroxylysine** are highly characteristic of collagen, and the collagen

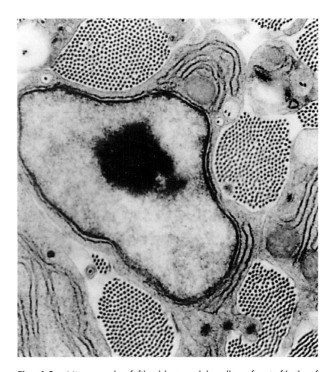

Fig. 4-3 Micrograph of fibroblast and bundles of unit fibrils of collagen in a developing tendon. Note the well-developed endoplasmic reticulum in these actively synthesizing fibroblasts. (Micrograph courtesy of D. Birk and R. Trelstad, J Cell Biology 103: 231, 1986.)

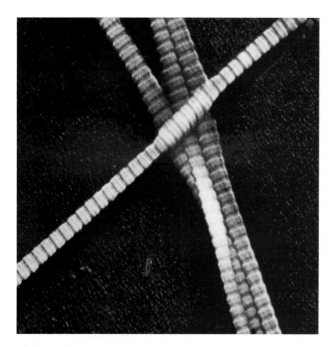

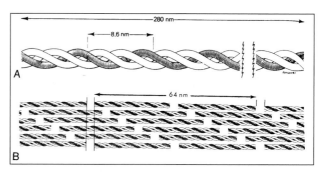

Fig. 4-5 (A) Each molecule of type-I collagen is composed of two alpha-1 polypeptide chains and one alpha-2 chain, intertwined in a triple helix. (B) Drawing of the arrangement of several rows of molecules in a collagen fibril. The molecules are aligned with a gap between their ends, and molecules of adjacent rows overlap in a stepwise fashion. At 64-nm intervals, the intermolecular gaps are in register across the fibril. Penetration of contrast medium into these is responsible for the dense cross-striations at these sites. (Modified from L.C. Junquiera and J. Carniero, Basic Histology, 3rd ed, Lange Medical Publications, 1980.)

Fig. 4-4 Shadowed electron micrograph of collagen fibers from human skin showing their characteristic 640 A cross-banding. (Courtesy of J. Gross and F.O. Schmitt.)

content of any given tissue can be quantitated by analysis for either of these amino acids. The polypeptide chains of tropocollagen are of two kinds, two alpha-1 chains and one alpha-2 chain (Fig. 4-5A). These have a left-handed helical configuration and are entwined to form a right-handed triple helix. In the assembly of a unit fibril of collagen, there is a short gap between the ends of successive tropocollagen molecules (Fig. 4-5B). At intervals of 64 nm along its length, certain of the intermolecular gaps are in register across the width of the fibril. Penetration of contrast medium into the gaps that are in register results in the uniformly spaced dark bands across the fibril. The light bands are regions in which molecular overlap prevents penetration of the stain.

Collagen synthesis depends on many different genes, and gene mutations may result in failure of assembly of specific collagens. In **osteogenesis imperfecta***, for example, the type-I alpha chains do not assemble into fibers. The bones are deficient in collagen and are extremely brittle, resulting in frequent fractures.*

Collagen was formerly thought to be a single protein, but it is now known to be a family of proteins that share some features of molecular organization but have alpha chains that differ in their amino acid composition and sequence. Twelve or more types of collagen have been discovered, but types I, II, III, and V are the most common. These all form fibrils and can be distinguished from one another by use of type-specific labeled antibodies. **Type-I**

collagen is the most ubiquitous, occurring in the connective tissue of the skin, in bone, tendon, fascia, and in the capsules of organs. It occurs in cross-striated fibrils and in fiber bundles with a wide range of sizes. **Type-II collagen** forms very thin fibers within an abundant ground substance. It occurs in cartilage, the nucleus pulposus of the intervertebral disks, and in the vitreous body of the eye. **Type-III collagen** forms the slender fibers traditionally called **reticular fibers**. Fibers of this kind are abundant in loose connective tissue, in the walls of blood vessels, in the stroma of various glands, and in spleen, kidney, and uterus. Collagens I, II, and III, which form fibers visible with the light microscope, are referred to as the **interstitial collagens** to set them apart from a larger group of collagens that are only detectable by use of specific antibodies. One of the group, **type-IV collagen**, is largely restricted to the basal lamina of epithelia, where, together with laminin and heparan sulfate proteoglycan, it forms a close meshwork that provides physical support for epithelia and is a selective filtration barrier to macromolecules.

The collagen fibers of loose connective tissue can be easily studied in spreads of an intact mesentery. Such preparations are thin enough to be studied without disturbing the arrangement of its fibrous components. The collagen, predominantly type I, is seen as randomly interwoven fibers of varying diameter and indefinite length (Fig. 4-2A). The largest, up to 15 μm in diameter, have a wavy course if not under tension. In electron micrographs, collagen fibers of all sizes are seen to be made up of varying numbers of **unit fibrils** of constant diameter (Fig. 4-3). In addition to relatively coarse type-I fibers, loose connective tissue contains networks of very thin (0.5–2.0 μm) **reticular fibers** consisting of type-III collagen. These are not ordinarily identifiable in thin spreads, but in histological sections, they can be selectively stained with silver salts and, therefore, are often described as **argyrophilic fibers** (Fig. 4-6). Reticular fibers are present in

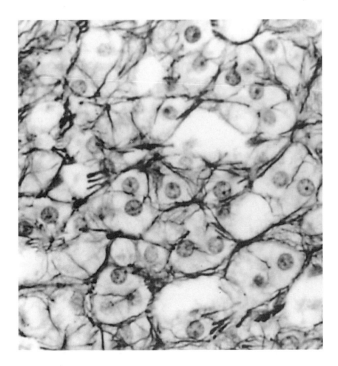

Fig. 4-6 Reticular fibers of the adrenal cortex. Reticular fibers are distinguished from other forms of collagen by their small size and blackening with silver stains.

connective tissue throughout the body. The flexible networks they form are very common around smooth muscle cells, and around the acini of glands. Reticular fibers are especially abundant in the connective tissue of hollow organs such as the bladder, intestine, and uterus that are subject to changes in volume.

Elastic Fibers

The **elastic fibers** of loose connective tissue are not readily identifiable in routine histological sections. In spreads of mesentery, selectively stained for **elastin** with resorcin-fuchsin, they are revealed as a network of slender branching fibers (Fig. 4-2B). Elastin is formed by polymerization of a precursor, **proelastin**, a globular molecule of 70,000 MW (molecular weight). The polymer is a rubberlike glycoprotein. Elastin contains two uncommon amino acids, **desmosine** and **isodesmosine**, which crosslink the molecules of elastin into a network of coiled chains that are responsible for its rubberlike properties. The fibers consist of a core of elastin with microfibrils of a glycoprotein, called **fibrillin**, embedded in its periphery. Elastin is synthesized by fibroblasts and smooth-muscle cells, and the fibers are assembled extracellularly. Elastic fibers can be stretched to one and a half times their original length and will return to their original length when the tension is relieved. When a fiber breaks, its ends quickly retract and coil up. Elastin may also form thin membrane-like sheets. In large arteries, for example, it takes the form of fenestrated elastic laminae arranged concentrically in

the wall of the vessel. The aorta, the large vessel which conducts the blood away from the heart, is distended by the outflow from each contraction of the ventricles, and elastic recoil of its wall is essential to maintain continuous flow from intermittent contraction of the heart.

Elastic fibers are especially abundant in the connective tissue of organs that must yield to externally or internally applied force. The lungs, for example, are expanded with each inspiration but must have sufficient resilience to return to their original volume during expiration. The connective tissue of the alveolar septa of the lung is rich in elastic fibers.

CELLS OF CONNECTIVE TISSUE

The cells of connective tissue are considered in two categories: **fixed cells** and **free cells**. The fixed cells are a relatively stable population of long-lived cells that includes the **fibroblasts**, which produce and maintain the extracellular components of connective tissue, and the **adipose cells**, which store lipids and release them into the blood for use as an energy source. The free cells are an ever-changing population of motile cells that wander through the ground substance. Most of these are short-lived and are continually replaced from a large pool of such cells circulating in the blood. This population includes **eosinophils, neutrophils, monocytes, lymphocytes, plasma cells,** and **mast cells**. Some of the free cells participate in short-term responses to injury or bacterial invasion, whereas others participate in the long-term immunological defenses of the body.

Fibroblasts

Fibroblasts are the dominant cell type of connective tissue and are responsible for production and maintenance of its fibrous and amorphous constituents. Their shape varies depending on their location. Where deployed along bundles of collagen fibers, they are usually fusiform, tapering toward both ends (Fig. 4-7). In other situations, they may be flattened stellate cells with several slender radiating processes. In electron micrographs, their long elliptical nucleus contains one or two nucleoli and small clumps of

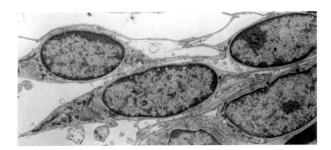

Fig. 4-7 Electron micrograph of relatively inactive connective-tissue fibroblasts, illustrating their fusiform shape and paucity of organelles.

chromatin. Long, slender mitochondria are found mainly in the perinuclear cytoplasm, but may extend a short way into the tapering cell processes. Endoplasmic reticulum is sparse in relatively inactive fibroblasts but may be more extensive in those of developing connective tissue. There is an inconspicuous juxtanuclear Golgi complex and a centrosome, from which microtubules radiate into the tapering cell processes.

The intracellular and extracellular events in synthesis of collagen by active fibroblasts are depicted in Figure 4-8. Polypeptide alpha chains are assembled on the polyribosomes of the endoplasmic reticulum and transfered to its lumen. These have an extra length of peptide, at either end, that is believed to ensure that the two kinds of alpha chains will assemble in the correct relation to one another. These added peptides also make the resulting **procollagen** molecules soluble and prevent their premature polymerization within the cell. The procollagen is exported from the cell into the extracellular matrix and, there, procollagen peptidases cleave the added peptides from the ends of the molecule to form **tropocollagen.** This polymerizes extra-

cellularly into unit fibrils of collagen. These then assemble into microscopically visible fibers. The synthesis, by fibroblasts, of proelastin and the glycosaminoglycans of the extracellular matrix has been less thoroughly studied.

***Scleroderma** is an inherited disease involving aberrant regulation of fibroblast growth and collagen synthesis. Excess connective tissue is formed and the thick, taut skin may interfere with flexure of the fingers. An increase in perivascular connective tissue may impair blood flow. Swallowing may be difficult due to thickening of the wall of the esophagus.*

Many fibroblasts are sessile (nonmotile) for long periods, but they are capable of moving through the extracellular matrix at a rate of about 1 μm/min, into an area of injury to participate in the repair process. Dividing fibroblasts are rarely seen in normal tissue. However, in responding to injury, they proliferate and become active in the synthesis of matrix components.

Adipose Cells

The **adipose cells,** or fat cells, are fixed cells of the connective tissue that synthesize and store large quantities of lipid. They arise from fusiform cells that initially develop a few isolated droplets of lipid in their cytoplasm. These increase in number and coalesce into larger droplets and, ultimately, into a single large drop. As the lipid accumulates, the cell takes on a spherical shape and may reach a diameter of 120 μm. Its nucleus becomes flattened and displaced to the periphery, and its cytoplasm is reduced to a thin film around a single huge drop of lipid (Fig. 4-9 [see Plate 4], and 4-10). Such cells may occur singly or in small

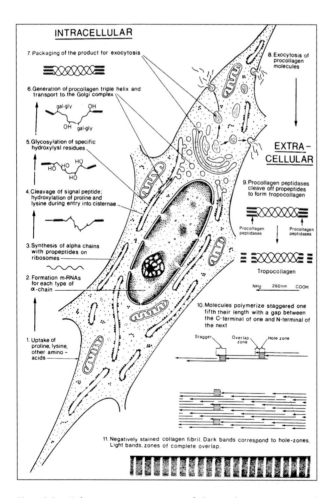

Fig. 4-8 Schematic presentation of biosynthetic events and organelle participation in the formation of collagen. On the left, the successive intracellular events are defined. On the right, the extracellular events leading to assembly of collagen fibrils. (From L.C. Junquiera, J. Carniero, Basic Histology, 3rd ed. Lange Medical Publications, 1980, with permission.)

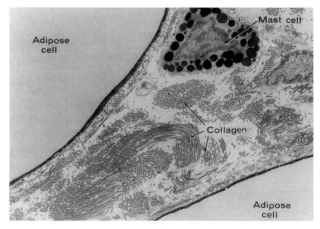

Fig. 4-10 Micrograph of portions of two adipose cells and the intervening tissue, containing a mast cell, a fibroblast, and numerous collagen fibers. Note the relatively enormous size of the adipose cells and their thin rim of cytoplasm around a large lipid droplet.

groups anywhere in loose connective tissue, but they tend to be concentrated along small blood vessels. Where they accumulate in such large numbers that they become the predominant cell type they form adipose tissue, which will be the subject of the next chapter.

FREE CELLS OF CONNECTIVE TISSUE

Macrophages (Histiocytes)

Macrophages (histiocytes) are phagocytic cells found throughout the connective tissue of the body. They arise by further differentiation of **monocytes** emigrating from the blood. In the unstimulated state, they may be fusiform or stellate cells adherent to the collagen fibers. They are distinguishable from fibroblasts by their slightly smaller and darker staining nucleus and by a cytoplasm that usually contains small vacuoles and a number of dense granules that are identifiable, in electron micrographs, as lysosomes. When stimulated, they round up and become actively motile, pleomorphic (having varying shape) cells with a remarkable capacity for phagocytosis. They participate in the normal maintenance of the connective tissue by ingesting dead cells, cellular debris, and any foreign particulate matter.

At sites of bacterial infection, they gather in large numbers and voraciously ingest and destroy the invaders with their lysosomal hydrolases. The mechanisms involved in their phagocytosis of bacteria have been thoroughly studied. Bacteria entering the tissues become coated with **immune globulins** (antibodies) and **serum complement** (a group of serum proteins which recognize matter foreign in the body). Binding of these proteins to the surface of the bacteria renders them more vulnerable to phagocytosis by macrophages, which have surface receptors for these serum proteins. Ingestion of a bacterium by a macrophage begins with a zipperlike progressive binding of receptors on its plasma membrane to the protein on the surface of the bacterium (Fig. 4-11). This proceeds until pseudopodia of the macrophage completely surround the bacterium. After fusion of the membrane at the leading edges of these encircling processes, the bacterium is enclosed in a **phagosome**, a membrane-limited intracellular vacuole. Lysosomes then fuse with the phagosome, discharging into it **lysozyme**, an enzyme that degrades the bacterial wall, and other hydrolases which complete the digestive process.

Phagocytosis is not the only role played by macrophages in the body's defenses against infection. They synthesize and release a variety of signaling molecules, collectively called **cytokines** (Fig. 4-12). Local diffusion and blood transport of these signaling molecules mobilize the body's resources for combating bacterial invasion. One of these, **interleukin-1**, is a chemo-attractant that causes large numbers of lymphocytes to gather at the site and stimulates their proliferation and antibody production.

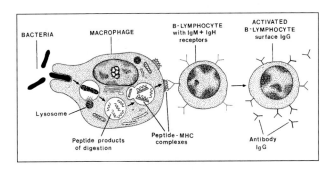

Fig. 4-11 B lymphocytes do not respond directly to antigen. Macrophages ingest bacteria, digest them, and combine an antigenic peptide of the bacteria with the MHC complex of "self". This complex is inserted into the membrane of the macrophage. B lymphocytes then bind to the antigen-MHC complex and are stimulated to produce specific antibody to that antigen.

SECRETORY PRODUCTS OF MACROPHAGES

Interleukin-1 (Il-1)
Interleukin-6 (Il-6)
Tumor necrosis factor (TNF)
Interferon
Colony stimulating factors
(M-CSF, G-CSF), GM-CSF)
Platelet derived growth factor (PDGF)
Fibroblast growth factor (FGF)
Transforming growth factor (TGF)
Erythropoietin

SURFACE RECEPTORS OF MACROPHAGES

Fc-receptors
Il-2-receptors
Complement receptors
Interferon receptors

Fig. 4-12 Partial listing of some of the surface markers and secretory products of macrophages.

It is also chemotactic for neutrophils, attracting them to the site to participate in phagocytosis of bacteria. Macrophages also have an essential role in initiating the body's immune response to an infection, by their intracellular processing of antigen (foreign protein) and its presentation to B lymphocytes in a form that is more immunogenic (Fig. 4-11).

By injecting the colloidal vital dye, Trypan Blue, into experiment animals, early histologists identified cells in many organs that took up the dye and were, therefore, believed to share the phagocytic properties of macro-phages. Among these were endothelial cells lining the sinusoids of certain organs, and various free cells bearing a resemblance to macrophages. The general term **reticuloendothelial system** was suggested for this heterogeneous group of cell types. This inclusive term is still used and strongly defended by its remaining proponents. However, the use of isotopic labeling to trace cell lineages, and of monoclonal antibodies

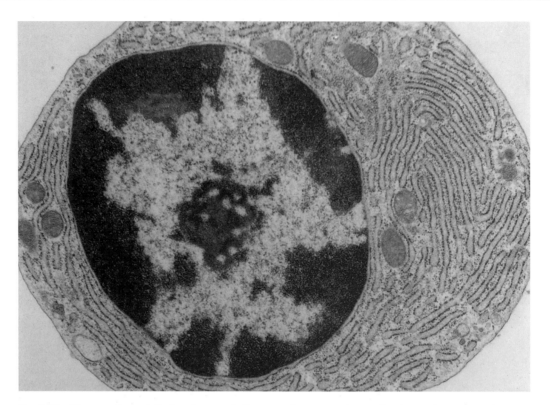

Fig. 4-13 Electron micrograph of a plasma cell illustrating the coarse pattern of its heterochromatin and its very extensive endoplasmic reticulum engaged in synthesis of immunoglobulins.

for recognition of specific surface markers has now made it possible to identify the legitimate members of this system with greater accuracy, and the term **mononuclear phago-cyte system** has become more widely accepted. This now includes all highly phagocytic cell types, of whatever shape or location, but it excludes the controversial sinusoidal endothelia, and certain other cells that take up small amounts of Trypan Blue by pinocytosis instead of phagocytosis. The principal members of the mononuclear phagocyte system, as currently interpreted, are monocytes, macrophages, alveolar phagocytes of the lungs, Kupffer cells of the liver, and the osteoclasts of bone.

Neutrophils

Neutrophilic leukocytes are not found in significant numbers in normal connective tissue, but they gather in great numbers at sites of infection. The mechanisms involved in their mobilization have recently been clarified. Cytokines liberated by macrophages at the site induce the endothelial cells of the local capillaries to synthesize and incorporate in their membrane a protein called **endothelial cell adhesion molecule-1 (ELAM-1)**. This makes the membrane sticky. Some of these same diffusable media-tors of inflammation apparently reach neutrophils in the blood, inducing them to synthesize and incorporate in their membrane **leukocyte adhesion molecules (LeuCAMs)**, which promote their adhesion to the sticky regions of the capillary endothelium. The neutrophils then migrate

through the wall of the capillaries and up the concentration gradient of cytokines diffusing from the site of inflamma-tion. These mechanisms ensure rapid mobilization of neu-trophils to join the macrophages in phagocytosis and digestion of bacteria.

Eosinophils

Eosinophils are relatively few in normal connective tis-sue, but they are increased in allergic conditions and in defense against parasites. They are especially numerous in the connective tissue beneath the epithelia of the respiratory and alimentary tracts where entry of foreign protein is most likely to occur. They do not phagocytize bacteria but are involved in damage control in allergic reactions, ingesting antigen–antibody complexes. They also release the enzymes **aryl sulfatase** and **histaminase** which destroy two of the main mediators of allergic reactions, histamine and heparin. In parasitic diseases, they secrete **cationic proteins** that form transmembrane pores in the parasites. They also release **superoxide ions** and **hydrogen peroxide**, which damage parasite membranes by lipid peroxidation.

Lymphocytes

Lymphocytes continually leave the blood and are nor-mally present in large numbers in loose connective tissue

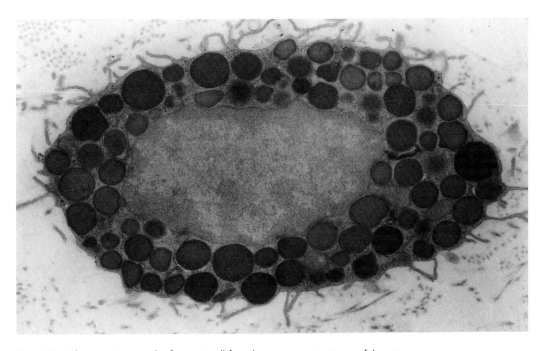

Fig. 4-15 Electron micrograph of a mast cell from loose connective tissue of the rat.

throughout the body, where they carry out their function of protective immunosurveillance. They gather in increased numbers at sites of inflammation. Lymphocytes cannot respond directly to foreign proteins (antigens). These are first ingested by macrophages that digest them and combine an antigenic peptide product of their hydrolysis with the major histocompatibility complex (MHC). This combination of molecules is inserted into their membrane. Presentation of an antigenic peptide to adherent lymphocytes stimulates their production of antibody to that antigen (Fig. 4-11). Three types of lymphocytes and their respective functions will be considered in a later chapter on the Immune System.

Plasma Cells

Plasma cells arise in the connective tissues by further differentiation of **lymphocytes.** They are major producers of antibodies and are widely distributed in the connective tissues of the body. They are large, spherical or ovoid cells having an eccentrically placed nucleus with a radial pattern of coarse clumps of heterochromatin. The cytoplasm is intensely basophilic and, in electron micrographs, is filled with closely spaced cisternae of rough endoplasmic reticulum (Fig. 4-13). No secretory granules are formed. Their product, **immune globulin** (antibody), is secreted continuously by exocytosis of small vesicles that shuttle between the Golgi complex and the cell surface. Occasional plasma cells have spherical inclusions 2–3 μm in diameter located within distended cisternae of the endoplasmic reticulum. Their significance is unclear, but it is speculated that they may be accumulations of defective products of antibody synthesis.

Mast Cells

Mast cells are the largest of the connective tissue cells measuring 20–30 μm in diameter. They are easily identified by the conspicuous, intensely basophilic granules that fill their cytoplasm, often obscuring the nucleus (Figs. 4-14 [see Plate 4] and 4-15). The granules stain metachromatically with Toluidine Blue, owing to their content of the sulfated glycosaminoglycan, **heparin**. They also contain **histamine** and the neutral proteases, **tryptase** and **chymase**. In electron micrographs, the mast cell contains short profiles of endoplasmic reticulum, a small Golgi, and a few mitochondria. The content of their granules varies in density. In the human, some granules have a cylindrical, scroll-like inclusion. In cross section, this appears to be made up of concentric laminae, each about the thickness of a lipid bilayer. In other mast cells, the granules have a denser matrix surrounding a paler central region that contains parallel linear densities. The significance of these variations is unknown.

Mast cells are sensitive sentinels for the immune system, detecting the entry of foreign proteins and rapidly initiating a local response. Their activation results in the prompt release of potent mediators of inflammation stored in their granules and this is followed by a slower release of **cytokines** that recruit other cell types to participate. Exocytosis of their granules is unusual in that the granules do not fuse with the cell membrane individually. Instead, several granules fuse with each other, with one opening at the cell surface. Thus, membrane-limited channels are created that extend some distance into the cytoplasm. This has been termed **compound exocytosis**. The stimulus evoking degranulation is the presence of an antigen to which the individual has been sensitized in a previous immune

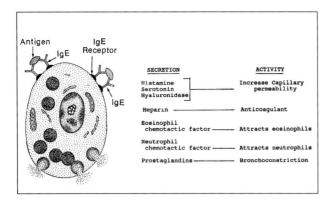

Fig. 4-16 Mast cells have surface receptors for IgE. Cross-linking of their surface IgE molecules by antigen causes their clumping and this triggers mast cell degranulation, with the release of several mediators of allergic reactions.

response (Fig. 4-16). The cells survive this massive discharge of their product and regenerate new granules.

Immunoglobulin-E (IgE) is a class of immunoglobulins produced by plasma cells that does not circulate in the blood in any significant amount. Instead, molecules of IgE of varying specificity bind to receptors on the mast cells. These cells are then primed to respond immediately when any of those antigens enter the tissues again. The response is usually mild and local, but some allergic individuals overreact to a second exposure, with consequences ranging from mild discomfort to very serious **anaphylaxis** (immediate intense hypersentivity). Such allergic individuals tend to produce antibodies of the IgE class to pollen and a host of other allergens. Upon re-exposure, these allergens bind to and crosslink IgE molecules on the surface of mast cells, triggering their degranulation and liberation of histamine and cytokines (Fig. 4-16). The response may be regional or general. In hay fever, histamine released by mast cells in the connective tissue of the nasal mucosa causes increased permeability of the capillaries and consequent swelling of the mucosa, accompanied by sneezing and nasal discharge. In asthma, the response is mainly in the lungs, where histamine plays a less important role than the cytokines. These cause a spasm of smooth-muscle cells in the wall of the bronchioles, making breathing difficult. In anaphylaxis, massive degranulation of mast cells along blood vessels releases histamine that is carried in the blood throughout the body, increasing capillary permeability with leakage of plasma into the tissues and a dramatic fall in blood pressure that may culminate in unconsciousness and, in rare instances, death.

The mast cell granules also contain ß-glucuronidase and aryl sulfatase, enzymes that have no role in the immune response but may degrade glycosaminoglycans of the extracellular matrix. This has led to the suggestion that, under normal conditions, mast cells may have a low level of secretory activity that contributes to the continual turnover of the ground substance of the connective tissue. This remains to be verified.

LOOSE CONNECTIVE TISSUE

Loose connective tissue is the most widespread of the connective tissues, occurring in sites where relatively little resistance to stress is required. It supports the epithelial parenchyma of the major organs and is the tissue through which their blood vessels are distributed. It occupies the spaces around and between muscles. It underlies the mesothelium lining the pleural and peritoneal cavities. There are, however, local differences in the relative proportions of its various fibrous and amorphous components, and some of these have led to their designation as distinct types of connective tissue.

Reticular Connective Tissue

Reticular tissue is a form of loose connective tissue in which a network of argyrophilic reticular fibers is the dominant fibrous component. The cells tend to be stellate with slender radiating processes deployed along the intersecting strands of the reticulum. They are not considered to be a distinct cell type but merely fibroblasts which synthesize type-III collagen and little or no type-I collagen. In addition, there is a large population of resident macrophages adhering to the reticular fibers. Reticular connective tissue forms the stroma of the bone marrow and that of the spleen, lymph nodes, and thymus. In the lymphoid organs, the spaces in the loose reticulum are packed with lymphocytes and, in the marrow, with precursors of the blood cells.

Mucous Connective Tissue

The distinctive feature of mucous connective tissue is a very large amount of amorphous ground substance that is unusually rich in hyaluronic acid. Collagenous and reticular fibers make up a very small portion of its volume. Its widely spaced cellular elements are fusiform or stellate fibroblasts and very few macrophages. This kind of connective tissue is rare in adults but common in the embryo. It is the principal component of the umbilical cord, where it was formerly called **Wharton's jelly** (Fig. 4-17A [see Plate 4]). Mucous connective tissue is also found in the pulp of developing teeth.

DENSE CONNECTIVE TISSUE

Dense connective tissue differs from loose connective tissue mainly in the great preponderance of its fibrous components with relatively few cells. Where the collagen fiber bundles are randomly oriented, the tissue is described as **dense irregular connective tissue.** Where the fibers are oriented parallel to one another or in some other ordered arrangement, it is called **dense regular connective tissue.**

Irregular Connective Tissue

Collagenous fibers make up the greater part of the volume of this tissue. The fiber bundles are relatively coarse and interwoven in a compact meshwork with little space occupied by cells and ground substance (Fig. 4-17B [see Plate 4]). A network of elastic fibers is usually interspersed among the collagen fibers. Fibroblasts are lodged between the bundles of collagen, but generally only their elongated nuclei are visible in histological sections. Macrophages are present in small numbers but are recognizable as such only after supravital staining. Free cells are very few. Dense irregular connective tissue is found in the dermis of the skin, the capsules of the spleen, liver, and lymph nodes, the tunica albuginea of the testis, the mammary gland (Fig. 4-17B [see Plate 4]), the dura mater of the brain, and the sheath of large nerves.

Regular Connective Tissue

This type of connective tissue occurs as robust cylindrical cords or flat sheets of closely approximated coarse collagen fibers that give the tissue a glistening white appearance in the fresh state. The fibers are oriented in the direction best suited to resist the mechanical stresses to which they are subjected. Tendons, which transmit the pull of muscles to the bones, are an example of this tissue type. They are made up of parallel type-I collagen fibers, closely packed, with very little intervening space for ground substance. The fibroblasts of tendons are aligned between fiber bundles, and most of their cytoplasm is in thin finlike processes that extend between, and partially surround, neighboring fiber bundles. Varying numbers of these primary bundles are assembled into larger secondary bundles that are surrounded by a very thin layer of loose connective tissue through which run small blood vessels and nerves. At the periphery of a tendon, a layer of dense irregular connective tissue forms the tendon sheath. The parallel collagen fibers of tendons create a structure that is quite flexible but offers great resistance to a pulling force.

> In **Ehler Danlos Syndrome** *there are molecular defects in collagens I and II that result in very lax ligaments and tendons. There is hyperextension of the joints and frequent dislocations. The loose skin can be stretched to an abnormal degree.*

Broad flat muscles do not have cylindrical tendons but are attached to their insertions by thin sheets of dense regular connective tissue, called **aponeuroses**. These consist of multiple layers of coherent fascicles of collagen fibers. Within any one layer, the fiber bundles are parallel, but their direction usually changes in successive layers. Separation of the layers is prevented by some fibers that crossover between layers.

ligaments

HISTOPHYSIOLOGY OF CONNECTIVE TISSUE

The ground substance of connective tissue contains a small amount of tissue fluid through which nutrients diffuse to the cells and waste products diffuse away. This fluid is continually renewed. Hydrostatic pressure at the arterial end of the capillaries causes water and electrolytes to pass through the vessel wall. Some of this fluid reenters the blood at the venous end of the capillaries where the hydrostatic pressure is lower, and some is returned to the blood via the lymphatics. Fluid normally enters and leaves the ground substance at the same rate. However, damage to the capillaries or obstruction of the lymphatics may result in accumulation of excess fluid in the ground substance, with consequent swelling (edema).

During the growth period, there is considerable turnover of the collagen fibers of connective tissue, but in the adult, they are relatively stable, except in bone, where they are broken down and reformed in the continuous remodeling of this tissue that goes on throughout life. The degradation of collagen fibers is carried out by specific collagenases and by other proteinases produced by fibroblasts, osteoblasts, and other cell types.

QUESTIONS*

1. Carbon black is almost "instantly" attacked when injected into the loose areolar tissues by which of the following cells?

   A. adult mesenchymal cells
   B. fibroblasts or fibrocytes
   C. histiocytes or connective tissue macrophages
   D. mast cells
   E. blood basophils

2. Which of the following substances is found in the basal lamina?

   A. collagen I
   B. collagen II
   C. collagen III
   D. collagen IV
   E. all of the above

3. Which statement is correct about plasma cells?

   A. contain a centrally located nucleus
   B. originate from T lymphocytes
   C. produce antibodies
   D. contain a well-developed smooth-surfaced endoplasmic reticulum
   E. are acidophilic

4. Find the **incorrect** statement about mast cells:

   A. contain a sulfated heparin proteoglycan
   B. contain histamine
   C. produce antibodies
   D. are actively phagocytic
   E. produce cytokines

5. Which statement is **incorrect** about macrophages?

   A. contain many lysosomes
   B. are phagocytic
   C. are formed from fibroblasts
   D. can form foreign-body giant cells
   E. none of the above

6. Mast cells have or are

   A. eccentrically located nuclei
   B. many lysosomes
   C. many basophilic granules
   D. phagocytic
   E. none of the above

7. Which of the following cells may be found in loose (areolar) connective tissue?

   A. plasma cells
   B. lymphocyte
   C. eosinophil
   D. macrophage
   E. all of the above

8. Elastin is synthesized by

   A. adipose cells
   B. fibroblasts
   C. mast cells
   D. plasma cells
   E. none of the above

9. All of the following regarding connective tissue lymphocytes are correct **except**

   A. may differentiate to form plasma cells
   B. involved in cell-mediated immunity
   C. may be of the B or T lymphocyte type
   D. their number is markedly increased at sites of inflammation
   E. are specifically effective in combating parasitic diseases

10. All of the following regarding reticular fibers are correct **except**

    A. consist of collagen fibrils
    B. are argyrophilic
    C. not discernable in H & E preparations
    D. generally observed as a network of slender branching fibers
    E. commonly abundant in connective tissue of hollow organs

*Answers on page 307.

5

ADIPOSE TISSUE

KEY WORDS

Adipocytes
Brown Adipose
   Tissue
Carotenoids
Chylomicrons
Lipase
Lipid
Lipoblasts

Lipoprotein Lipase
Lipoproteins: VLDL
Mesenchymal Cells
Panniculus Adiposus
Thermogenin
Triglycerides
White Adipose Tissue

Mammals feed intermittently but consume energy continuously. Therefore, it is advantageous to have a site of temporary storage of energy-rich material. The most favorable substance for this purpose is **lipid,** because it weighs less and occupies less volume per calorie of stored chemical energy than carbohydrate or protein. Adipose tissue (fat) is a form of connective tissue specialized for storage of lipid. By accumulating intracellular lipid in periods of food intake and releasing fatty acids in periods of fasting, adipose tissue is able to provide the body with a stable supply of energy-rich fuel.

There are two types of adipose tissue which differ in color, vascularity, metabolic activity, and distribution in the body. One is the familiar **white adipose tissue,** which is widespread and makes up the bulk of the body fat. The other, called **brown adipose tissue,** is less abundant and is restricted to certain regions. The cells of white adipose tissue contain a single large droplet of lipid and are described as **unilocular** fat cells. Those of brown adipose tissue contain many smaller droplets of lipid and are described as **multilocular** fat cells.

UNILOCULAR ADIPOSE TISSUE

The **unilocular adipose tissue** varies in color from white to yellow in the fresh state, depending, in part, on the abundance of **carotenoids** (a group of yellow-red pigments) in the diet. The cells are typically spherical, but where closely packed together, they may take on a polyhedral shape due to mutual deformation. Most of their volume is occupied by a single large drop of stored lipid that displaces the nucleus to one side of the cell and flattens it against the plasmalemma. The cytoplasm is reduced to a thin rim around the lipid droplet and accounts for only about one-fortieth of the cell volume. During their development, unilocular fat cells may contain multiple lipid droplets, but these coalesce into a single droplet as the cell matures.

If unfixed adipose tissue is stained with the lipid soluble dye, Sudan Black, it appears as a mosaic of large lipid drops that are polygonal in outline and of nearly uniform size (Fig. 5-1A). In the preparation of histological sections, the lipid is extracted from the cells, leaving behind only their thin rim of cytoplasm, containing the greatly flattened nucleus. In well-preserved specimens, the polygonal shape of the mutually deforming cells is retained and the tissue appears as a network with large polygonal meshes (Fig. 5-1B). However, during dehydration of a specimen prior to embedding, the thin rims of cytoplasm often collapse to varying degrees, giving the cells an irregular outline that does not accurately represent their form in vivo. Fat cells are 50–150 μm in diameter, four or five times the diameter of the capillaries found in the angular intercellular spaces (Fig. 5-2). Each cell is surrounded by a loose network of reticular fibers, and the tissue as a whole is partitioned by thin connective tissue septa into lobules that are discernible with the naked eye. This lobulation is most obvious in subcutaneous tissue such as that over the but-

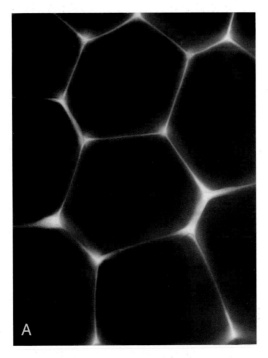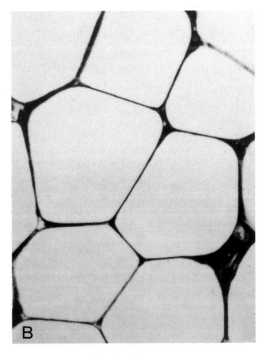

Fig. 5-1 (A) A thin spread of unilocular adipose tissue stained with Sudan Black without previous dehydration. The lipid has been retained and is stained by the fat-soluble dye while the surrounding cytoplasm is unstained. (B) Unilocular adipose tissue prepared by the routine method involving dehydration before staining. The lipid has been extracted and only the thin rim of cytoplasm remains.

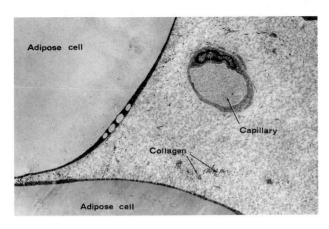

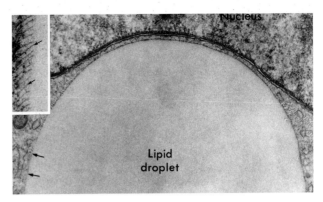

Fig. 5-2 Electron micrograph of portions of two adipose cells and a cross section of capillary. Note the very large size of the adipose cells relative to the diameter of the capillary.

Fig. 5-3 Electron micrograph of a portion of a developing fat cell. The lipid has been retained and is only slightly stained by the osmium of the fixative. The lipid is not surrounded by a membrane. The inset shows the regularly spaced vimentin filaments that surround the lipid droplet.

tocks, where the adipose tissue has a cushioning or shock-absorbing function.

In electron micrographs, a small Golgi complex, a few filamentous mitochondria, and occasional fenestrated cisternae of rough endoplasmic reticulum can be found in the thicker region of cytoplasm around the nucleus. The lipid drop is not enclosed by a membrane but may be surrounded by a layer of 10-nm intermediate filaments consisting of vimentin (Fig. 5-3, inset). The thin peripheral layer of cytoplasm contains many small vesicles that are believed to arise in pinocytosis. There may also be small lipid droplets that have not yet fused with the main lipid drop. These are usually not seen in sections examined with the light microscope. The membrane of each adipose cell is surrounded by a thin layer of glycoprotein resembling the basal lamina of epithelia.

Development and Distribution

In the 1800s, adipose tissue was considered to be merely loose connective tissue in which many of the fibroblasts had accumulated excess lipid. In this interpretation, any area of connective tissue could become adipose tissue. Although it is true that **adipocytes** may occur in loose connective tissue anywhere, they tend to develop in large numbers in preferred sites. This would be hard to explain if adipocytes could arise from fibroblasts wherever they occur. It is now generally accepted that adipose cells arise from precursors, **lipoblasts,** that differentiate from mesenchymal cells. The development of adipose tissue in some sites and not in others is attributed to the persistence of varying numbers of these precursor cells in different regions. Verification of this interpretation is difficult because fibroblasts, mesenchymal cells, and lipoblasts are not easily distinguishable in the connective tissues of the adult.

In the human infant, there is a continuous subcutaneous layer of adipose tissue, the **panniculus adiposus.**

This later thins out in some areas, and, although subcutaneous fat is still widespread in the adult, it exhibits quantitative regional differences that are influenced by age and sex. The characteristic differences in body form of males and females is due, in large measure, to different sites of predilection for fat deposition. In the male, the principal regions are in subcutaneous tissue over the nape of the neck, over the deltoid and triceps muscles, in the lumbosacral region, and the buttocks. In the female, subcutaneous fat is most abundant in the breasts, buttocks, in the region over the trochanter of the femur, and on the anterior and lateral aspects of the thighs. With advancing years, the male tends to accumulate fat over the anterior abdominal wall. In addition to these subcutaneous deposits, there are large accumulations of fat in the omentum, mesenteries, and retroperitoneal region of the body cavity, in both sexes.

Histophysiology of White Adipose Tissue

After a meal, the lipids in the diet are degraded in the duodenum by the pancreatic enzyme **lipase,** yielding fatty acids and glycerol. These are taken into the intestinal epithelial cells and there recombined to form **triglycerides** (neutral fats) that are released at the basolateral membrane of the cells and carried via the lymph to the bloodstream, in the form of minute (2–3 µm) particles called **chylomicrons,** which consist of triglycerides surrounded by a layer of apolipoproteins and phospholipids. Triglycerides synthesized in the liver are carried in the blood in the form of **very-low-density lipoprotein (VLDL)** particles, smaller than chylomicrons. Upon reaching the capillaries of adipose tissue, the enzyme **lipoprotein lipase,** in the luminal membrane of the capillary endothelium, breaks down the chylomicrons and VLDL, liberating fatty acids (Fig. 5-4). These traverse the endothelium and surrounding areolar tissue and are taken

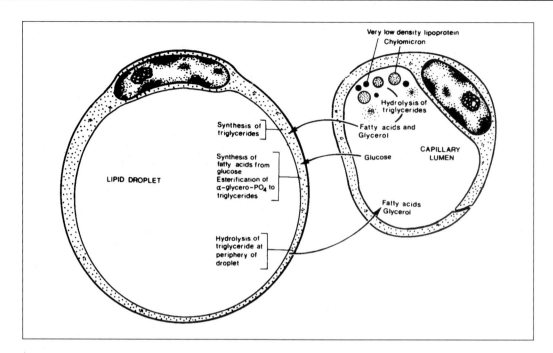

Fig. 5-4 Schematic representation of metabolic exchange between a capillary (right) and a white fat cell (left). Chylomicrons and very-low-density lipoprotein particles in the plasma are hydrolyzed by a lipoprotein lipase to fatty acids and glycerol, which diffuse into the fat cell where they are reesterified to triglyceride and stored. Blood glucose diffusing from the capillary to the fat cell can also be used in the synthesis of lipid from carbohydrate. Upon neural or hormonal stimulation, cyclic AMP is elevated, activating a cytoplasmic lipase that hydrolyzed triglyceride at the periphery of the droplet, yielding fatty acids and glycerol which diffuse back into the capillary and are carried to other tissues in the blood.

up by the adipose cells and combined with endogenous glycerol phosphate to form triglycerides that are added to the store already in the lipid drop. Fat cells can also synthesize triglycerides from absorbed glucose. In adipose cells of an animal fed after a period of fasting, glycogen is stored transiently in the thin rim of cytoplasm around the lipid droplet (Fig. 5-5). This is subsequently broken down to yield glucose, from which glycerol and fatty

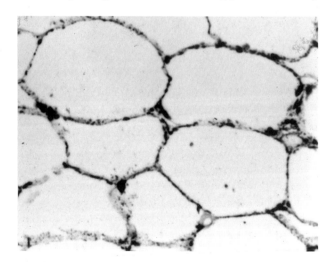

Fig. 5-5 White adipose tissue of a rat refeeding after a period of fasting. The dense granules around the periphery of the fat droplet are glycogen, which would disappear as this carbohydrate was used in the synthesis of triglycerides.

acids are synthesized and combined to make additional triglyceride.

Adipose tissue is not an energy reserve that is drawn on only in times of fasting. Isotopic tracer studies have clearly established that the stored lipid is continually being broken down and renewed, even in an individual in caloric balance. In laboratory rodents, the half-life of depot lipids is about 8 days, which means that almost 10% of the fatty acid in adipose tissue is replaced each day. Continuous renewal also occurs in humans, but the exact rate of turnover of fatty acid is not known.

In addition to its lipid-storing function, the subcutaneous adipose tissue has long been regarded as an insulating layer that helps to conserve body heat. It is now known that its chemical reactions also generate a small amount of heat. The insulating function of adipose tissue is best exemplified in aquatic mammals; they have a very thick layer of subcutaneous fat (blubber) to minimize loss of heat to the cold water in which they live.

MULTILOCULAR ADIPOSE TISSUE

The **brown adipose tissue** ranges in color from tan to reddish brown. Its color is due, in part, to its rich vascularity and, in part, to cytochromes in its exceptionally abundant mitochondria. The cells are polygonal in section and considerably smaller than those of white adipose tissue.

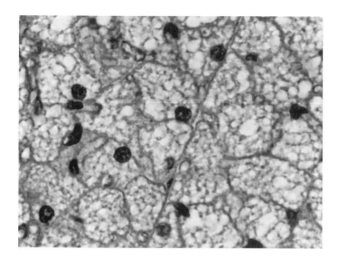

Fig. 5-6 Photomicrograph of typical multilocular adipose tissue (brown fat). The polygonal cells contain many small droplets of lipid instead of a single large droplet.

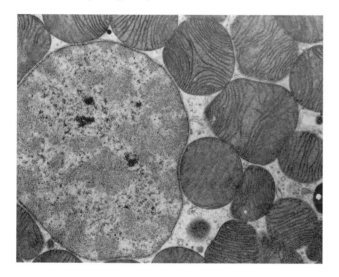

Fig. 5-7 Electron micrograph of the juxtanuclear portion of a brown fat cell in an animal recently aroused from hibernation. No lipid remains. Note the very large spherical mitochondria characteristic of this tissue.

Their cytoplasm is relatively abundant and contains multiple lipid droplets of varying size (Fig. 5-6). The spherical nucleus is eccentric in position but is not displaced to the periphery of the cell, as in white fat. In electron micrographs, large spherical mitochondria occupy a large part of the cytoplasm between lipid droplets (Fig. 5-7). They have numerous cristae that often traverse the entire width of the organelle. Rough endoplasmic reticulum is virtually absent, but there are occasional tubular profiles of smooth endoplasmic reticulum. Free ribosomes and variable amounts of glycogen are also present.

Brown fat has a lobular organization, and the pattern of distribution of its blood vessels is reminiscent of that of a gland. In animals subjected to prolonged fasting, their brown fat gradually loses lipid, becoming more deeply colored and reverting to a glandlike mass of epithelioid cells

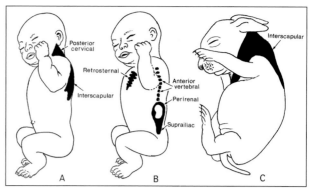

Fig. 5-8 The distribution of brown adipose tissue. (A) In newborn human there are superficial deposits in the posterior triangle of the neck and in a pair of interscapular fat bodies. (B) The deeper deposits include fat pads in the retrosternal region and along the anterior surface of the vertebral column. There are also sizable deposits around the kidneys and extending downward in the suprailiac region. (C) In the newborn rabbit, there are large deposits of brown fat around the neck and between the shoulder blades. (Redrawn and modified from D. Hull, British Medical Bulletin, 221:92, 1966.)

that bear no resemblance to fibroblasts of connective tissue.

The blood supply of brown adipose tissue is very rich and its connective tissue stroma is sparse. Its cells are, therefore, in more intimate relation to one another and to the capillaries than in white fat. Silver stains and electron micrographs reveal numerous small unmyelinated nerves in brown adipose tissue. Their axons are frequently found in close apposition to the surface of the cells. This contrasts with the nerves in white adipose tissue which appear only to innervate the blood vessels.

Development and Distribution

Brown adipose tissue is found in most mammalian species. It is always prominent in the newborn, but in adults it is most conspicuous in those species that hibernate. In the common laboratory rodents, brown adipose tissue occurs in two symmetrical interscapular fat bodies, in lobules between muscles around the shoulder girdle, and in the axillae. It occupies the costovertebral angle and forms slender lobules along either side of the aorta and in the hilus of the kidneys. In the human, it occurs in the posterior triangle of the neck, in the substernal and interscapular regions, intra-abdominally along the vertebral column, and around the kidneys (Fig. 5-8).

The embryological origin of brown adipose tissue is not well understood, but it is commonly thought that **mesenchymal cells** give rise to two types of **lipoblasts,** one that differentiates into unilocular adipose tissue and one that develops into multilocular brown fat (Fig. 5-9). Brown fat accounts for 5–6% of the body weight in the newborn rabbit and only 2% in the human newborn. In rodents, it retains its multilocular character in adult life. In humans, it

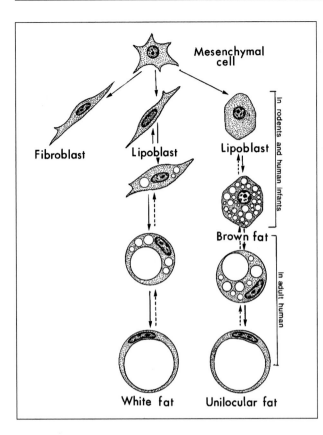

Fig. 5-9 In the development of adipose tissue, mesenchymal cells give rise to fibroblasts and two types of fusiform lipoblasts. One of these differentiates into unilocular white fat, the other into multilocular brown fat. The latter persists, as such, in rodents, but in the human, its multiple droplets gradually coalesce, and it comes to resemble white adipose tissue.

consists of typical multilocular adipose cells at birth and in early childhood, but as children grow older, the lipid droplets tend to coalesce, and in the adult, the cells come to resemble those of white adipose tissue. However, there is compelling evidence that two physiologically distinct types adipose tissue still exist, even though they may be difficult to distinguish in well-nourished adults. In near-starvation, or in the elderly suffering from chronic wasting diseases, multilocular fat again becomes apparent in the same regions in which it is found in the newborn. Further support for two types of fat comes from the observation that there are two types of tumors of fat, called lipomas.

The cells of one type resemble those of unilocular adipose tissue and those of the other resemble brown fat.

Histophysiology of Brown Adipose Tissue

Brown adipose tissue serves as an energy reserve but has little or no insulating function. One of its major functions is heat generation. Its very numerous mitochondria give it an unusual capacity for generating heat by oxidation of fatty acids. The rate of substrate oxidation by brown fat cells, in vitro, is as much as 20 times that of white fat cells. Each milliliter of oxygen consumed in the process contributes about 5 calories of body heat. Brown fat cells are activated in a cold environment and may treble their heat production.

Adult animals in a cold environment produce heat as a by-product of the muscular activity involved in shivering. Newborn and very young animals are unable to shiver and rely on their brown adipose tissue for nonshivering thermogenesis. Upon exposure to cold, sensory receptors in the skin send nerve impulses to the temperature-regulating center in the brain, which relays impulses along sympathetic nerves to the brown adipose tissue. Some of these nerves act upon the blood vessels to increase blood flow; others, terminating on brown adipose cells, release norepinephrine which activates the enzyme that splits triglycerides to fatty acids and glycerol, thereby triggering a heat-producing cycle of fatty acid oxidation and triglyceride regeneration, which converts chemical-bond energy to heat energy. This is made possible by a unique uncoupling protein, **thermogenin,** in the inner membrane of brown fat mitochondria that permits the energy generated in the above reactions to be dissipated as heat instead of being used in the synthesis of ATP, which is its fate under other circumstances. The heat warms the blood flowing through the brown adipose tissue and this heat is carried in the circulation to other parts of the body.

Brown adipose tissue is especially abundant in animal species that hibernate. Its heat production is believed to be essential for their rapid warming during arousal from the torpid state. In the adult human, a physiological role for brown fat in temperature regulation is less well established, but in the newborn and in young infants, it is believed to be essential for maintenance of normal body temperature.

QUESTIONS*

1. Which of the following cells stain with osmium tetroxide or Sudan Black to show small multilocular globules?

   A. white fat cells
   B. brown fat cells
   C. yellow fat cells
   D. ovarian tissue
   E. none of the above

2. Find the **incorrect** statement. Brown fat cells

   A. are found mainly in fetuses
   B. are unilocular
   C. can be stimulated by sympathetic nervous system
   D. mitochondria have no elementary particles
   E. are less numerous than white fat cells

3. Which **one,** if any, of the following functions is characteristic of brown adipose tissue?

   A. filler
   B. cushion
   C. insulation
   D. energy production
   E. none of the above

4. All of the following regarding white adipose tissue are correct **except**

   A. is in a continual state of formation and degradation
   B. serves effectively as an insulator
   C. adipocytes contain numerous fat droplets
   D. also termed unilocular adipose tissue
   E. adipocytes exhibit "signet ring" appearance

5. The two types of adipose tissue differ in

   A. color
   B. vascularity
   C. metabolic activity
   D. body distribution
   E. all of the above

6. Unilocular adipocytes

   A. contain sperical centrally located nuclei
   B. may contain multiple lipid droplets
   C. are activated in a cold environment
   D. have abundant cytoplasm
   E. occur only in specific limited areas of the body

7. Brown fat

   A. serves as an energy reserve
   B. is often called panniculus adiposus
   C. is composed of cells which contain few mitochondria
   D. contain peripherally located nuclei
   E. has a very poor blood supply

8. All of the following are involved in the process of storing lipids in adipose tissue following a meal **except**

   A. triglycerides
   B. lipoprotein lipase
   C. chylomicrons
   D. glucose
   E. very high-density lipoproteins (VHDL)

*Answers on page 307.

6

CARTILAGE

KEY WORDS

Annulus Fibrosis	Intervertebral Disk
Chondrocyte	Isogenous
Chondrofication	Keratan Sulfate
Chondroitin Sulfate	Lacunae
Chondronectin	Nucleus Pulposis
Elastic	Osteoblast
Epiphyseal Plate	Perichondrium
Glycosaminoglycans	Somatomedin-C
Hyaluronic Acid	Somatotrophin
Interterritorial Matrix	Territorial Matrix

Cartilage is a specialized form of connective tissue in which cells, called **chondrocytes,** are sparsely distributed in a firm, gellike, extracellular matrix. It is not penetrated by blood vessels. Its cells, isolated in small cavities, called **lacunae,** are nourished by diffusion of metabolites through the aqueous phase of the matrix, from capillaries in the surrounding connective tissue. The unique viscoelastic properties of the matrix give cartilage great firmness and resiliency, and it is able to retain these properties while rapidly growing. This makes cartilage an ideal skeletal material for the developing embryo. Most of the skeleton is initially formed of cartilage that is replaced by bone later in development. In postnatal life, cartilage becomes more restricted in its distribution, but it continues to play an important role in the growth in length of the bones of the extremities throughout childhood. By the time adult stature has been attained, all cartilage has been replaced by bone, except on the joint surfaces of the long bones, the ventral ends of the ribs, the intervertebral disks of the spine, the tracheal rings, and in the nose and larynx.

Three types of cartilage are distinguished on the basis of the relative abundance of collagen and elastin in the matrix: **hyaline cartilage, elastic cartilage,** and **fibrocartilage.** Of these, hyaline cartilage is the most common, and elastic and fibrocartilage can be regarded as variants with properties adapted to specific local needs.

HYALINE CARTILAGE

Histogenesis

At sites of cartilage formation in the embryo, mesenchymal cells withdraw their processes and form dense aggregations that constitute **centers of chondrification** (Fibs. 6-1A and 6-1B). Other mesenchymal cells differentiate to form an ensheathing layer of fusiform cells and collagen fibers, the **perichondrium.** Proliferation and further differentiation of the cells of this layer adds cells to the periphery of the center of chondrification, contributing to its **appositional growth.** Cells more deeply situated in the center of chondrification continue to secrete additional hyaline matrix around themselves. The accumulation of matrix moves the cells apart, with each occupying its own small **lacuna,** within the matrix (Fig. 6-1D). These are initially distributed singly in the matrix. However, the chondrocytes retain, for some time into postnatal life, the ability to divide, and after each division a small amount of additional matrix is secreted between the daughter cells. As a result of this **interstitial growth,** the cells in cartilage of adults occur in pairs or groups of four or six (Figs. 6-2 and 6-3 [see Plate 5]). The cells of each group are said to be **isogenous** because they represent the progeny of a single chondrocyte. Interstitial growth is transient, and after a few divisions, the cells cease to divide and remain quiescent throughout adult life.

Chondrocytes

In histological sections of cartilage, the lacunae near the perichondrium are elliptical, with their long axis parallel to the surface. Those in isogenous groupings, deeper in the matrix, are hemispherical or roughly triangular. In vivo, the chondrocytes conform to the shape of their lacu-

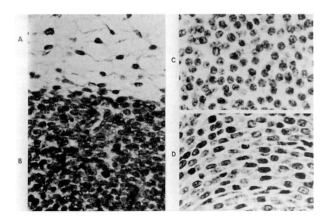

Fig. 6-1 Early stages in the histogenesis of cartilage. (A) Mesenchymal cells (top) withdraw their processes and aggregate as shown in (B), an area of precartilage. (C) The cells are moved apart by the deposition of cartilage matrix between them. (D) The cells then become more fusiform.

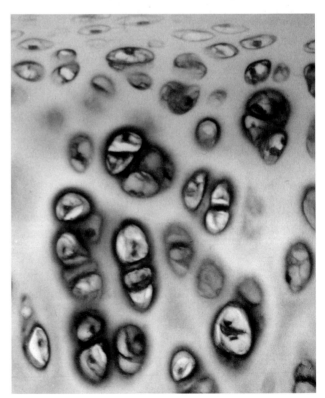

Fig. 6-2 Hyaline cartilage of the trachea. Note that the cells immediately beneath the perichondrium (top), recently added in appositional growth, are single and elongate. Those below are in isogenous groups resulting from interstitial growth.

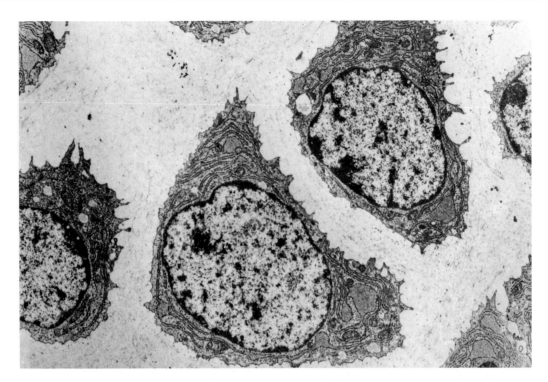

Fig. 6-4 Electron micrograph of unusually well-preserved chondrocytes and intervening matrix. Note the irregular outlines of the cells, and their well-developed endoplasmic reticulum. Reprinted with permission from R. Seegmiller, C. Ferguson, and H. Sheldoh, Journal of Ultrastructure Research, 38:288, 1972.)

na, but during preparation of histological sections, they retract from the wall of the lacuna and often appear stellate. The matrix immediately surrounding each cluster of isogenous cells stains more intensely with basic dyes and is termed **territorial matrix.** Between cell groups it is less basophilic and is called the **interterritorial matrix** (Figs. 6-2 and 6-3 [see Plate 5]). In preparation of cartilage for electron microscopy, there is less cell shrinkage and chondrocytes fill their lacunae. The nucleus is well preserved, and a Golgi complex, a few mitochondria, and cisternae of rough endoplasmic reticulum can be seen in the cytoplasm (Fig. 6-4). The organelles are larger and more numerous in chondrocytes actively engaged in synthesis of matrix components.

Chondrocytes secrete and maintain the surrounding matrix. They are also able to depolymerize and remove the adjacent matrix to enlarge their lacunae. This can be observed in the early stages of replacement of cartilage by bone in the process of **endochondral ossification.** The chondrocytes hypertrophy at the expense of the surrounding matrix, which is reduced to thin plates or spicules between the enlarged lacunae. These become sites of deposition of calcium phosphate. The chondrocytes then degenerate and their coalesced lacunae are invaded by blood vessels from the perichondrium, accompanied by cells that differentiate into bone-forming cells, **osteoblasts.** Near the ends of the cartilage models of the long bones (viz. femur or tibia), the proliferating chondrocytes become arranged in longitudinal columns parallel to the long axis of the cartilage model and, in so doing, form the cartilaginous **epi-**

physeal plates between the epiphysis and the shaft of a developing long bone (Figs. 6-5 [see Plate 5]) and 6-6). Growth in length of the bone depends on continuing chondrocyte proliferation at the distal end of the epiphyseal plate, followed by their maturation, hypertrophy, and ultimate degeneration at the other side of the plate where their place is being taken by bone-forming osteoblasts. This will be explained in more detail in the chapter on Bone.

*The **chondrodystrophies** are a group of diseases characterized by disturbance of cartilage growth and its replacement by bone. One of the more common examples is **achondroplasia,** an inherited disorder in which there is reduced proliferation of the chondrocytes in the epiphyseal plate of long bones, resulting in a form of dwarfism in which the trunk is of normal length but the extremities are very short.*

Cartilage Matrix

Like the extracellular matrix of connective tissue, the matrix of hyaline cartilage consists of collagen fibers in an amorphous matrix, rich in proteoglycans. Collagen makes up 40% of its dry weight, but this is not apparent in histological sections, for the collagen fibers and the matrix have about the same refractive index. The arrangement of the

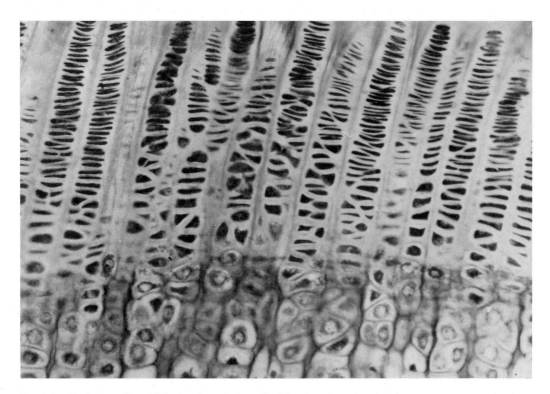

Fig. 6-6 Hyaline cartilage of the epiphyseal plate of rabbit tibia. Here the chondrocytes are arranged in long parallel columns. From above downward, one can identify zones of proliferation, maturation, hypertrophy, and degeneration.

collagen fibers can be studied with polarization optics in sections from which the proteoglycans have been extracted. Type-II collagen predominates and occurs in cross-striated fibers 15–45 nm in diameter that do not assemble into coarse bundles. Fibers at the smaller end of this range form a loose three-dimensional network throughout the matrix. The larger fibers are deployed in a pattern suggesting that their orientation is adapted to resist the strains to which that particular cartilage is normally subjected. Collagen types IX, X, and XI have been identified in cartilage, in small amounts, and these may serve to stabilize the network of type-II collagen fibers.

The proteoglycans are present in higher concentration than in any other connective tissues and they form a much firmer gel. They consist of a core protein 200–300 nm in length, from which many glycosaminoglycan molecules radiate in a bottle-brush configuration. The principal glycosaminoglycans of cartilage are **chondroitin sulfate** and **keratan sulfate.** The proteoglycans of cartilage are among the largest molecules produced by cells, having molecular weights ranging up to 3.5×10^6 Da. Proteoglycan molecules of the matrix are bound at their globular head to a long molecule of **hyaluronic acid** and are spaced along its length at intervals of 30 nm, forming a large **proteoglycan aggregate.** A single molecule of hyaluronic acid may have as many as 100 proteoglycan molecules linked to it. These aggregates interact with specific sites on the cross-banded collagen fibers. In electron micrographs prepared by high-pressure freezing, freeze-substitution and low-temperature embedding, it is possible to see what appear to be the core proteins of the proteoglycans, and around these a network of thin filaments that are believed to be their glycosaminoglycan side chains. Chondrocytes also synthesize **chondronectin,** a large molecule involved in the adherence of the chondrocytes to the collagen fibers of the surrounding matrix.

ELASTIC CARTILAGE

Elastic cartilage is found in the external ear, in the wall of the external auditory and eustachian canals, and in certain small cartilages of the larynx. It differs from hyaline cartilage in its greater opacity, yellowish color, and its greater flexibility. Its chondrocytes are indistinguishable from those of hyaline cartilage and are housed in lacunae that are scattered singly or in pairs. The matrix is somewhat less abundant and a significant fraction of its substance consists of branching fibers of **elastin.** In histological sections stained for elastin, the fibers deep in the cartilage may be so closely packed that the amorphous components of the matrix are not apparent (Fig. 6-7). Nearer the periphery of an elastic cartilage, the network of elastic fibers is looser and fibers can be seen to continue into the perichondrium.

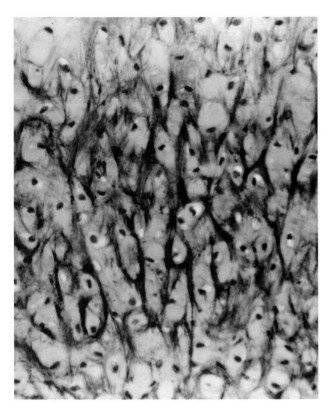

Fig. 6-7 Photomicrograph of elastic cartilage from the epiglottis of a child. Note the dark-staining bundles of elastic fibers in the matrix between groups of chondrocytes.

As in hyaline cartilage, the mechanical properties of elastic cartilage are dependent on the proteoglycans of its matrix. If the enzyme papain is injected intravenously into a rabbit, its ears soon collapse as the enzyme degrades the proteoglycans of their elastic cartilage. The chondrocytes quickly respond by secretion of proteoglycans and other matrix components, and the ears are restored to their erect position in 48 h.

FIBROCARTILAGE

Fibrocartilage is found in the vertebral column, the pubic symphysis, and at sites of insertion of ligaments and tendons into bone. It resembles dense regular connective tissue, and the two are often continuous without any clear line of demarcation. Chondrocytes, surrounded by a small amount of matrix, are aligned in rows between coarse parallel bundles of type-I collagen fibers. A thin basophilic territorial matrix can be identified around the lacunae, but the interterritorial matrix is largely replaced by the bundles of collagen. The tissue as a whole is acidophilic. A well-defined perichondrium is usually lacking.

Fibrocartilage with a somewhat different organization is found in the **intervertebral disks** between successive vertebrae. In the center of the disk, there is a soft viscous **nucleus pulposus.** This consists of a small population of cells in a semifluid matrix rich in hyaluronic acid and type-II collagen fibers. This is surrounded by a thick ring of fibrocartilage, called the **annulus fibrosus,** made up of multiple concentric lamellae of collagen fibers. Some of these terminate in a thin layer of hyaline cartilage on the surface of the vertebrae above and below the disk. A few chondrocytes can be found between the lamellae of the annulus. The orientation of the collagen fibers in successive lamellae changes, giving the fibrocartilage the ability to resist any forces that would tend to displace the vertebrae with respect to one another.

> *In the common clinical condition,* **herniated intervertebral disk,** *the annulus fibrosus has been torn, permitting the nucleus pulposus to herniate into the vertebral canal and press on the spinal nerves. This results in severe pain and neurological disturbances in the region supplied by those nerves.*

HISTOPHYSIOLOGY OF CARTILAGE

In adult life, the firm extracellular matrix of the articular cartilages at joints enables them to withstand great compressive forces, and their smooth surface permits frictionless joint movement. In children, growth in stature depends on the rapid interstitial growth of epiphyseal cartilage and its replacement by bone. Such growth is indirectly controlled by **somatotrophin,** the growth hormone of the anterior pituitary. This regulates the liver's production of another hormone, **somatomedin-C,** which stimulates the proliferation of the chondrocytes in the epiphyseal plates of the long bones.

Cartilage is an avascular tissue, and cartilages are limited in size by the distance that small molecules can diffuse through the matrix to nourish the chondrocytes. The matrix is also a barrier to the entry of lymphocytes, and immunoglobulins (antibodies) cannot diffuse into the matrix. This property is of clinical importance for cosmetic and reconstructive surgery, for cartilage can be transplanted from one individual to another without fear of rejection by the immune system.

QUESTIONS*

1. Find the best answer: The matrix of hyaline cartilage

   A. contains primarily type-II collagen
   B. contains hyaluronic acid
   C. contains proteoglycans
   D. contains glycosaminoglycans with sulfated hexosamines
   E. all of the above

2. Fibrocartilage

   A. is composed primarily of coarse parallel bundles of type-II collagen fibers
   B. has a well-developed perichondrium
   C. exhibits well-developed isogenous groupings
   D. contains multiple concentric lamellae of collagenous fibers
   E. is located in long bones

3. Chondrocytes are nourished by

   A. closely associated capillary plexuses
   B. the rich vascularity of cartilage
   C. diffusion of metabolites through the matrix
   D. intrachondral canals
   E. capillaries directly open to lacunae

4. Isogenous groupings of lacunae are most commonly seen in

   A. fibrocartilage
   B. elastic cartilage
   C. perichondrium
   D. hyaline cartilage
   E. all of the above

5. The major element(s) of cartilage is (are)

   A. blood vessels
   B. chondrocytes
   C. chondroblast
   D. osteocytes
   E. extracellular matrix

6. The primary element of the hyaline cartilage matrix is

   A. collagen
   B. chondrocytes
   C. triglycerides
   D. elastic fibers
   E. lacunae

7. The most common type of cartilage is

   A. fibrocartilage
   B. hyaline
   C. tropocollagen
   D. elastic
   E. chondrocartilage

8. Elastic cartilage differs from hyaline cartilage because elastic cartilage

   A. has more chondrocytes per unit area of matrix
   B. has a soft viscous center
   C. has a much more abundant matrix
   D. is more flexible
   E. is less opaque

*Answers on page 307.

7

BONE

Bone consists of cells and fibers in an amorphous ground substance containing crystals of **hydroxyapatite** ($Ca_{10}[PO_4]_6[OH]_2$), a complex calcium salt. The calcification of the matrix makes bone a hard, unyielding substance ideally suited for its protective and supportive role in the skeleton. Bones provide attachment and levers for muscles involved in locomotion; they protect the vital organs of the cranial and thoracic cavities; and they constitute a mobilizable store of calcium which can be drawn upon in the homeostatic regulation of the concentration of this ion in the blood and tissue fluids.

A connective tissue sheath, the **periosteum,** covers the outside of bones, and a similar, but thinner layer, the **endosteum,** lines their interior. Both of these layers contain **osteoprogenitor cells,** cells that can be reactivated to form bone in the repair of fractures. The cells within bone include **osteoblasts,** which secrete the organic components of bone, **osteocytes,** which reside in lacunae within the matrix, and **osteoclasts,** which participate in the continual resorption and remodeling of bone.

MACROSCOPIC STRUCTURE

In considering this complex tissue, it may be helpful, at the outset, to describe certain features of the gross structure of a typical long bone. In a longitudinal section, the shaft, or **diaphysis,** consists of a thick wall of dense bone, the **substantia compacta,** around a voluminous central **medullary cavity.** Toward the ends of the diaphysis, the compact bone becomes thinner and the medullary cavity contains a three-dimensional network of branching bone spicules (trabeculae), forming the **substantia spongiosa,** also described as **cancellous** bone (Fig. 7-1). The central cavity of the shaft contains the blood-forming tissue, **bone marrow,** and it extends some distance into the

labyrinthine system of spaces among the trabeculae of cancellous bone at either end. At the ends of a long bone, where it forms movable joints with other bones of the appendicular skeleton, the thin layer of compact bone is covered by a layer of hyaline cartilage, the **articular cartilage.**

In the growing bones of children, regions at either end, called the **epiphyses,** are separated from the diaphysis by a thin zone of hyaline cartilage called the **epiphyseal plate** (Fig. 7-2). This is the principal site of growth in the length of the bone. When adult stature is attained, this layer of cartilage is eliminated and the epiphyses and the diaphysis become continuous. In the flat bones of the skull, compact bone forms outer and inner layers, generally referred to as the **outer table** and **inner table.** A thin zone of spongy bone between them is called the **diploë.**

MICROSCOPIC STRUCTURE

Osteoprogenitor Cells

In the **periosteum** on the outer surface of a bone and in the **endosteum** lining the shaft and covering the trabeculae of spongy bone, there are inconspicuous fusiform **osteo-**

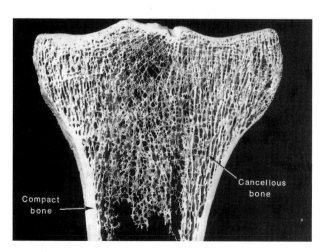

Fig. 7-1 A thick ground section of the proximal end of the tibia, illustrating the cortical compact bone of the shaft and the lattice of trabeculae of cancellous bone in the interior.

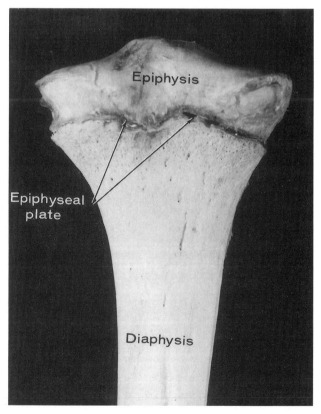

Fig. 7-2 Photograph of the upper half of the tibia, showing the epiphysis at the proximal end, the cartilaginous epiphyseal plate, and the diaphysis.

progenitor cells. Their elongated nucleus is pale staining and the cytoplasm is acidophilic or faintly basophilic. These cells are the inactive precursors of the principal osteogenic cells of growing bones, the **osteoblasts.** The osteoprogenitor cells can be reactivated in adult life to proliferate and differentiate into osteoblasts needed in the repair of fractures.

Osteoblasts

During active deposition of new bone matrix, **osteoblasts** are cuboidal cells aligned on the surface of bone (Fig. 7-3). They do not form a typical epithelium but are attached to one another at the ends of short lateral processes. Their nucleus is in the rounded end of the cell, away from the bone. The cytoplasm is intensely basophilic and reacts positively with the histochemical reaction for acid phosphatase. In electron micrographs, they have the appearance one would expect in a cell actively engaged in protein synthesis. Rough endoplasmic reticulum is abundant and there are many free ribosomes. A number of small vacuoles, associated with the juxtanuclear Golgi complex, contain an amorphous or flocculent material of appreciable density. Osteoblasts synthesize the type-I collagen, glycoproteins and proteoglycans of bone matrix, and some of its

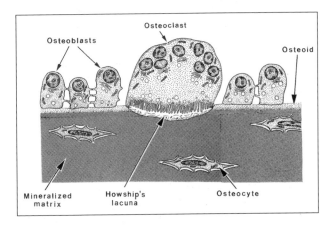

Fig. 7-3 Drawing of the three principal cell types of bone and their relationship to a trabecula of mineralized bone matrix.

minor components (**osteocalcin, osteonectin,** and **osteopontin**). They have surface receptors for certain hormones, vitamins, and cytokines that influence their activity. When their synthetic activity declines, they become flattened against the bone, and their basophilia and content of endoplasmic reticulum are reduced.

The release of matrix components by osteoblasts is not confined to their basal pole, for on an expanding bony surface, some of their number gradually become enveloped by

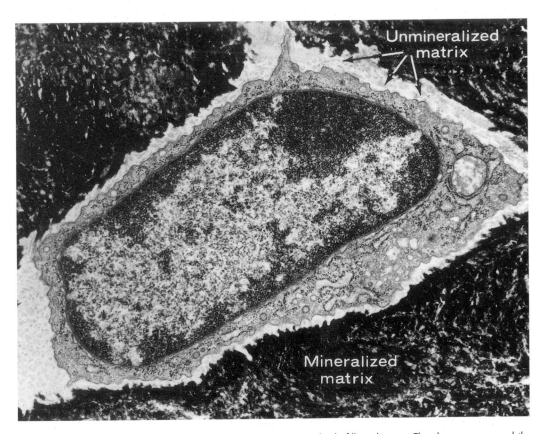

Fig. 7-4 Electron micrograph of an osteocyte. Note that it completely fills its lacuna. The clear area around the cell is occupied by collagen fibers and unmineralized matrix. The mineralized matrix is black, due to electron scattering by the apatite crystals. (Courtesy of Marie Holtrop.)

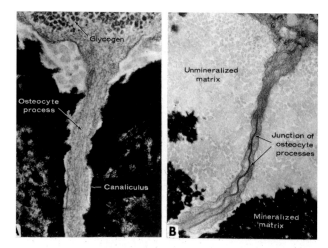

Fig. 7-5   (A) Micrograph of an osteocyte process extending from the cell body (top) into a canaliculus. (Micrograph courtesy of M. Holtrop.) (B) Micrograph of two osteocyte processes traversing the unmineralized matrix and entering a canaliculus. Note the gap junction between the overlapping processes. (Courtesy of M. Holtrop and M. J. Wenger.)

their own secretions and are transformed into **osteocytes,** imprisoned in lacunae within the newly deposited matrix.

Osteocytes

The **osteocytes** are the principal cells of adult bone. They reside in lacunae within the calcified matrix (Figs. 7-3 and 7-4). The cell body is somewhat flattened, the nucleus elongate, and there are numerous long cell processes that radiate from it. Osteocytes have a more heterochromatic nucleus than osteoblasts, and their cytoplasm contains less endoplasmic reticulum and a smaller Golgi complex. Although they do not have the appearance of a synthetically active cell, there is evidence that they play an active role in the maintenance of the surrounding matrix.

Because the osseous matrix is deposited around the cell, the shape of the lacuna conforms to that of the cell. Radiating from it are slender **canaliculi** that are occupied by the slender processes of the osteocyte (Fig. 7-5A). The ends of the processes of neighboring osteocytes meet within the canaliculi and have gap junctions at their site of contact (Fig. 7-5B). Thus, unlike the cells of cartilage, osteocytes are not completely isolated within the matrix but are in communication with one another via a system of junctions that permit the flow of ions and small molecules from cell to cell. The diffusion of nutrients through the calcified matrix is very limited, but there is probably some exchange of metabolites between the cells and the blood via the film of extracellular fluid occupying the narrow space between the cells and the walls of the lacunae and canaliculi.

The canaliculi are not visible in routine histological preparations, but if a section of dried bone is ground down

to a thin translucent sheet and then examined with the microscope, the air-filled lacunae and their radiating canaliculi are clearly visible (Fig. 7-6). Such a preparation is described as a ground section of bone.

Osteoclasts

Throughout adult life, bone undergoes a continuous process of internal remodeling and renewal that involves removal of bone matrix and its replacement by newly deposited bone. In this process, the agents of bone resorption are the **osteoclasts,** huge cells up to 15 μm in diameter with as many as 50 nuclei. They occupy shallow concavities in the surface, called **Howship's lacunae.** These are produced by the degradation of bone by enzymes that osteoclasts secrete onto the underlying bone (Fig. 7-4). The osteoclasts exhibit an obvious polarity with their nuclei congregated near their smooth contoured free surface. The other end, next to the bone, has a striated appearance and, in electron micrographs, the cell membrane there is deeply infolded to delimit a large number of clavate (club-shaped) or foliate (leaflike) cell processes (Fig. 7-7). These are more variable in shape and closer together than microvilli. Cinematographic studies of living osteoclasts document frequent changes in their shape as they are extended and retracted. The term **ruffled border** is now used to distinguish this surface specialization from the more stable and orderly brush-border of some epithelia. The plasmalemma of the border bears a knap of exceedingly fine bristlelike appendages 15–20 nm long and spaced about 20 nm apart. This bristle-coat makes the membrane of the border appear thicker than the rest of the plasma membrane. Around the circumference of the ruffled border, the membrane is very closely applied to the underlying bone, and the subjacent cytoplasm is unusually rich in actin filaments. This specialization, termed the **sealing zone,** bounds a closed space between the ruffled border of the osteoclast and the underlying bone. The ultrastructure of osteoclasts is unremarkable except for their numerous nuclei and their specialized border. There are multiple Golgi complexes and pairs of centrioles. The cytoplasm near the ruffled border contains many mitochondria, a few profiles of rough endoplasmic reticulum, and numerous lysosomes.

Osteoclasts secrete H⁺ ions into the underlying lacuna acidifying its contents to dissolve the bone mineral. They also secrete collagenase and other hydrolytic enzymes to digest the organic components of the matrix. Crystals of calcium salts and disintegrating collagen fibers can be identified in the subosteoclastic compartment.

Traditionally, osteoclasts were regarded as the sole agents of bone resorption. However, they are only effective when they are directly adherent to mineralized bone matrix and the matrix is usually covered by a thin layer of unmineralized matrix called **osteoid.** It is now believed that the

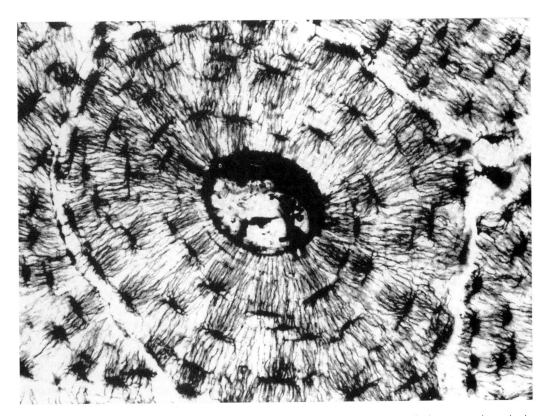

Fig. 7-6 Photomicrograph of a typical haversian system in a ground section of bone. The lacunae and canaliculi appear black, and the surrounding mineralized matrix is white.

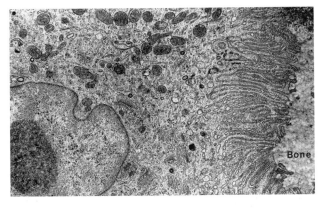

Fig. 7-7 Electron micrograph of a portion of an osteoclast including part of a nucleus at the lower left, and at the right, the ruffled border closely applied to an area of bone matrix being resorbed. (Courtesy of M. Garrant.)

osteoblasts on bone surfaces participate in bone resorption by secreting enzymes that remove the layer of osteoid, exposing the mineralized matrix to attack by osteoclasts.

Osteoclasts were long thought to arise by coalescence of monocytes reaching the bone in the blood. There is now evidence that they arise from a precursor that resembles the monocyte but differs from it in having a distinctive tartrate-resistant acid phosphatase.

Bone Matrix

Collagen accounts for 90% of the organic material of bone matrix. In the first bone deposited **(primary bone),** the fibers are randomly oriented, but in mature lamellar bone (*secondary bone*), they have a highly ordered arrangement, with those in each lamella parallel in their orientation. The proteoglycans of bone have a shorter core protein than those of cartilage and fewer side chains. Among the glycosaminoglycans are chondroitin sulfates and keratan sulfate. Matrix proteins specific for bone are **osteocalcin** and **osteopontin,** which bind tightly to the mineral hydroxyapatite and have binding sequences that are thought to be involved in the binding of osteoblasts and osteoclasts to the matrix.

The inorganic matter of bone consists of **hydroxyapatite,** which is essentially identical in composition to a component of geological deposits of calcium phosphate. Although some bone mineral may be amorphous, the great bulk of it is in the form of rodlike hydroxyapatite crystals 40 nm in length and 1.5–3 nm in thickness. These recur at regular intervals of 60–70 nm along the length of the collagen fibers. Bone matrix also contains significant concentrations of citrate ($C_6H_5O_{73}^-$) and carbonate (CO_{33}^-) ions. A layer of water and ions **(hydration shell)** surrounds each hydroxyapatite crystal and is believed to facilitate the exchange of ions between the crystals and the body fluids.

ORGANIZATION OF LAMELLAR BONE

Compact bone of adults is largely composed of cylindrical subunits called **haversian systems** or **osteons,** each composed of 4–15 lamellae of calcified matrix arranged concentrically around a **central canal** containing a capillary or postcapillary venule (Fig. 7-8). The haversian systems may branch, with the bifurcation of the blood vessel in their central canal. The collagen fibers within each lamella are parallel to each other and have a helical course along the length of the osteon. However, the pitch of the helix changes in successive lamellae, so that at any given point along the osteon, the fibers in adjacent lamellae are oriented nearly at right angles to one another. Thus, when haversian systems are viewed in cross section with the polarizing microscope, bright, birefringent lamellae alternate with dark isotropic lamellae (Figs. 7-9A and 7-9B). The central canals of the haversian systems communicate with each other and with the marrow cavity via occasional oblique channels that traverse the surrounding lamellae. These are called **Volkmann's canals.** Unlike the central canals, they are not surrounded by concentric lamellae.

Between the haversian systems, there are angular areas of parallel lamellae of varying size and shape, called the **interstitial lamellae.** These are remnants of preexisting haversian systems that have been largely eroded away by osteoclasts in the continual internal remodeling of bone. The boundary of each haversian system is sharply outlined by a thin refractile layer called a **cement line.** Thus, in cross sections, compact bone appears as a mosaic of circular and angular subunits held together by a thin intervening layer of cement (Fig. 7-9A).

Immediately beneath the periosteum, on the shaft of a bone, there are a number of lamellae that extend, without interruption, around the entire circumference of the shaft. These are called the **outer circumferential lamellae.** Comparable lamellae beneath the endosteum are designated the **inner circumferential lamellae** (Fig. 7-8). The periosteum is fixed to the outer circumferential lamellae by bundles of collagen fibers, called **Sharpey's fibers,** that penetrate these lamellae and extend a short distance deeper into the bone.

HISTOGENESIS OF BONE

Bone always develops by replacement of a preexisting connective tissue. In the embryo, two different modes of osteogenesis are observed. Where bone is formed by replacing primitive connective tissue (mesenchyme), the process is called **intramembranous ossification.** Where bone formation takes place in preexisting cartilage, it is called **endochondral ossification.** The flat bones of the skull develop by intramembranous ossification, whereas the long bones of the appendicular skeleton develop by endochondral ossification. In both, the deposition of bone matrix is essentially the same, but in endochondral ossification, the bulk of the cartilage matrix must be removed before bone deposition begins. In both methods, bone is first laid down as a network of trabeculae, called the **primary spongiosa** (Fig. 7-10 [see Plate 5]), which is subsequently transformed into compact bone by filling in the interspaces between trabeculae.

Intramembranous Ossification

In this mode of ossification, the embryonic mesenchyme first condenses into a richly vascularized layer of primitive connective tissue. Its stellate cells are in contact with one another via long cell processes, and the intercellular spaces are occupied by a ground substance containing randomly oriented collagen fibers. Certain of the mesenchymal cells then aggregate and differentiate into osteogenic cells that deposit bone matrix around themselves. This process results in thin tabeculae of eosinophilic bone matrix. These tend to form equidistant between neighboring blood vessels, and because the blood vessels form a network, the trabeculae in the **primary spongiosa** also have a branching and anastomosing pattern (Fig. 7-10 [see Plate 5]). Other cells of the mes-

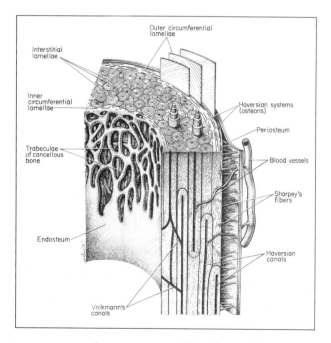

Fig. 7-8 Drawing of a sector of the shaft of a long bone, showing the disposition of the lamellae in the osteons, the interstitial lamellae, and the outer and inner circumferential lamellae. (Redrawn from A. Benninghoff, Lehrbuch der Anatomie des Menschen, Urban and Schwartzenberg, Berlin, 1935).

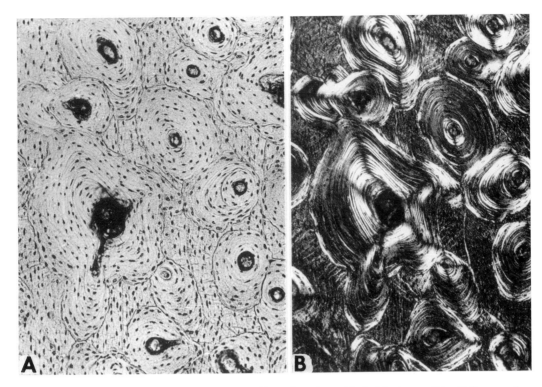

Fig. 7-9 (A) Photomicrograph of a ground section of bone from the midshaft of the human tibia. (B) Same section photographed through the polarizing microscope. The alternating light and dark concentric layers in the haversian systems result from differing orientation of the collagen fibers in successive layers. (Micrograph courtesy of R. Amprino.)

enchyme enlarge and become intensely basophilic **osteoblasts** that gather on the surface of the primary trabeculae. Their secretion of additional matrix results in the trabeculae becoming longer and thicker. As osteoblasts become incarcerated in lacunae within the matrix as **osteocytes,** they are replaced at the surface of the trabeculae by further differentiation of osteoprogenitor cells in the perivascular connective tissue. The area of the sheet of primitive connective tissue wherein these events take place is designated a **primary center of ossification.** In portions of the primary spongiosa destined to become compact bone, progressive thickening of the trabeculae encroaches upon the perivascular spaces until they are relatively narrow. Where spongy bone will persist in postnatal life, the thickening of the trabeculae does not progress as far, and the connective tissue between them is gradually transformed into bone marrow. In the flat bones that develop by intramembranous ossification, the collagen fibers are initially random in their orientation. Later, in early postnatal life, the primary bone is replaced by lamellar bone in which the collagen fibers in successive lamellae of the haversian systems are precisely oriented. The portion of the original layer of primitive connective tissue that does not undergo ossification condenses to form the periosteum and endosteum. Bones so formed are said to be made up of **membrane bone,** a term used to distinguish them from bone that develops in preexisting cartilage (Figs. 7-11A and 7-11B).

ENDOCHONDRAL OSSIFICATION

Long bones, such as the humerus and femur, develop in the embryo from cartilages of roughly similar shape, commonly referred to as their **cartilage models.** The first indication of the formation of a **center of endochondral ossification** is a local enlargement of the chondrocytes in the middle of the cartilage model (Fig. 7-12). As their lacunae enlarge, the intervening cartilage matrix is gradually reduced to irregularly shaped spicules. The hypertrophied chondrocytes then die and small aggregations of calcium phosphate crystals form within the remaining trabeculae of cartilage matrix. While these changes are occurring in the interior of the cartilage, osteoprogenitor cells in the perichondrium become activated and deposit a thin **periosteal collar** of bone around the middle of the shaft of the cartilage model. At the same time, capillaries and associated osteoprogenitor cells invade the spaces left behind by the degeneration of hypertrophied chondrocytes. The vessels branch and grow toward either end, forming loops that extend into the blind ends of cavities in the calcified cartilage (Figs. 7-13A through 7-13E [See Plate 6]). Osteoprogenitor cells, accompanying the invading blood vessels, differentiate into osteoblasts that congregate on the surface of the spicules of calcified cartilage and begin to deposit bone matrix on them. The resulting trabeculae have a mottled appearance due to the difference in staining properties of the core of cartilage and the coating of bone.

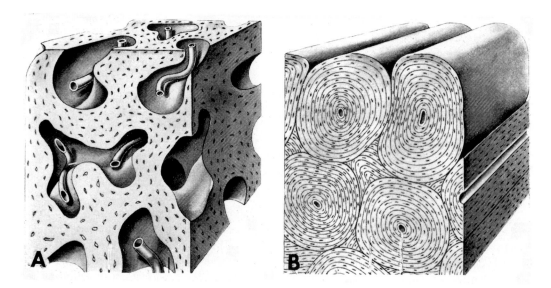

Fig. 7-11 Three-dimensional representation of the differences between (A) primary woven bone and (B) mature lamellar bone. (From N. M. Hancox, Biology of Bone, Cambridge University Press, 1972.)

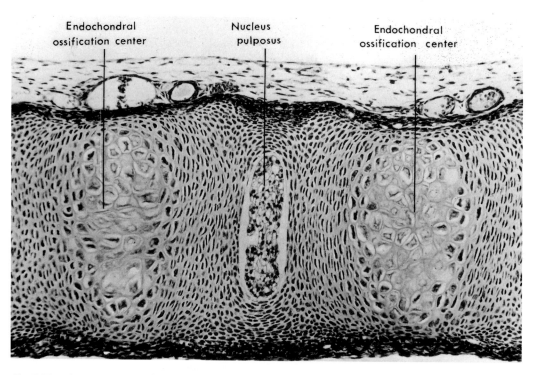

Endochondral ossification center   Nucleus pulposus   Endochondral ossification center

Fig. 7-12 Photomicrograph of two vertebrae of a mouse embryo. In each, there is a central area of hypertrophied cartilage cells. This appearance represents a very early stage in formation of a center of endochondral ossification.

This stage of development is usually reached by the third month of fetal life. The developing long bones have expanded ends **(epiphyses)** of hyaline cartilage and a shaft **(diaphysis)** consisting of an hour-glass-shaped region of endochondral ossification surrounded by a collar of bone of periosteal origin (Fig. 7-13F [See Plate 6]). The term **primary center of ossification** embraces all of the events described above and is intended to distinguish the diaphyseal center of ossification, which develops first, from **secondary centers of ossification** that develop much later in the epiphyses.

Growth in Length of Long Bones

While cartilage is being replaced by bone in the expanding diaphyseal center of ossification, interstitial and appositional growth of the cartilage of the epiphyses continues, and the chondrocytes near the diaphysis become arranged in longitudinal columns separated by columns of cartilage matrix (Figs. 7-14 and 7-15 [see Plate 7]). As ossification progresses, the chondrocytes in the longitudinal columns undergo changes similar to the early events in the primary center of ossification. Four zones become recognizable along their length. At their epiphyseal ends, there is a **zone of proliferation,** where frequent mitosis of the chondrocytes ensures continuing elongation of the cartilage model. Below this is a **zone of maturation,** in which the cells undergo significant enlargement, which reaches its peak in a **zone of hypertrophy,** where the cells are very large and highly vacuolated. The matrix between columns in this zone is undergoing calcification (Fig. 7-16 [see Plate 8]. Therefore, this region is also referred to as the **zone of provisional calcification.** Finally, at the diaphyseal end of the columns is the **zone of degeneration,** where the hypertrophied chondrocytes are dying and the open ends of their vacated lacunae are being invaded by capillary loops and associated osteoprogenitor cells from the marrow cavity. The osteoprogenitor cells differentiate into osteoblasts that deposit bone matrix on the spicules of calcified cartilage that remain between the cell columns (Figs. 7-15 and 7-16 [see Plates 7 & 8]).

Shortly after birth, chondrocytes in the centers of the two epiphyses hypertrophy, heralding the formation of **secondary centers of ossification** at both ends of the long bone (Figs. 7-13G and 7-13H [see Plate 6]). Their development proceeds, as in the primary center, except that there is no associated subperichondrial deposition of bone. In the subsequent expansion of the secondary centers, all of the epiphyseal cartilage is finally replaced by bone except for a layer at the end that persists as the **articular cartilage** and a thin transverse disk between the epiphysis and the diaphysis, the **epiphyseal plate.** All subsequent growth in length of the long bones during childhood is attributable to proliferation of chondrocytes in the epiphyseal plate and their replacement by bone. At the end of the growing period, proliferation of the cartilage cells slows and finally ceases. Replacement of cartilage by bone continues resulting in obliteration of the epiphyseal plate (Figs. 7-13I and 7-13J [see Plate 6]). This **closure of the epiphyse**s occurs at the age of 18–20 years. Thereafter, no further growth is possible.

Growth in Diameter of Long Bones

While growth in length of the long bones is occurring at the epiphyseal plate, growth in the diameter of the diaphysis is progressing by circumferential deposition of membrane bone beneath the periosteum. The resulting thickening of the shaft is accompanied by mobilization of osteoclasts on its inner surface. These resorb bone there and thus enlarge the marrow cavity. Deposition of bone on the outside and resorption of bone on the inside of the shaft continues until the diameter of the adult bone is attained. Early in this process, all of the spicules of endochondral bone formed in the primary center of ossification are removed by osteoclasts in the enlargement of the marrow cavity and, thereafter, the entire shaft consists of membrane bone deposited by the periosteum. The respective rates of deposition of bone on the outside and osteoclastic

erosion of bone on the inside of the shaft are such that the thickness of the wall soon reaches its definitive thickness, and thereafter remains nearly constant.

Surface Modeling of Bones

Throughout their growth, long bones retain approximately the same external form. Obviously, this would not be true if new bone were deposited at a uniform rate at all points beneath the periosteum. Instead, the shape of a bone during its growth is maintained by a continual modeling or sculpturing of its surface that involves subperiosteal bone deposition in some areas and bone resorption in other areas. This can be demonstrated if a bone-seeking radioisotope is given to a growing rat and autoradiographs are then made of longitudinal sections of its tibia. The sites of new bone formation are disclosed by the distribution of silver grains in the overlying photographic emulsion. In the conical regions toward the ends of the bone, the grains are aligned immediately beneath the endosteum, whereas in the cylindrical midportion of the shaft, they are found beneath the periosteum. Study of parallel histological sections reveals numerous osteoclasts beneath the periosteum of the conical region and beneath the endosteum in the cylindrical shaft. Thus, it is clear that in surface modeling of this bone, the periosteum plays opposite roles in the two regions of the bone: subperiosteal bone deposition occurring in the cylindrical shaft while subperiosteal bone resorption is taking place in the conical region toward the ends. Thus in the bone, as a whole, the diverging walls of the conical region are being straightened and are contributing, at their lower end, to the lengthening of the cylindrical portion of the shaft. How these local variations in function of the endosteum and periosteum are controlled in space and time so as to continually mold the shape of the bone is a fascinating unsolved problem in morphogenesis.

Internal Reorganization of Bone

As described above, the progressive thickening of the primary lattice of bone spicules largely obliterates the perivascular spaces, converting the primary spongiosa to compact bone. In this process, bone is deposited in ill-defined concentric layers. True haversian systems are first formed during the internal reorganization involved in secondary bone formation.

In this process, **absorption cavities** appear in primary compact bone due to osteoclast activity. The long cylindrical cavities so formed are invaded by blood vessels and accompanying osteoprogenitor cells from the bone marrow. When bone resorption ceases, the osteoclasts lining the cavities are replaced by osteoblasts that deposit concentric lamellae of bone on the inner aspect of the absorption cavity. These lamellae have the ordered arrangement of collagen fibers characteristic of the haversian systems of adult bone. From the age of 1 year onward, only lamellar bone of this character is deposited in the shafts of long bones and this secondary bone ultimately replaces all of the primary bone.

Internal bone reconstruction does not end with the replacement of primary bone by secondary bone but continues throughout life. Resorption cavities continue to appear and to be filled with third, fourth, and higher orders of haversian systems. Interstitial lamellae of adult bone represent persisting fragments of earlier generations of haversian systems. This continuous turnover provides the plasticity that enables bone to alter its internal architecture to adapt to new mechanical stresses.

In histological preparations of bone, all of the haversian systems look alike, regardless of their age. However, calcification of their lamellae proceeds much more slowly than their deposition, and recently deposited osteons can be distinguished from older ones in historadiograms produced by placing a ground section of bone between an X-ray source and a photographic film. In the resulting image, the recently formed haversian systems, with a low calcium content, appear dark; older ones are lighter and interstitial lamellae are white (Fig. 7-17).

Repair of Fractures

The osteogenic potential of cells of the periosteum and endosteum can be evoked again after the cells have been quiescent for many years. After a fracture, the blood clot formed at the site is soon invaded by cells and a **fibrocartilaginous callus** is formed between the bone fragments. Previously quiescent cells of the periosteum are reactivated and form a **bony callus,** a meshwork of trabeculae of membrane bone that ultimately bridges the gap between fragments. At the same time, the callus of fibrocartilage is eroded away and replaced by bone deposited by reactivated cells of the endosteum. Over the following weeks, the spongy bone uniting the fragments is transformed into compact bone. Subsequent resorption of excess bone reestablishes continuity of the marrow cavity and restores the normal surface contours to the bone.

HISTOPHYSIOLOGY OF BONE

Calcium Homeostasis

In addition to its obvious supportive and protective function, bone is a mobilizable store of calcium. The importance of calcium in the body cannot be overemphasized. Calcium ions are essential for the activity of many enzymes: for maintenance of cell cohesion and the regulation of membrane permeability; for the coagulation of blood; for contraction of smooth and striated muscle; and

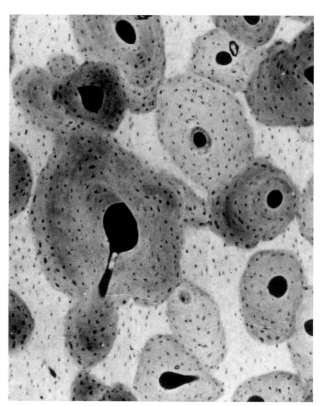

Fig. 7-17 A historadiogram of the same field shown in Figure 7-9A. The differing shades of gray, from nearly white to nearly black, reflect the differing concentrations of calcium. The most recently deposited haversian systems are incompletely calcified and appear dark gray, whereas the older ones, containing a higher concentration of calcium, are lighter. (Courtesy of R. Amprino.)

for many other vital functions. Homeostatic mechanisms have evolved to keep the plasma calcium concentration remarkably constant, in the range of 9–11 mg/100 ml.

The simplest and most rapid mechanism for mobilization of calcium is simple diffusion of calcium ions from the hydrated shell around the hydroxyapatite crystals of bone to the interstitial fluid, and then to the blood. This is adequate to maintain a low calcium level in the plasma (7 mg/100 ml). The most labile calcium is in the recently formed and incompletely mineralized osteons. The continual remodeling of adult bone ensures that there is always a pool of young osteons that can respond to homeostatic demands for calcium.

Another important mechanism for maintaining calcium levels involves the absorption of bone by osteoclasts. The cells of the parathyroid gland are sensitive to changes in blood calcium level. When it falls significantly, they increase their release of **parathyroid hormone** which acts upon osteoblasts to suppress their deposition of bone and to induce their secretion of the **osteoclast-stimulating factor.** The activated osteoclasts then resorb bone-liberating calcium to restore the normal blood level. The parathyroid hormone also acts upon the kidney to increase the rate of resorption of calcium from the glomerular filtrate. This renal effect of the hormone prevents a continual loss of calcium in the urine that would ultimately deplete the calcium stores in the bones.

The peptide hormone **calcitonin,** secreted by the parafollicular cells of the thyroid, has an effect opposite to that of parathyroid hormone. A **rise** in plasma calcium concentration stimulates release of calcitonin, just as a **fall** in plasma calcium induces secretion of parathyroid hormone. The hormone acts directly on osteoclasts to inhibit bone resorption.

Effect of Hormones on Bone Growth

Several hormones have significant effects on skeletal growth and bone remodeling. A childhood deficiency of **somatotrophin,** the growth hormone of the pituitary, results in **dwarfism.** An excess of the hormone, prior to epiphyseal closure, results in **gigantism.** In adults, an excess of somatotrophin leads to **acromegaly,** characterized by unsightly thickenings of the bones of the face.

The gonadal hormones **estrogens** and **androgens** influence the time of fusion of the epiphyses. In precocious sexual development, skeletal maturation is accelerated and growth stunted. The decline of hormone secretion in the aging disturbs the balance between bone deposition and bone resorption resulting in fragile bones.

> *An influence of gonadal hormones on bone becomes clinically apparent after age 50. The normal balance between deposition and absorption is disturbed and there is a slow, progressive reduction in bone mass per unit volume. This occurs in both sexes but is accelerated in women after menopause and often leads to* **osteoporosis,** *in which the reduction in trabeculae and thinning of the cortex makes the bones fragile. Nearly a third of women who live to 80 will have had fractures of hips or compression of vertebrae. Administration of estrogens is thought to slow the process of bone resorption.*

Nutritional Effects

Normal growth of the skeleton is dependent on an adequate intake of protein, minerals, and essential vitamins in the diet. A gross deficiency of calcium leads to rarifaction of the bones and increased risk of fractures. A deficiency of **vitamin D** in children may lead to **rickets,** a condition in which there is a disorderly arrangement of the cartilage cells of the epiphyseal plate and of the incompletely calcified bone in the metaphysis. Such bones are deformed by weight-bearing, leading to bowlegs. **Vitamin** C is essential for collagen synthesis. A deficiency of this vitamin leads to retardation of growth and delayed healing of fractures.

JOINTS

Bones of the skeleton are joined together at articulations (joints) of two major types: **diarthroses,** in which there is movement between the bones, and **synarthroses,** in which little or no motion is permitted. The articulations at the hip and knee are typical diarthroses.

Diarthroses

In diarthroses, the apposed surfaces of the bones are covered by hyaline cartilage that lacks a perichondrium, and they are enclosed in a loose **joint capsule** that permits a wide range of movement. The capsule consists of an outer **fibrous layer** and an inner **synovial layer** which is more cellular (Figs. 7-18 and 7-19). In areas subject to stress, the synovial layer (**synovium**) rests directly on the fibrous layer. Elsewhere, it is separated from it by a layer of loose connective tissue containing numerous adipose cells. The fibrous layer is continuous with the periosteum of the two

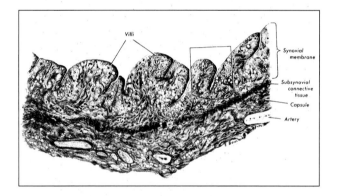

Fig. 7-18 Drawing of a section through the capsule of the knee joint, showing the synovial villi of varying size. The appearance of the area in the box, at higher magnification, is shown in Figure 7-19.

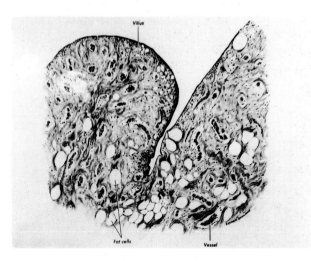

Fig. 7-19 Drawing of the synovium of the knee joint of a young adult. Note the concentration of cells near the free surface of the villus and the irregular distribution of adipose cells near the fibrous layer.

bones and may be thickened by ligaments that serve to maintain contact between the articulating surfaces.

The misleading term "synovial membrane" is often applied to the inner layer of the capsule although it does not have a continuous lining of adherent cells. Two types of cells, **type A** and **type B** are identifiable in it. The occurrence of cells of intermediate appearance suggests the possibility that these may be different functional phases of the same cell type. The type-A synovial cells are situated at, or near, the free surface and have surface filapodia and numerous micropinocytotic vesicles. Their cytoplasm contains many mitochondria and a prominent Golgi complex, but little endoplasmic reticulum. In some areas, there are gaps between these cells where the extracellular matrix is directly exposed to the fluid that fills the joint cavity. Elsewhere, they may be in contact and deeply interdigitated. The type-B cells are more deeply situated and resemble fibroblasts. Tubular and cisternal endoplasmic reticulum is abundant in their cytoplasm. Glycogen is present in a moderate amount in both synovial cell types. The **synovial fluid,** in the joint cavity, is a transudate of blood plasma to which the synovial cells add **hyaluronate** and **lubricin,** which contribute to its viscoelastic and lubricating properties. Histochemical studies indicate that type-A cells are probably the site of synthesis of these compounds.

Synarthroses

Three types of synarthrosis are distinguished according to the nature of the tissue joining the bones: **synostosis, synchondrosis,** and **syndesmosis.** The sutures between bones of the skull are about the only examples of synostoses. There, the interdigitating surfaces of the two bones are covered by periosteum with their collagen fibers intermingling to form the **sutural ligament.** After appositional growth at the sutures ends, bone matrix is gradually deposited in the sutural ligament and the bones become continuous. A **syndesmosis** is an articulation in which closely applied bones are joined by an interosseous ligament, a layer of connective tissue that permits a very small amount of movement. In a **synchondrosis,** such as the pubic symphysis, the bones are united by a disk of fibrocartilage.

QUESTIONS*

1. Concerning bone, all of the following are true **except**

   A. it is constantly renewed
   B. it is responsive to endocrine and nutritional factors
   C. it is avascular
   D. it may develop from mesenchyme
   E. it may grow by appositional growth

2. Canaliculi are found in

   A. articular cartilage
   B. perichondrium
   C. compact bone
   D. bone marrow
   E. none of the above

3. Concerning Volkmann's canals, which one, if any, of the following statements is correct?

   A. connect osteocytes
   B. are absent from long bones
   C. contain blood vessels and nerves
   D. are created by calcium deficiency
   E. none of the above

4. Concerning outer circumferential lamellae which one, if any, of the following statements is correct?

   A. are formed by the periosteum
   B. line the inner surface of long bones
   C. disappear during bone formation
   D. are typical of spongy bone
   E. none of the above

5. Concerning osteoclasts, all of the following statements are correct **except**

   A. can be considered to be specialized foreign-body giant cells
   B. derive from monocytes
   C. are typically found on the inner (closer to brain) side of the fetal cranium
   D. are restricted to immature bone
   E. create Howship's lacunae

6. Concerning canaliculi which one, if any, of the following statements is correct?

   A. connect lacunae in cartilage
   B. connect lacunae in bone
   C. contain nerve fibers
   D. contain blood vessels
   E. none of the above

7. Osteogenic tissue is found in

   A. bone marrow
   B. endosteum
   C. tendon
   D. hyaline cartilage
   E. none of the above

8. Which of the following are true about osteoblasts?

   A. reside in lacunae within the matrix
   B. are typically multinucleated
   C. are active in resorption of bone
   D. are part of the haversian systems
   E. are aligned along the surface of bone

9. Epiphyseal plates

   A. separate two epiphyses
   B. are easily observed in bones of children
   C. are composed of spongy bone
   D. contain Volkmann's canals
   E. separate two diaphyses

10. As bone grows

    A. it changes its external form
    B. haversian systems remain unaltered
    C. continual deposition and resorption of matrix is involved
    D. the periosteum plays an active dual role
    E. the epiphyses play essentially no rule

*Answers on page 307.

8

HEMOPOIESIS

CHAPTER OUTLINE

Bone Marrow
Hemopoiesis
    Hemopoietic Stem Cells
    Erythropoiesis
    Granulocytopoiesis
    Monocytopoiesis
    Thrombocytopoiesis
    Lymphopoiesis
Histophysiology of Bone Marrow

KEY WORDS

Basophilic	Monocyte
Colony Forming Unit	Myeloblast
(CFU)	Myelocyte
Diapedesis	Normoblast
Endomitosis	Orthochromatic
Erythroblast	Phagocytin
Erythrocyte	Platelet
Erythropoietin	Polychromatophilic
Granulocyte	Proerythroblast
Hemoglobin	Prolymphocyte
Hepatic Phase	Promyelocyte
Lymphoblast	Promonocyte
Lymphocyte: T, B	Red Marrow
Megakaryocyte	Reticulocyte
Mesoblastic phase	Stem Cell
Metamyelocyte	Thromboplastid
Monoblast	Yellow Marrow

Blood cells are short-lived, having life spans ranging from a few days to several weeks, and they must be continually replaced by new cells formed in the generative process called **hemopoiesis.** The numbers produced are astonishing. In the adult human, approximately 10^{10} red blood cells (erythrocytes) and 4×10^8 white blood cells (leukocytes) are produced per day. The principal site of hemopoiesis in the adult is the **bone marrow,** which occupies the medullary cavities of long bones and interstices in the spongiosa of vertebrae, ribs, and sternum.

Early in prenatal life when the skeleton is entirely cartilaginous, there are no marrow cavities and the earliest blood cell production, the **mesoblastic phase** of hemopoiesis, occurs in small islands of cells in the yolk sac and body stalk of the embryo. At about 6 weeks of gestation, round basophilic precursors of erythrocytes can be found in the primordium of the liver, initiating the **hepatic phase** of hemopoiesis. Later in gestation, after medullary cavities develop in the long bones, blood formation is initiated there, establishing the **myeloid phase** of hemopoiesis which continues throughout adult life.

BONE MARROW

Bone marrow occurs in two forms: **red marrow,** which is active in hemopoiesis, and **yellow marrow,** which is inactive and consists mainly of adipose cells which give it its yellow color. At birth, red marrow is found throughout the skeleton, but after age 6, it is gradually replaced by yellow marrow in many of the bones. By age 20, red marrow persists only in the vertebrae, ribs, pelvis, and the proximal ends of the humerus and femur. There is some evidence that yellow marrow can revert to red marrow in response to unusual demands for blood cells.

Active red marrow is a soft, highly cellular tissue consisting of the precursors of the blood cells supported by a stroma of reticular cells and associated reticular fibers. It is

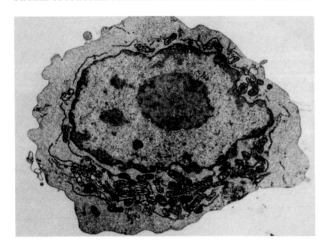

Fig. 8-1 Electron micrograph of a member of the pool of stem cells, showing its euchromatic nucleus, large nucleolus, and numerous mitochondria.

permeated by a network of venous sinusoids 50–70 µm in diameter, lined by a fenestrated endothelium with a discontinuous basal lamina. Closely packed blood-forming cells occupy the interstices of a loose meshwork of reticular cells that are joined at the ends of their broad thin processes. The reticular cells synthesize the collagen of the stromal reticular fibers. They, as well as the macrophages of the marrow, are believed to release cytokines, called **colony-stimulating factors,** which promote proliferation and differentiation of the blood cell precursors.

HEMOPOIESIS

Hemopoietic Stem Cells

Blood cell formation depends on the existence of **hemopoietic stem cells** in the marrow (Fig. 8.1). The proliferation of these pluripotential cells and the differentiation of their progeny generate all of the types of blood cells. They make up a very small fraction of the total population of nucleated cells in the marrow. According to the best estimates, they represent between 1 in 10,000 and 1 in 100,000 bone marrow cells. At any one time, the majority of them are dormant, but they are capable of resuming division in response to demands for new blood cells of any type. Stem cells that are cycling may either undergo **self-renewing divisions** to maintain the pool of pluripotential stem cells, or they may undergo **differentiating divisions** that give rise to cells that proliferate and differentiate into **progenitor cells** of four kinds (Fig. 8-2, above dashed line). These are all similar in appearance. They all have a euchromatic nucleus, a prominent nucleolus and varying amounts of intensely basophilic cytoplasm.

Much of our knowledge of the kinds of progenitor cells and their developmental potentialities has come from animal experiments that took advantage of the fact that the spleen provides an environment sufficiently similar to that of the bone marrow to permit hemopoiesis. A suspension of mouse hemopoietic cells is injected into a syngeneic mouse that has been subjected to X-irradiation sufficient to prevent proliferation of its own cells. The injected cells home individually into different sites in the spleen. There, they proliferate and differentiate. After a few days, grossly visible cell colonies have formed. The cell types in a colony are then examined. If all cell lineages are represented in the colony, the single cell of origin was a **pluripotential hemopoietic stem cell.** If only developmental stages of neutrophils and monocytes are present, the cell of origin was a bipotential progenitor cell which has been designated the **colony-forming unit granulocyte–monocyte (CFU-GM).** On the other hand, if the colony contains only stages in the development of erythrocytes, the precursor cell was a **colony-forming unit erythrocyte (CFU-E),** and so on for the three other lineage-specific precursor cells. Thus, the

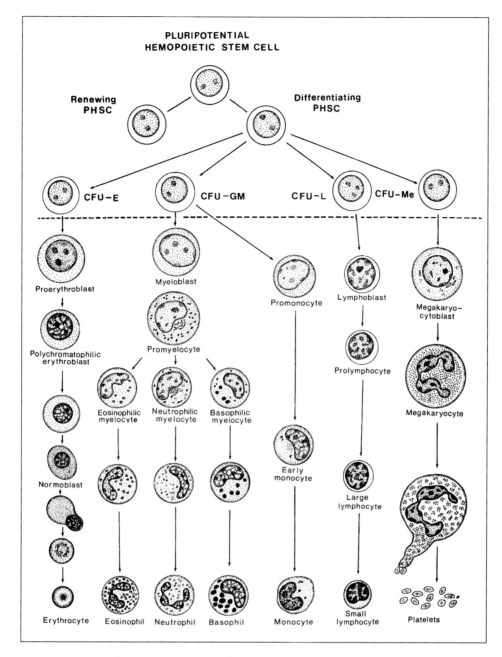

Fig. 8-2 Drawing of various stages in the differentiation of the blood cell types from the pluripotential hemopoietic stem cell of the marrow. The stem cell types above the dashed line are not readily identifiable with the light or electron microscope. Those below the line can be distinguished in bone marrow preparations.

spleen assay method is the basis for the widely used terminology for the several kinds of committed precursor cells: **CFU-E,** giving rise to erythrocytes; **CFU-GM,** forming monocytes and granulocytes; **CFU-L,** forming lymphocytes; and **CFU-Me,** developing into megakaryocytes (Fig. 8-2). These progenitor cells are not morphologically distinguishable, but in their further differentiation, each progresses through a series of intermediate stages that are morphologically identifiable. The appearance of some of these stages in bone marrow smears is illustrated in Figures 8-3 and 8-4 [see Plates 9 & 10]. The identifying charac-

teristics of the intermediate stages for each cell lineage will be described below.

Erythropoiesis

In the early embryo, the erythrocytes develop from precursors in the yolk sac, and they retain their nucleus (Fig. 8-4 [see Plate 10]). In postnatal life, they develop in the bone marrow from committed precursors called **erythroblasts** that undergo several divisions and their daughter

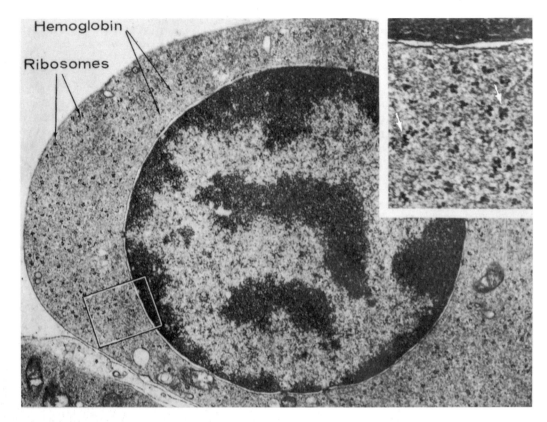

Hemoglobin

Ribosomes

Fig. 8-6 Electron micrograph of a late polychromatophilic erythroblast from guinea pig bone marrow, showing the coarse blocks of heterochromatin in the nucleus and a cytoplasm consisting mainly of hemoglobin and persisting polyribosomes. In the inset, at higher magnification, polyribosomes (at arrows) can be distinguished from the smaller, less-dense particles of hemoglobin.

cells differentiate further and synthesize the oxygen-carrying protein **hemoglobin.** Before entering the blood, the immediate precursors of the erythrocytes expel their nucleus and organelles and are reduced to membrane-limited corpuscles containing hemoglobin in solution.

The first recognizable stage of the erythrocyte lineage, in the bone marrow, is the **proerythroblast.** It is a round cell up to 16 μm in diameter, with a rim of moderately basophilic cytoplasm around a large nucleus containing two or three nucleoli. This stage undergoes several divisions and its progeny, called **basophilic erythroblasts,** are slightly smaller and have an intensely basophilic cytoplasm around a slightly more heterochromatic nucleus (Figs. 8-5A and 8-5B [see Plate 10]. In electron micrographs, polyribosomes are abundant in its cytoplasm and a few less-dense particles of hemoglobin can be resolved. The hemoglobin particles greatly increase in the next stage of differentiation, called the **polychromatophilic erythroblast** (Figs. 8-4 [see Plate 10] and 8-6). It is a still smaller cell, easily identified by its intensely stained heterochromatic nucleus that lacks a nucleolus and by the color of the cytoplasm, which ranges from blue-gray to olive green. With a further increase in hemoglobin and a relative decrease in number of polyribosomes, the cell becomes an **orthochromatic erythroblast,** with pinker cytoplasm. Chromatin condensation has progressed further and the

nucleus is considerably smaller. This cell type is also commonly called a **normoblast.** Toward the end of this stage, the cell extrudes its nucleus, with a thin coating of adherent cytoplasm (Figs. 8-5 and 8-7 [see Plate 11]). The remainder of the cell then assumes the biconcave discoid shape of an erythrocyte. It has a slightly blue tint due to the persistence of the small numbers of polyribosomes in its cytoplasm. If stained with the dye, Brilliant Cresyl

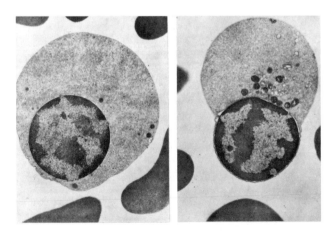

Fig. 8-8 Electron micrographs of human orthochromatic erythroblasts (normoblasts). The cell at the right is in the process of extruding its nucleus.

Blue, the remaining polyribosomes aggregate into a loose blue-staining network in an otherwise acidophilic cytoplasm. Such immature erythrocytes are commonly called **reticulocytes.** The last of the polyribosomes are ultimately eliminated by intracellular digestion and the cells are then mature **erythrocytes.** These traverse the wall of the marrow sinuses by diapedesis and enter the circulation.

---

*Anemia is the term applied to any significant reduction in erythrocyte numbers or their content of hemoglobin that results in reduced oxygen-carrying capacity. In **pernicious anemia,** certain cells in the gastric mucosa fail to secrete a sufficient intrinsic factor, a protein necessary for absorption of vitamin B₁₂. Deficiency of this vitamin results in inadequate production of erythrocytes. Iron is also necessary for hemoglobin synthesis. Deficiency of iron in the diet may result in **iron-deficiency anemia.** In an inherited disease, **sickle cell anemia,** a molecular abnormality of the hemoglobin, results in its crystalization and deformation of erythrocytes to a crescentic form in low-oxygen tensions.*

Granulocytopoiesis

Among the several progenitor cell types, the bipotential colony-forming unit granulocyte–monocyte (CFU-GM) gives rise either to granulocytes or to monocytes (Fig. 8-2). The first morphologically identifiable precursor of the neutrophil lineage is the **myeloblast,** a round cell about 16 μm in diameter, with a large euchromatic nucleus containing three or more nucleoli. The cytoplasm is moderately basophilic and devoid of granules. Division of the myeloblast produces daughter cells, called **promyelocytes,** that attain a larger size. These are the largest cells of this lineage (20 μm). The nucleus is still euchromatic, and the cytoplasm is basophilic. Electron micrographs reveal a few mitochondria, numerous azurophilic granules, and scattered profiles of rough endoplasmic reticulum (Figs. 8-8 and 8-4 [see Plate 10]). The progeny of the promyelocytes differentiate into **myelocytes** that are considerably smaller. Their chromatin is more condensed and azurophilic granules are more numerous (Fig. 8-4 [see Plate 10]). It has been the traditional view that promyelocytes give rise to myelocytes of three kinds destined to develop into neutrophils, eosinophils, or basophils. Many hematologists now believe that eosinophils and basophils arise from

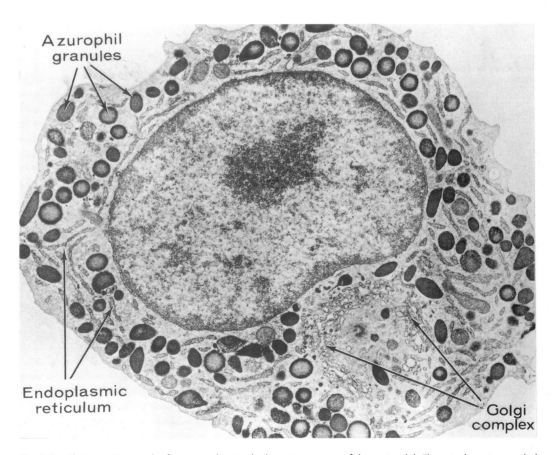

Fig. 8-9 Electron micrograph of a promyelocyte, the largest precursor of the neutrophil. The cytoplasm is crowded with peroxidase-positive azurophil granules, and a positive reaction is evident in the endoplasmic reticulum. The specific granules have not yet formed. (Reprinted with permission from D. Bainton, J. Ullyot, and M. Farquhar, Journal of Experimental Medicine 134:907, 1971.)

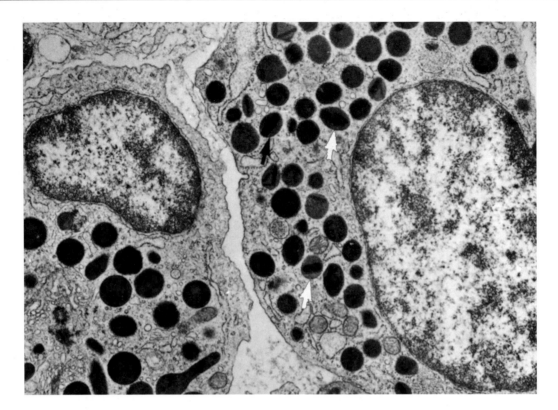

Fig. 8-10   Electron micrograph of a pair of late eosinophilic myelocytes from rat bone marrow. Endoplasmic reticulum is less extensive and crystals are forming in the specific granules (arrows) but are difficult to see due to the density of the surrounding matrix.

precursor cells distinct from those of neutrophils, but students need not be concerned with these conflicting interpretations. In clinical medicine, one only relies on stages beyond the promyelocyte that can be distinguished in marrow and blood smears.

From stem cell to the early myelocyte stage, the precursors of neutrophils, eosinophils, and basophils are difficult to distinguish in marrow smears. Their separate paths of differentiation are first detectable with the appearance of their specific granules. The earliest identifiable stage of the neutrophil lineage, the **neutrophilic metamyelocyte,** has a deeply indented nucleus and a cytoplasm containing both azurophilic and specific granules. The latter stain very faintly in blood smears. In electron micrographs, they are less dense than the azurophilic granules and are often elongate in shape. The azurophilic granules are lysosomes containing peroxidase, acid phosphatase, esterase, ß-glucuronidase, and 5-nucleotidase. The specific granules contain alkaline phosphatase, collagenase, lysozyme, and basic proteins collectively called **phagocytins.** In subsequent maturation of the metamyelocyte, the specific granules increase in number, and the nucleus becomes slender and elongated. Because of the shape of its nucleus, such cells are often referred to as **band-forms.** In the mature **polymorphonuclear neutrophil,** the elongated nucleus is constricted in several

places along its length, resulting in multiple nuclear lobules joined by very slender segments (Fig. 8-4 [see Plate 10]).

The specific granules of **eosinophil myelocytes** are larger than those of neutrophils, and in rodents, they contain a crystal (Figs. 8-4 [see Plate 10] and 8-10). The nucleus is indented in the metamyelocyte and bilobed in mature **eosinophils,** but it never attains the degree of lobulation seen in neutrophils. **Basophilic myelocytes** are rarely seen in marrow preparations because of their small numbers and the difficulty of preserving their granules. In mature **basophils,** the nucleus is deeply indented or bilobed, and the cytoplasm contains a relatively small number of large, intensely basophilic specific granules.

The transit time from stem cell to mature neutrophil, eosinophil, or basophil is about 18 days, and it is estimated that the rate of production of granulocytes of all types is about 1.6×10^4/kg/day, of which the great majority are neutrophils. A large reserve of neutrophilic band-forms and mature neutrophils is retained in the marrow, perhaps as many as 10 times the daily production. These can be mobilized quickly in case of infection anywhere in the body. After leaving the marrow, some neutrophils do not immediately circulate but adhere for several hours to the endothelium of small vessels. These are termed the **marginated pool** of neutrophils. These are very rapidly mobilized if needed. Those circulating in the blood are predominantly mature neutrophils, but during an infection, many band-forms are also released into the blood. After circulating for about 15 h, neutrophils migrate into the connective tissues where they spend the last 4 or 5 days of their short life span.

*Leukemia is a form of cancer due to malignant transformation of the hemopoietic precursors of the leukocytes. Leukemias are classified as **lymphocytic leukemia** or **myelogenous leukemia** according to whether lymphocytes or granulocytes are principally involved. These diseases may occur in an acute form leading to death within a matter of months, or in a more chronic form with a slower course.*

Monocytopoiesis

Monocytes develop from the bipotential progenitor CFU-GM. The first morphologically recognizable precursor is the **monoblast,** a large basophilic cell devoid of specific granules. Its division gives rise to somewhat smaller **promonocytes.** Some of these proliferate rapidly and produce numerous **monocytes** that enter the circulation as rapidly as they are produced. Other promonocytes form a reserve of more slowly proliferating precursors that remain in the marrow. Their proliferation can be accelerated to meet an increased need for circulating monocytes. The transit time from stem cell to monocyte is about 55 h. Monocytes probably remain in the circulation no more than 36 h before migrating into the tissues, where they increase in size, acquire many lysosomes, and become actively phagocytic **macrophages.** The life span of macrophages may be as long as several months.

Thrombocytopoiesis

The blood of all vertebrates contains cellular elements that promote blood clotting to prevent excessive blood loss from injured blood vessels. In lower vertebrates, these are nucleated cells called **thrombocytes.** In mammals, the functional equivalent of thrombocytes are the **blood platelets (thromboplastids).** These small, anucleate, membrane-limited bits of cytoplasm are cast off by large polymorphonuclear cells called **megakaryocytes** situated near the sinuses in the bone marrow. These originate from a unipotential progenitor, **colony-forming unit megakaryocyte** (CFU-Me). The first morphologically identifiable precursor is the **megakaryocytoblast,** a large cell, ranging from 15 to 50 µm in diameter, with a reniform nucleus containing multiple inconspicuous nucleoli. The cytoplasm is basophilic and devoid of specific granules. In the course of its further differentiation,

the CFU-Me undergoes multiple nuclear divisions without cytoplasmic division, a process called **endomitosis.** Thus, they become giant polyploid cells containing 8–32 sets of chromosomes. The megakaryocytes are the largest cells of the marrow, measuring 50–100 µm in diameter (Fig. 8-11). They are roughly spherical and have a remarkably pleiomorphic nucleus with multiple lobes connected by narrower segments. The early megakaryocyte contains many small, round azurophilic granules uniformly distributed in the central cytoplasm. In mature megakaryocytes, these granules are found throughout the cytoplasm, but they are now clustered in small groups, separated by aisles of granule-free cytoplasm. In electron micrographs, pairs of membranes, separated by a narrow space, are oriented in intersecting planes, partitioning the cytoplasm into units 1–3 µm in diameter, each containing a cluster of azurophilic granules (Figs. 8-11 and 8-12). The pairs of membranes surrounding the units are formed as invaginations of the cell membrane that elongate and penetrate deep into the cytoplasm where they ramify to form a labyrinthine system of so-called **platelet demarcation channels** (Fig. 8-12). Large cell processes called **proplatelets** are extended by mature megakaryocytes into the lumen of a neighboring sinusoid. These may contain as many as 1000 platelet subunits. Fragmentation of these processes along the platelet demarcation channels releases membrane-bounded individual **platelets** into the bloodstream. A megakaryocyte may be able to release as many as 8000 platelets before it degenerates and is replaced.

*Thrombocytopenia is a term applied to any disorder in which there is a deficiency in the number of circulating platelets. **Thrombocytopenic purpura** is a chronic autoimmune disease in which antibodies bind to platelets and interfere with their function. Patients have multiple black-and-blue spots after minimal trauma, and prolonged bleeding from lacerations.*

Lymphopoiesis

As stated in the chapter on blood, the lymphocytes are not a single cell type, but a family of morphologically similar cells that can only be distinguished by immunocytochemical detection of specific marker molecules on their surface. The stem cells of the bone marrow give rise to unipotential lymphocyte precursors, CFU-L that give rise to **lymphoblasts.** The daughter cells of the two or three lymphoblast divisions, called **prolymphocytes,** are smaller cells with condensed chromatin and a basophilic cytoplasm containing a few azurophilic granules. At this stage,

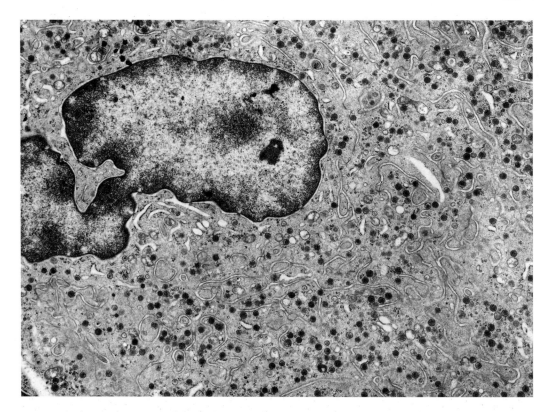

Fig. 8-11 Electron micrograph of a megakaryocyte from rat bone marrow. It is a very large, polyploid cell with a multilobulate nucleus. The small granules seen throughout the cytoplasm are the azurophilic granules of future platelets.

they do not yet have any of the surface markers of T or B lymphocytes. Some prolymphocytes remain in the marrow and proliferate there, producing lymphocytes throughout fetal and postnatal life. Prolymphocytes make up about 30% of the nucleated cells of the marrow. However, a great number of prolymphocytes enter the circulation and their further differentiation into B lymphocytes takes place in the spleen, lymph nodes, and lymphoid nodules of the gastointestinal tract.

Lymphoblasts and prolymphocytes destined to become T lymphocytes are carried in the blood to the cortex of the thymus. There, they proliferate and differentiate as they move through the cortex toward the medulla. In the course of this differentiation, they acquire the surface markers characteristic of the subsets of T lymphocytes. We will return to this subject in the chapter on the immune system and lymphoid organs.

HISTOPHYSIOLOGY OF BONE MARROW

The life-sustaining function of the erythrocytes is the transport of oxygen from the lungs to the other tissues and organs. The rate of their production is regulated, in part, by **erythropoietin,** a glycoprotein hormone produced by certain cells in the kidney. These cells are sen-

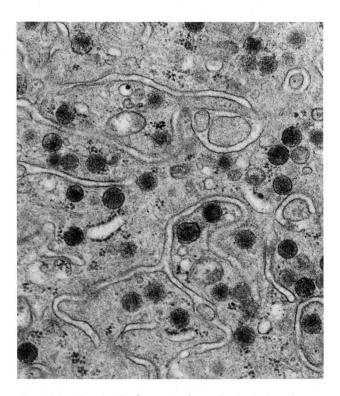

Fig. 8-12 Micrograph of an area of megakaryocyte cytoplasm at higher magnification, showing the platelet demarcation channels outlining future platelets.

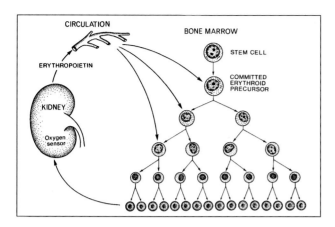

Fig. 8-13 Diagram of the mechanism for control of erythropoiesis. Hypoxia, due to reduced numbers of erythryocytes, is detected by a sensor in the kidney that secretes erythropoietin, which acts upon committed precursors of erythrocytes in the marrow, inducing their proliferation and differentiation.

sitive to deficient oxygen saturation of the blood (hypoxia), whether this is due to anemia or high altitude. They respond by releasing erythropoietin into the circulation. Reaching the marrow, it binds to specific receptors on committed erythroid precursors, stimulating erythropoiesis. The production of erythropoietin is increased or decreased in direct proportion to the degree of hypoxia (Fig. 8-13).

The production and release of granulocytes from the marrow normally occurs at a replacement rate. However, the rate of neutrophil release from reserves in the marrow is influenced by **interleukin-1** and **interleukin-3,** cytokines liberated by cells at sites of inflammation and carried in the blood to the bone marrow.

QUESTIONS*

1. Platelets arise

   A. as cytoplasmic separations from megakary-ocytes
   B. by differentiation of a stem cell plateletoblast
   C. as noncellular aggregations of blood-borne precursor substances
   D. by budding from monocytes
   E. as granules extruded from neutrophils

2. As cells undergo hemopoiesis,

   A. the nucleus decreases in size
   B. the nucleocytoplasmic ratio increases
   C. the cell enlarges
   D. the nucleoli become more prominent
   E. the chromatin becomes finer and more disperse

3. You would expect a 4-month old conceptus to have

   A. an established bone marrow with ongoing hemopoiesis
   B. multiple circulating plasma cells
   C. nucleated erythrocytes
   D. multiple circulating myelocytes
   E. multiple circulating megakaryocytes

4. Azurophilic granules in the granulocytic lineage of cells

   A. are related to phagocytosis
   B. contain peroxidase
   C. contain hemoglobin particles
   D. are lysosomes
   E. are directly related to blood clot promotion

5. All of the following about bone marrow are true **except** one statement. Which one?

   A. Bone marrow occurs in two forms.
   B. It is composed primarily of haversian systems.
   C. It may contain variable amounts of adipose cells.
   D. It is an active part of hemopoiesis.
   E. It is found throughout the skeleton in newborns.

6. Reticulocytes

   A. typically exhibit a dense compact nucleus
   B. have a basophilic cytoplasm
   C. arise from immature monocytes
   D. exhibit dense cytoplasmic granulation
   E. contain polyribosomes in aggregations

7. Thromboplastids

   A. are a type of granulocyte
   B. are actively involved in phagocytosis
   C. are plasma-limited bits of cytoplasm
   D. derive from proerythroblasts
   E. are part of the lymphopoietic cell line

8. All of the following statements are true about the erythrocytic cell line **except** one. Identify the false statement.

   A. They contain numerous fine cytoplasmic granules.
   B. They are produced under control by erythropoietin.
   C. The cells change their cytoplasmic staining characteristics as they mature.
   D. They arise from primordial cells in the fetal liver.
   E. They are actively involved in oxygen transport.

9. Granulopoiesis

   A. give rise to monocytes as well as granulocytes
   B. results in mature red blood cells
   C. is produces blood platelets
   D. when stimulated, produces enormous numbers of proerythroblasts
   E. is not influenced by cytokines

10. Concerning blood cell formation, all of the following are true **except**

   A. Formation is stem cell dependent.
   B. most stem cells are dormant at any one time.
   C. stem cells are euchromatic with basophilic cytoplasm.
   D. stem cells are the major component of cells in marrow.
   E. stem cells can divide.

*Answers on page 307.

9

MUSCLE

CHAPTER OUTLINE

KEY WORDS

A-Band	Myofibril
Actin, G-, F-	Myofilament
Anisotropic	Myoglobin
Atrium	Myoneural Junction
Atrioventricular Node	Myosin
Calmodulin	Pacemaker
Calsequestrin	Perimysium
Cardiodilatin	Purkinje Fiber
Corbular Reticulum	Sarcolemma
Dyad	Sarcomere
Dystrophin	Sarcoplasm
Endomysium	Sinoatrial Node
Epimysium	Smooth Muscle
Fields of Cohnheim	Striated Muscle
H-Band	T-tubule
I-Band	Terminal Cisterna
Internodal	Titin
Isotropic	Triad
Lipochrome	Troponin
M-Band	Tropomyosin
Motor End-Plate	Ventricle
Motor Unit	Z-Line
Myocyte	Zeugmatin
Myoendocrine Cell	

Contractility is a property exhibited, in varying degree, by nearly all cells. In muscle, this ability to convert chemical energy into mechanical work has become highly developed. The locomotion of animals, the beating of their hearts, and the movements of the stomach and intestine depend on three types of muscle, each specialized for the kind of force required. The types of muscle are **smooth muscle, skeletal muscle,** and **cardiac muscle.** The contraction of smooth muscle is slow and is not subject to voluntary control. Contraction of skeletal muscle is rapid and under voluntary control. Contraction of cardiac muscle is forceful, rhythmic, and involuntary. The smooth muscle that generates movement in the viscera is controlled by the autonomic nervous system. Skeletal muscle is activated by nerves of the cerebrospinal system. Cardiac muscle is endowed with an intrinsic mechanism for generating rhythmic contractions but receives additional input from the cerebrospinal nervous system that influences the frequency of heartbeat.

SMOOTH MUSCLE

Microscopic Structure

Smooth muscle forms a major portion of the wall of the alimentary tract, from the middle of the esophagus to the sphincter of the anus. Smooth muscle provides the motive force for mixing the ingested food with digestive enzymes and for its propulsion through the tract. Circumferentially oriented smooth muscle also occurs in the walls of blood vessels and controls their caliber. It forms

the wall of the oviducts and uterus and is found in many other sites in the body.

Smooth muscle is made up of long fusiform (spindle-shaped) cells with an elongated nucleus situated in their wider central portion. They vary greatly in length, ranging from 20 µm in small blood vessels to 500 µm in the pregnant uterus. Where smooth muscle is organized in bundles or layers, the individual cells are offset so that their wide portions are adjacent to the thin tapering ends of neighboring cells. Therefore, in transverse sections, smooth muscle appears as a mosaic of polygonal profiles, varying from one to several microns in diameter, with a nucleus found only in the largest profiles (Figs. 9-1 and 9-2). The major cell organelles are confined to the conical regions of cytoplasm at the poles of the elongated nucleus. The rest of the cytoplasm generally appears rather homogeneous under the light microscope, but longitudinal bundles of the contractile components, called **myofilaments,** can be detected by their birefringence when examined with the polarizing microscope. Each smooth muscle cell is enveloped by a thin **external lamina,** resembling the basal lamina of epithelia. Outside of this, there is a network of reticular fibers that bind the cellular units together so that their contraction produces a coordinated force. Neighboring cells are in contact only at gap junctions, which provide the cell-to-cell communication necessary for integrated contraction throughout the layer of smooth muscle.

In electron micrographs, the juxtanuclear region of the smooth-muscle cell contains a small Golgi complex, a few long mitochondria, and short profiles of endoplasmic reticulum (Fig. 9-3). The peripheral cytoplasm, containing the contractile elements, appears rather homogeneous, and **myofilaments** are identifiable only at high magnification.

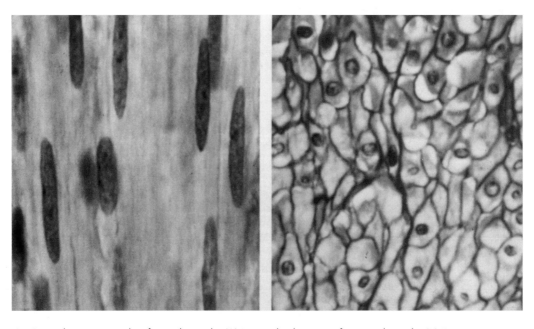

Fig. 9-1   Photomicrographs of smooth muscle. (A) Longitudinal section of intestinal muscle. (B) Transverse section stained with the periodic–Shiff reaction, which stains the lamina externa, accentuating the cell outline.

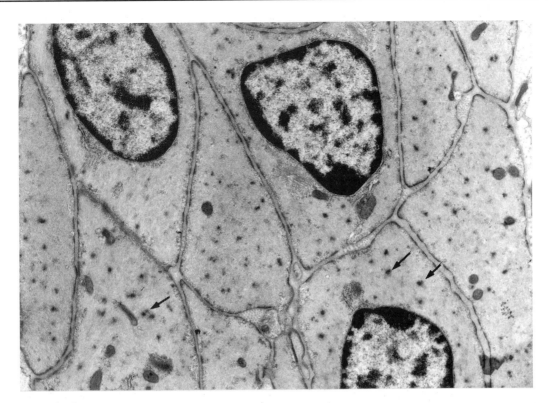

Fig. 9-2 Electron micrograph of smooth muscle in cross section. The cells are separated by intercellular spaces containing a delicate network of reticular fibers. Scattered through the cytoplasm are densities (arrows) that are sites of lateral bonding of actin filaments and filaments of the cytoskeleton. Densities at the cell periphery are sites of attachment of filaments to the cell membrane.

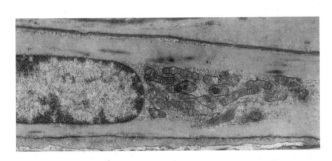

Fig. 9-3 Electron micrograph of a longitudinal section of a smooth-muscle cell. The organelles are concentrated in conical regions of cytoplasm extending from the poles of the elongate nucleus. The remainder of the cytoplasm is occupied by myofilaments that are not resolved at this magnification.

A cytoskeleton, consisting of a network of longitudinal and oblique bundles of 10-mm intermediate filaments can be demonstrated by using labeled antibodies to **desmin.**

At high magnification, parallel filaments of **actin,** 4.5 μm in length and 4–8 nm in diameter, form bundles oriented longitudinally or obliquely in the cytoplasm. Intermingling with the actin filaments of the bundles are **myosin** filaments 1.5 μm in length and 15 nm in diameter (Fig. 9-4). The ratio of actin filaments to myosin filaments is about 12 to 1. The filament bundles terminate in dense bodies located at nodal points of the cytoskeletal network or in subplasmalemmal dense plaques (Figs. 9-4 and 9-5).

The cytoplasmic dense bodies and the plaques contain the actin-binding protein α-actinin. The plaques also bind labeled antibodies against a second actin-binding protein, **vinculin.**

Histophysiology

Contraction of smooth muscle is relatively slow, but it can be sustained for long periods. The cells can shorten to one-quarter of their resting length and can generate a force, per cross-sectional area, comparable to that of striated muscle, while consuming far less energy. Contraction is believed to involve a sliding of the actin filaments with respect to the myosin filaments that results in a shortening of the filament bundles. However, a sliding mechanism of shortening is more difficult to validate in smooth muscle than in striated muscle. Myosin can interact with actin only if its light chain is phosphorylated. Smooth-muscle contraction is initiated by an influx of calcium which binds to a calcium-binding protein, **calmodulin.** The calcium–calmodulin complex binds to **myosin light-chain kinase,** activating this enzyme, which catalyzes the phosphorylation of myosin light chains, enabling them to interact with actin filaments and cause contraction.

Smooth muscle differs in its mode of activation in different organs. Intestinal smooth muscle, an example of

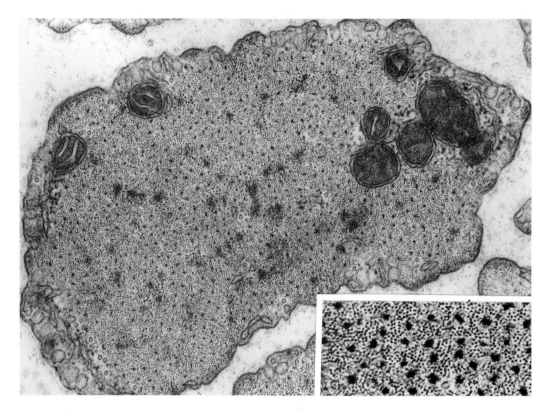

Fig. 9-4 Electron micrograph of a vascular smooth-muscle cell in cross section. Clearly visible are thick and thin filaments. These are shown at higher magnification in the inset. (Courtesy of A.P. Somlyo, E. Devine, and A.V. Somlyo, Vascular Smooth Muscle, Springer-Verlag, 1972.)

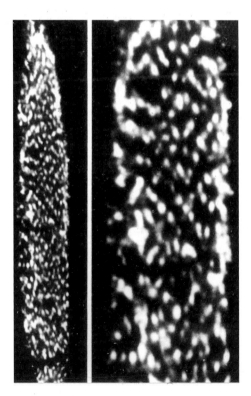

Fig. 9-5 Confocal images of contracted isolated smooth-muscle cells labeled with fluorescent antibody to the alpha actinin of the cytoplasmic dense bodies indicated by arrows in the previous figures. (Courtesy of A. Draeger, W.B. Amos, M. Ikebe and J.V. Small, Journal of Cell Biology 11, 2463, 1990).

unitary smooth muscle, has an autorhythmicity. Intrinsically generated stimuli are conducted, via gap junctions, throughout a large area of smooth muscle that contracts in unison, and waves of contraction (peristalsis) then sweep along the intestine to advance its contents. The type of smooth muscle in large arteries, in the ducts of the male reproductive tract, and in the ciliary body of the eye is designated **multiunit smooth muscle.** In muscle of this kind, there is little evidence of impulse conduction from fiber to fiber via gap junctions. Instead, each fiber is innervated, and contraction is more rapid than in unitary smooth muscle. Adrenergic and cholinergic nerves to smooth muscle of this type act antagonistically.

SKELETAL MUSCLE

Microscopic Structure

The units of organization of **skeletal,** or **striated, muscle,** are not individual cells, but are long, cylindrical, multinucleate syncytia, formed by fusion of multiple myoblasts during embryonic development. These so-called **muscle fibers,** 0.1 mm in diameter and several centimeters in length, are arranged in bundles (fasicles) large enough to be visible with the naked eye. The muscle, as a whole, is surrounded by a thin layer of dense connective tissue

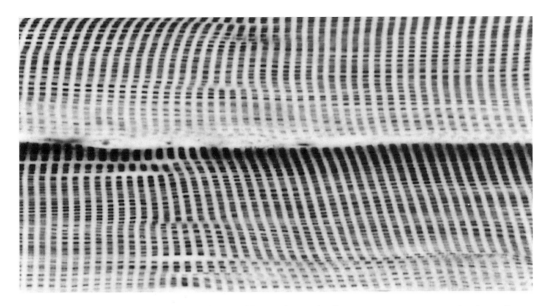

Fig. 9-6 Photomicrograph of two skeletal muscle fibers in longitudinal section. Preparation stained with iron hematoxylin to show the alternating dark A-bands and light I-bands.

forming the **epimysium.** Thin, branching connective tissue septa extend inward from the epimysium and envelop each of the fasicles of muscle fibers. These constitute the **perimysium.** A delicate network of reticular fibers around the individual muscle fibers is the **endomysium.** This delicate network binds the contractile units together but permits some motion between them.

The plasma membrane of skeletal and cardiac muscle fibers has traditionally been called the **sarcolemma,** and their cytoplasm is referred to as the **sarcoplasm.** The sarcolemma of each muscle fiber is coated with a thin amorphous layer, the **external lamina,** that resembles the basal lamina of epithelia but is thinner. The inner surface of the sarcolemma bears a thin layer of a 400-kDa protein, **dystrophin,** that is not found in other cells. It is believed to provide the membrane with an internal reinforcement against the stresses developed in muscle contraction, relaxation, and stretching, but it may have other functions yet to be discovered.

> *In the hereditary disease, **muscular dystrophy,** there is a defect in the gene for **dystrophin,** that normally coats the inside of the sarcolemma. Muscular weakness is evident by age 5, and by age 12 the patient is confined to a wheelchair. The disease is sex linked, affecting only males.*

Under the light microscope, muscle fibers have a closely spaced cross-striation which is the basis for the term "striated muscle," commonly used to distinguish skeletal and cardiac muscle from smooth muscle. Within each muscle fiber, the thousands of contractile **myofibrils,** are also cross-banded, with their bands normally in register (Fig. 9-6) and this accounts for the cross-striation of the fiber as a whole.

The column of myofibrils in the sarcoplasm occupies the greater part of the cross section of a muscle fiber, displacing its many nuclei to the periphery, where they are flattened against the sarcolemma (Fig. 9-7). Their long elliptical profiles are regularly spaced along the length of the fiber. Their exact number cannot be specified, but in a fiber several centimeters in length, they would number in the hundreds. Their peripheral location is helpful in distinguishing skeletal muscle from cardiac muscle, where the nuclei are located in the center of the fiber. All of the common organelles are present in the sarcoplasm. A small Golgi is associated with one pole of many of the nuclei. Long mitochondria are found in the juxtanuclear sarcoplasm and are also deployed in longitudinal rows between bundles of myofibrils, where they provide the energy for contraction. Lipid droplets are found in small numbers among the organelles at the poles of the nuclei, and glycogen particles are distributed throughout the sarcoplasm. In addition to these microscopically visible components, the sarcoplasm contains **myoglobin** in solution. This oxygen-binding protein is largely responsible for the brown color of muscle. Oxygen dissociates from myoglobin, as required, and becomes available for oxidative reactions.

In transverse sections of striated muscle, the myofibrils are resolved as fine dots, either uniformly distributed or aggregated in polygonal areas, that were formerly called the **fields of Cohnheim.** The bulk of the evidence now favors a uniform distribution of myofibrils in vivo and suggests that the fields of Cohnheim are an artifact of specimen preparation. In longitudinal sections, dark bands alternate with relatively light bands (Fig. 9-6). When viewed with the polarizing microscope, the dark bands are **anisotropic** and are therefore designated the **A-bands,** whereas the light bands are **isotropic** and are called

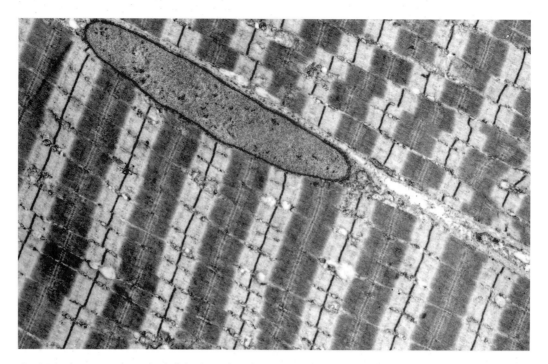

Fig. 9-7 Electron micrograph of skeletal muscle in longitudinal section. Note the uniform diameter of the myofibrils and the location of the nucleus immediately beneath the sarcolemma. The corresponding bands of the myofibrils are normally in register across the entire muscle fiber. At the upper right, where they are out of register, is a preparation artifact.

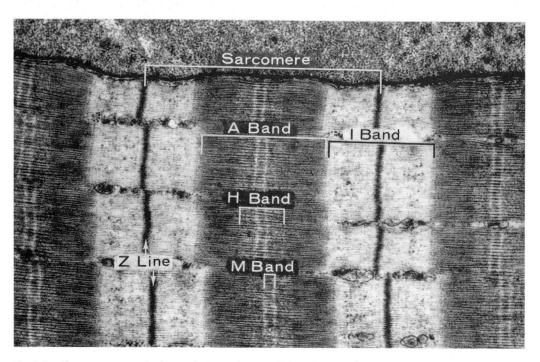

Fig. 9-8 Electron micrograph of several juxtanuclear myofibrils of skeletal muscle, labeled to identify the various bands in the pattern of cross-striations in relaxed muscle.

I-bands. The relative length of the bands depends on the state of contraction of the muscle. The I-bands are very short during contraction and longer in relaxation. The length of the A-bands remains constant in all phases of contraction. Each I-band is bisected by a narrow transverse line, the **Z-line,** or **Z-disk.** The segments between successive Z-lines are called the **sarcomeres,** and all morphological changes in the contractile cycle are described with reference to this subunit. Each sarcomere includes an A-band and half of the two contiguous I-bands. The A-bands, I-bands, and Z-disks are ordinarily the only cross-striations visible with the light microscope.

Ultrastructure of Myofibrils

The A-band, I-band and Z-disks are more clearly resolved in electron micrographs, and two additional bands can be made out: a paler-staining **H-band** in the middle of the A-band, with a thin **M-band**, or M-line traversing its center (Fig. 9-8). At high magnification, the myofibrils are seen to be made up of myofilaments of two kinds: thin **actin filaments** and thicker **myosin filaments** (Fig. 9-9). Myosin filaments are the major constituent of the A-band of the sarcomere. They are 1.5 μm in length and 15 nm in diameter and are arranged parallel, with a space of about 45 nm between them. They are held in lateral register by

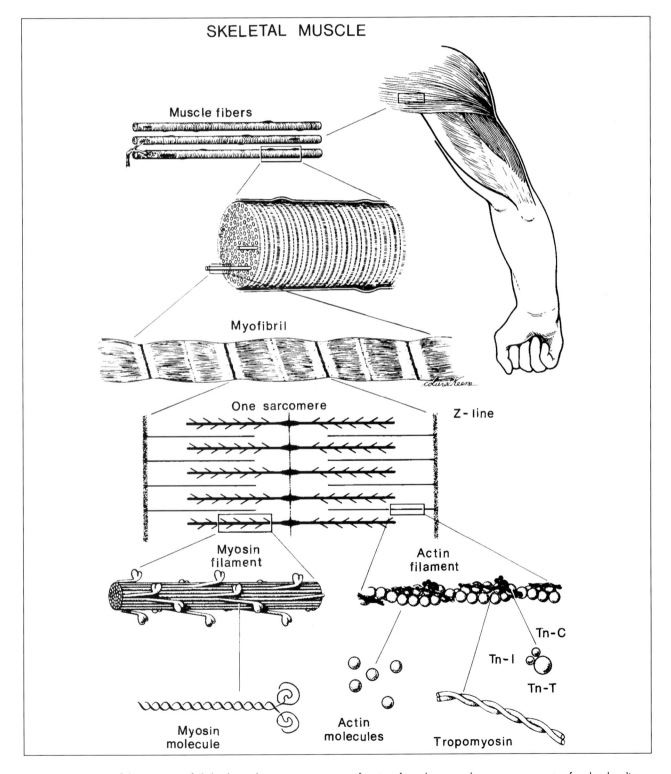

Fig. 9-9 Drawing of the structure of skeletal muscle at increasing magnifications from the gross down to components of molecular dimensions. The interdigitating myosin and actin filaments of one sarcomere are depicted diagramatically in the center of the figure. (Drawing by Sylvia Collard/Keene.)

slender cross-links located at the midpoint of the A-band. The transverse alignment of these links is responsible for the linear density identified as the M-line.

Actin filaments are the dominant component of the I-band, and they extend for a variable distance into the A-band, interdigitating with the myosin filaments. Therefore, in cross sections of myofibrils at the level of the I-band, only punctate profiles of actin filaments are seen, and in sections through the middle of the A-band, only the larger cross-sectional profiles of myosin filaments are found. However, in cross sections nearer the ends of the A-band where actin and myosin filaments interdigitate, both kinds of filaments are found, with cross sections of the thin actin filaments arranged in a hexagonal pattern around each myosin filament. In longitudinal sections, the space between interdigitating thick and thin filaments is traversed by regularly spaced **cross-bridges** that radiate from each myosin filament toward the surrounding actin filaments.

Information on the substructure of the thick filaments has been obtained by mechanical dissociation of isolated filaments. Each filament yields about 350 myosin molecules. These, in turn, consist of two polypeptide chains entwined to form the rodlike tail of the molecule. At one end, globular regions of the peptide chains form two diverging heads. The heads of the myosin molecules are the cross-bridges that project from the myosin filaments toward the actin filaments (Fig. 9-9). The actin-binding property of the heads of the myosin molecules is essential for muscle contraction. In forming the thick filaments, myosin molecules assemble in an overlapping antiparallel fashion with their rodlike tails toward the middle of the A-band. A central region of the band therefore consists only of the smooth rod segments of the molecules and is devoid of cross-bridges. These regions are in lateral register across the myofibril forming the H-band in the middle of the sarcomere (Fig. 9-9).

Isolated thin filaments have a beaded appearance at high magnification. They arise by polymerization of globular monomers of **G-actin,** 5.6 nm in diameter. The polymers, **F-actin,** form two helically entwined strands in which each gyre of the helix is about 36 nm in length. A consistent orientation of the actin subunits gives the thin filaments a definite polarity, and the actin filaments on either side of the Z-disk are of opposite polarity. Associated with the actin filaments are long molecules of **tropomyosin** arranged end-to-end in the grooves between the helically entwined F-actin chains. Bound to each molecule of tropomyosin is a complex of three **troponin** peptides designated **Tn-T, Tn-I,** and **Tn-C.** Tn-T binds the complex to tropomyosin, Tn-C has a binding site for the calcium that initiates contraction, and Tn-I inhibits the binding of the myosin heads to actin in the resting muscle. These submicroscopic components of the actin filaments have key roles in the mechanism of muscle contraction that will be discussed below.

A recently discovered muscle protein called **titin** is the largest protein known. It is a single chain of nearly 27,000 amino acids with a molecular weight of about 3 million. Its molecules are about 1 µm long and span the distance between the M-line and the Z-disk (Fig. 9-10). They are probably attached to the adjacent thick filaments. The elastic properties of the titin molecules are thought to be responsible for the ability of a muscle to spring back to resting length after being stretched.

The myofilaments of successive sarcomeres are linked end-to-end at the Z-disk, but just how is difficult to observe because of the density of the disk and the superimposition of its components. The actin filaments appear to end at the edge of the disk. There, each filament is attached to four diverging Z filaments which course obliquely across the disk to attach to four actin filaments of the next sarcomere. Filaments of one sarcomere are slightly offset with respect to those approaching the disk from the other side. Therefore, in longitudinal sections, the connecting Z filaments form a zigzag pattern across the myofibril. Much of the density of the Z-disk is attributable to α-actinin, the same actin-binding protein that is involved in end-to-end linkage of actin filaments in the cytoplasmic dense bodies of smooth muscle. Another protein, **zeugmatin,** is localized at the boundaries of the disk. Its exact role has yet to be discovered.

Mechanism of Contraction

Ultrastructural studies of the myofibrils have led to a widely accepted **sliding filament hypothesis** to explain striated-muscle contraction. In this hypothesis, it is assumed that, when a muscle contracts, the thick myosin filaments and the thin actin filaments maintain the same length as in the resting muscle, but the thin actin filaments slide more deeply into the A-bands, thus shortening the sarcomeres along the entire length of the myofibrils (Fig. 9-11). This accounts for the change in breadth of the H-band in different phases of the contractile cycle. Its width is defined as the distance between the ends of the actin filaments extending into the sarcomere

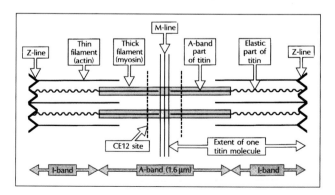

Fig. 9-10 Diagram illustrating the probable arrangement of titin molecules within the sarcomere. The elastic part of the molecule is shown only in the I-band. (From J. Trinick, Current Opinion in Cell Biology 8:112, 1991.)

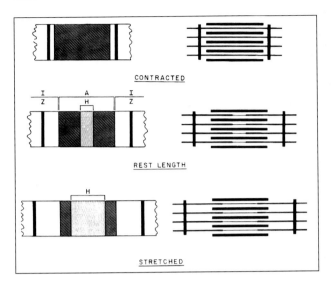

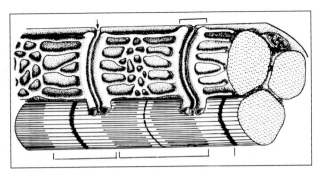

Fig. 9-12 Drawing of the sarcolemma and three subjacent myofibrils, illustrating the location of the triads of the reticulum at the A–I junctions with the longitudinal elements of the reticulum between successive triads. Also shown is the continuity of the membrane of the T-tubules with the sarcolemma.

Fig. 9-11 Diagram of the changing appearance of the cross-striations of skeletal muscle in different phases of contraction (at left) and (at right) the corresponding changes in the degree of interdigitation of the thick and thin filaments of the sarcomeres.

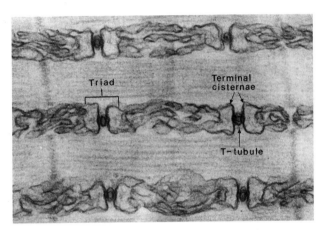

Fig. 9-13 Sarcoplasmic reticulum of a fish striated muscle. It is basically similar to that of mammals, with repeating transverse triads connected by longitudinal tubules of the reticulum. In the mammal, the triads are located at the junction of the A-bands with

from opposite ends. It is widest in resting muscle and becomes narrower in contracted muscle, due to the deeper penetration of the actin filaments into the A-band. Sliding of the filaments is initiated by an influx of calcium ions into the muscle fibers. Calcium storage and release to the myofibrils is the function of the **sarcoplasmic reticulum,** a specialization of endoplasmic reticulum unique to muscle.

The Sarcoplasmic Reticulum

Most of the organelles of muscle fibers do not differ significantly from those of other cells and need not be described again. The only exception is the sarcoplasmic reticulum, which corresponds to the endoplasmic reticulum of other cells but has acquired physiological properties not typical of that organelle. It is the site of sequestration of calcium during muscle relaxation and release of calcium into the sarcoplasm to trigger muscle contraction. It consists of a network of membrane-bounded tubules surrounding each myofibril, and it exhibits a repeating pattern related to specific regions of the sarcomeres. The tubules are largely devoid of associated polyribosomes. Their prevailing orientation is longitudinal, but there are lateral branches that form a closed-meshed network around the myofibril at the level of the H-band of each sarcomere. Over each junction of an A-band with an I-band, the longitudinal sarcotubules are confluent with a pair of parallel transverse tubules of larger caliber, called the **terminal cisternae.** Thus, along the myofibrils, two pairs of parallel terminal cisternae are associated with each sarcomere (Figs. 9-12 and 9-13). Between each pair of terminal cisternae there is a slender transverse tubule, commonly called the **T-tubule,** which is not an integral part of the sarcoplasmic reticulum but is a tubular invagi-

nation of the sarcolemma that extends inward from the surface of the fiber, crossing many myofibrils. Its membrane is continuous with the sarcolemma, where its lumen is open to the extracellular space. The two parallel terminal cisternae and the intervening T-tubule form a complex referred to as the **triad.** To distinguish the terminal cisternae from the longitudinal elements of the reticulum, they are often referred to as the **junctional reticulum.** The lumen of the terminal cisternae contains an amorphous material of low density consisting mainly of **calsequestrin,** a 55-kDa protein that can bind 300 nM of calcium per milligram and is believed to serve as a sequestering agent for the storage of calcium within the junctional reticulum. In that portion of the membrane of the terminal cisternae that adjoins the T-tubule there are clusters of intramembranous particles, each surrounding a calcium channel in the membrane. These particles are believed to contain the Ca^{2+}–Mg^{2+}-ATPase that is responsible for transport of Ca^{2+} from the sarcoplasm back into the lumen of the transverse tubules during the relaxation phase of the contractile cycle.

Histophysiology

Stimulation of muscle begins at the **myoneural junction** with the generation of an action potential that spreads over the sarcolemma and along the membrane of the T-tubules to the interior of the muscle fibers. This initiates events at the interface between the T-tubules and the terminal cisternae that result in the rapid release of the sequestered calcium ions into the sarcoplasm. In resting muscle, the binding sites for myosin on the thin filaments are blocked by the **tropomyosin–troponin complexes.** Release of calcium into the sarcoplasm is followed by its binding to troponin C of each unit along the actin filaments. This results in a conformational change in the complex that drives it deeper into the groove of the actin helix, exposing the myosin-binding sites. Binding to heads of the myosin molecules of the adjacent thick filaments then activates myosin ATPase. This, in turn, releases energy that induces flexion of the heads of the myosin molecules with a force sufficient to slide the neighboring actin filaments a short distance toward the middle of the A-band. The myosin heads then detach and reattach to the next set of binding sites on the actin filament for a new cycle of bridge making and bridge breaking (Fig. 9-14). Hundreds of such cycles take place to produce the observed displacement of the actin filaments. This continues until calcium is taken up and sequestered in the terminal cisternae of the sarcoplasmic reticulum and the tropomyosin–troponin complexes again cover the myosin-binding sites on the actin filaments, restoring the resting state of the muscle.

Innervation of Muscle

See also p. 113

Skeletal muscles are innervated by axons of nerve cells located in the spinal cord. At the muscle, the nerve divides into multiple branches that penetrate into its interior via the perimyseal septa. Individual axons then ramify in the endomyseum and form endings on a variable number of the muscle fibers (Figs. 9-15 [see Plate 12] and 9-16). A single motor neuron may innervate from 1 to over 100 muscle fibers. The axon and the muscle fibers it innervates constitute a **motor unit.** The activation of a single axon will result in a muscle tension proportional to the number of muscle fibers innervated by that axon. In the graded response which is possible in whole muscles, the strength of contraction depends on the number of motor units that are activated.

At its junction with a muscle fiber, an axon loses its myelin sheath and branches into several short axon terminals (terminal boutons) that occupy shallow depressions in the surface of the fiber. Together, these structures constitute a **motor end-plate** or **myoneural junction** (Fig. 9-16). The sarcolemma beneath the end-plate is infolded to form a number of **synaptic clefts** that serve to increase the area of sarcolemma exposed to neurotransmitter. The axoplasm of the nerve terminal contains a few mitochondria and a large number of 40–60nm synaptic vesicles that contain the neurotransmitter acetylcholine (Fig. 9-17). In impulse transmission, the content of these vesicles is released into the space between the axon terminals and the muscle fiber. **Acetylcholine** diffusing across the cleft reaches acetylcholine receptors in the sarcolemma. In freeze-fracture preparations viewed at very high magnification, these appear as clusters of five intramembrane particles around

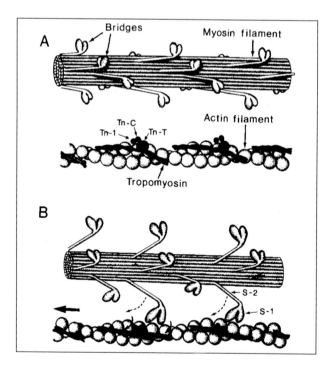

Fig. 9-14 (A) Schematic representation of the arrangement of filaments in a segment of a thick filament of skeletal muscle and the neighboring double helical actin filament with its associate tropomyosin and troponin complexes. (B) Calcium binding causes a change in configuration of the tropomyosin–troponin complexes, exposing myosin-binding sites on the actin filament. The myosin heads, energized by ATP, change their angle and move the actin filaments.

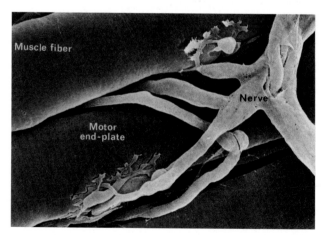

Fig. 9-16 Scanning electron micrograph of a motor nerve and two end-plates on adjacent muscle fibers. (Courtesy of J. Desaki and Y. Uehara, Journal of Neurocytology 10:101, 1981.)

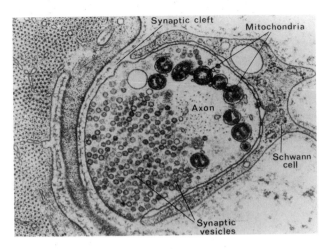

Fig. 9-17 Electron micrograph of a nerve ending on a muscle fiber (at left), showing an accumulation of mitochondria in the axoplasm and a large number of synaptic vesicles. (Courtesy of T. Reese.)

a central ion channel. Binding of acetylcholine to the receptors opens their channels transiently, permitting sodium ions to enter the sarcoplasm. Influx of sodium depolarizes the postsynaptic membrane, initiating an action potential that is propagated over the sarcolemma and into the T-tubules, activating the release of calcium that triggers muscle contractions.

> *Myasthenia gravis is an autoimmune disease characterized by muscular weakness and fatigability. For unknown reasons, antibodies are formed against the acetylcholine receptors in the postsynaptic membrane of the muscle fibers. Failure of transmission of the nerve impulse at many neuromuscular junctions results in weak contractions.*

Muscle Fiber Diversity

The fibers that make up a given muscle are not all identical. They vary in color, diameter, and in cytochemical and physiological properties. Traditionally, three types have been described: **red fibers, white fibers,** and **intermediate fibers.** The red fibers (**slow twitch fibers**) are smaller in diameter and have a dark color. The deeper color is attributable to their greater content of myoglobin and to the cytochromes in their unusually large and abundant mitochondria. Lipid droplets are common in their sarcoplasm and the Z-bands are wider than in the other fiber types. They are innervated by slender axons with relatively simple motor end-plates. Motor units consisting of red fibers contract relatively slowly but are more resistant to fatigue than other types because of their greater ability to regenerate ATP. These properties make muscles that are rich in red fibers well suited for postural maintenance.

White fibers (**fast twitch fibers**) are the largest of the fiber types. Their subsarcolemmal mitochondria are smaller than those of red fibers, and mitochondria between the myofibrils are relatively few. Their generation of ATP depends on anaerobic glycolysis of glucose derived from glycogen in their sarcoplasm. They are innervated by large axons that have motor end-plates about twice the size of those of red fibers. They contract rapidly and generate a large force, but they fatigue rapidly. They are best suited for brief bursts of intense muscle activity. As their name implies, the intermediate fibers have characteristics intermediate between the red and white fibers. The disposition of their mitochondria is similar to that of red fibers, except that thick interfibrillar columns of mitochondria are seldom found.

Histochemical reactions are often used to distinguish fiber types: ATPase, succinic dehydrogenase, NADH dehydrogenase activities, and neutral fat content are all low in white fibers and high in red fibers. Glycogen is abundant in white fibers and sparse in red fibers.

CARDIAC MUSCLE

Microscopic Structure

Unlike skeletal muscle, cardiac muscle consists of separate cellular units, **cardiac myocytes,** which are about 80 μm in length, 15 μm in diameter, and are joined end-to-end at junctional specializations called **intercalated disks** (Figs. 9-18 [see Plate 12] and 9-19). Although the cell columns thus formed are predominantly parallel, the individual myocytes branch and form oblique interconnections with neighboring columns. This results in a complex three-dimensional organization that is quite different from the precise parallel arrangement of the cylindrical fibers in skeletal muscle.

Cardiac myocytes have an oviod, centrally placed nucleus (Fig. 9-18 [see Plate 12]) surrounded by myofibrils having a pattern of cross-striations similar to that of skeletal muscle. These diverge around the nucleus, outlining a fusiform central region of sarcoplasm rich in organelles and inclusions. A small Golgi complex is found near one pole of the nucleus. Lipid droplets are common in this region and, in elderly individuals, granular deposits of **lipochrome** pigment may be abundant, constituting up to 20% of the dry weight of the myocardium.

Ultrastructure

The principal identifying features of cardiac myocytes are the centrally placed single nucleus and the occurrence of transverse intercalated disks, at intervals along the length of the myofibers. These are specialized junctions between cardiac myocytes. An intercalated disk may extend straight across the fiber, but, more commonly, seg-

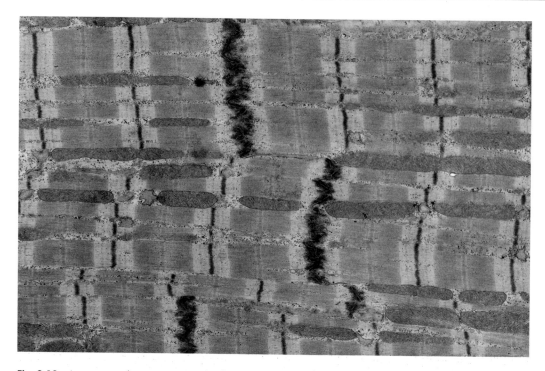

Fig. 9-19 Low-power electron micrograph of cardiac muscle in longitudinal section, including examples of intercalated disks where cellular units of the muscle join end-to-end. Longitudinal portions of the interface are smooth and have no associated dense material.

p. 23

ments of it are slightly offset longitudinally, giving it a staircaselike configuration. The dense transverse portions of the disk are sites of attachment of the myofilaments to the sarcolemma. In the transverse portions of a disk, the opposing membranes are highly interdigitated. This feature may be partially obscured, in histological sections, by a dense subsarcolemmal amorphous component of the junction, but it is apparent in electron micrographs. The intercalated disk is comparable to the zonula adherens of epithelial junctions. Its dense material includes the actin-binding proteins α-actinin and vinculin. In the pattern of cross-striations, the transverse portions of the intercalated disks invariably occur at the level of the I-band. Where the transverse segments of the intercalated disk are offset, the membranes of the connecting longitudinal segments have no associated dense material and are unspecialized, except for the presence of occasional gap junctions.

A distinctive feature of cardiac muscle in cross section is the absence of distinct, polygonal myofibrils of uniform size. The bulk of the cross section is occupied by a continuum of myofilaments, interrupted here and there by rows of circular profiles of tubules of the sarcoplasmic reticulum and by mitochondria (Fig. 9-20). In longitudinal sections, the sarcomeres are normally in register across the whole fiber. The continuity of the cross-striations across the fiber is interrupted only by longitudinally oriented mitochondria and tubules of the sarcoplasmic reticulum. Rows of **glycogen** particles are occasionally found between myofilaments in the I-bands.

As noted above, the slender T-tubules of skeletal muscle are located at the level of the A–I junctions. In cardiac muscle, they are of larger caliber and occur at the level of

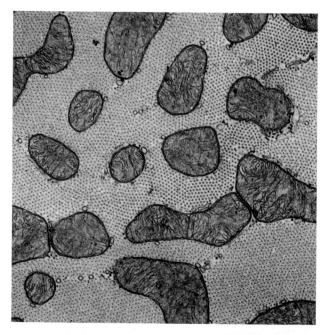

Fig. 9-20 Electron micrograph of a portion of a cardiac muscle cell in cross section. Note that the myofilaments are not associated in distinct myofibrils with clearly defined limits, as in skeletal muscle. They form a more-or-less continuous mass interrupted by mito-chondria and elements of the sarcoplasmic reticulum.

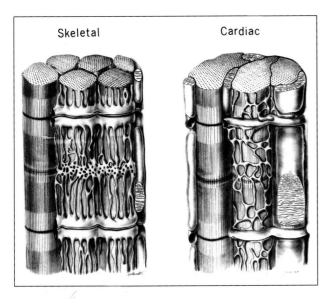

Fig. 9-21 Drawings comparing the sarcoplasmic reticulum of amphibian skeletal and mammalian cardiac muscle. In cardiac muscle, extensive terminal cisternae are replaced by small local dilatations of the reticulum, and the T-tubules, at the level of the Z-band, are of larger caliber than those of skeletal muscle.

the Z-disks (Fig. 9-21). They are not flanked by long terminal cisternae. Therefore, triads are lacking. The tubules of the sarcoplasmic reticulum are less numerous than those of skeletal muscle. They form a subsarcolemmal network of tubules 25–35 nm in diameter, called the **corbular reticulum,** that continues into deep clefts within the column of myofilaments. The reticulum is close-meshed adjacent to A-bands and more loosely organized at I-bands. The functional counterparts of the terminal cisternae are relatively small saccular dilatations of certain longitudinal tubules of the reticulum that establish close contact with the T-tubules at the level of the Z-disks. These complexes are called **dyads.** Transduction of excitation takes place in these structures via rows of transmembrane particles called **feet,** or **spanning proteins,** bridging the gap between the T-tubule and the junctional saccule of the reticulum. In addition, there are small expansions of the subsarcolemmal reticulum that are connected directly to the sarcolemma by junctional feet. The calcium-binding protein **calsequestrin** can be localized in the junctional saccules and neighboring tubules of the reticulum. Owing to its less extensive junctional reticulum, cardiac muscle has limited intracellular reserves of calcium. During depolarization of the sarcolemma and of the membrane of the T-tubules, an influx of extracellular calcium is thought to supplement the intracellular reserves in the reticulum. Filament sliding is evidently activated by calcium from both sources.

There are differences in size of the myocytes in different regions of the heart. Those of the atria tend to be smaller than those of the ventricles, and transverse tubules are shorter. Indeed, they are seen only in the largest atrial fibers. It is likely that there is less need for transverse

tubules for inward conduction of excitation in fibers of small diameter.

Myocardial Endocrine Cells

There are specialized myocytes in the right and left atrial appendages that secrete peptide hormones. These are involved in the regulation of blood volume and the electrolyte composition of the extracellular fluid. The **myoendocrine cells** resemble working myocytes in having myofilaments that diverge around a central nucleus. The organelles do not differ significantly from those of myocytes elsewhere. Their most distinctive feature is the presence of many membrane-bounded secretory granules, 0.3–0.4 µm in diameter in the core sarcoplasm that extends in either direction from the poles of the nucleus. The granules contain the precursor of a family of peptides, collectively called **cardiodilatins** or **atrial natriuretic peptides.** These peptides are released into the blood and cause peripheral vasodilatation and consequent lowering of blood pressure. They also constrict the efferent arteriole of the renal glomeruli resulting in diuresis (increased urine) and increased excretion of sodium.

Myocardial Conduction Tissue

For the heart to function as an efficient pump, contraction of the atria must be completed shortly before the onset of ventricular contraction. The precise timing of these events of the cardiac cycle depends on myocytes that are specialized for initiation and conduction of excitation to the different regions of the myocardium at a rate that will ensure their activation in the correct sequence. The **sinoatrial node,** at the junction of the superior vena cava with the right atrium, is considered the **pacemaker** of the heart. It consists of pale-staining, highly branched nodal myocytes containing relatively few myofilaments, and these are inconsistent in their orientation. The node is richly vascularized, contains considerable connective tissue, and is innervated by both divisions of the autonomic nervous system. The **nodal myocytes** have an inherent rhythm of depolarization and repolarization that is faster than that of the working myocardium. Their spontaneous depolarization initiates waves of excitation that spread, via gap junctions, through the atria and ventricles, determining their rate of contraction. However, the inherent rhythm of the node can be modified by input from the autonomic nervous system. Sympathetic nerve impulses accelerate the heart rate and parasympathetic nerve impulses slow the heart beat.

Internodal tracts conduct the wave of depolarization from the sinoatrial node to the **atrioventricular node,** situated in the lower part of the **interatrial septum.** The histological appearance of this node is similar to that of the

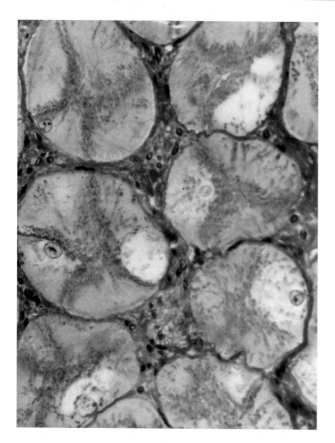

Fig. 9-22 Cross sections of Purkinje fibers of the ox heart. Myofilaments occupy only the small dark areas of the sarcoplasm. The paler intervening areas are rich in glycogen.

sinoatrial node. From there, the wave of depolarization is conducted from cell to cell in a tract called the **atrioventricular bundle (bundle of His).** This divides into right- and left-bundle branches that course beneath the **endocardium** on either side of the **interventricular septum** toward the apex of the heart, where they turn back and branch into multiple small bundles. These communicate, through gap junctions, with many ordinary cardiac muscle cells in the wall of the ventricle, first at the apex and later nearer the base. The specialized myocytes of the atrioventricular bundle and its branches are called **Purkinje fibers.** They are wider than ordinary ventricular fibers and have their myofilaments arranged peripherally around a clear core of sarcoplasm containing the nucleus and a large amount of glycogen (Fig. 9-22). This distribution of the conducting tissue results in the stimulus for contraction reaching the apex of the heart first and progressing toward the base, a sequence essential for efficient ejection of blood into the aorta.

QUESTIONS*

1. Krause's "Z"-line is found in which of the following?

   A. the "I"-band
   B. the "A"-band
   C. the "M"-band
   D. the "H"-band
   E. none of the above

2. A sarcomere is the area between two of which of the following structures?

   A. two A-bands
   B. two I-bands
   C. two Z-lines
   D. two M-lines
   E. two H-bands

3. Which of the following **best** characterizes a cardiac muscle cell?

   A. triads are rare
   B. large T-tubule
   C. T-tubule at Z-line
   D. central, "swollen" nuclei
   E. all of the above.

4. Elongated, centrally located nuclei are found in which of the following cells?

   A. smooth muscle
   B. skeletal muscle
   C. cardiac muscle
   D. endomysial connective tissue
   E. all of the above

5. Which of the statements about myocardial cells is/are **true?**

   A. have many large mitochondria with abundant cristae
   B. have centrally located nuclei
   C. contain lipofuscin
   D. all of the above
   E. none of the above

6. Which is true about the I-band of the skeletal muscle myofibril?

   A. there are only myosin filaments
   B. there are both actin and myosin filaments
   C. there are only actin filaments
   D. contains mitochondria
   E. none of the above

7. Which is **incorrect** when the skeletal muscle fiber contracts?

   A. H-band disappears
   B. Z-bands are closer together
   C. myosin filaments slide into the I-band
   D. actin filaments slide into the A-band
   E. the sarcomere becomes thicker

8. Which of the following proteins found in the skeletal muscle fiber bind calcium?

   A. myosin
   B. myoglobin
   C. meromyosin
   D. troponin
   E. actin

9. During voluntary contraction of skeletal muscle, the sarcomere

   A. stays the same length
   B. gets longer
   C. gets shorter
   D. the I-bands within the sarcomere get longer
   E. none of the above

10. Sarcoplasmic reticulum surrounds which of the following?

    A. skeletal muscle actin filaments
    B. skeletal muscle myosin filaments
    C. skeletal muscle fiber
    D. skeletal muscle myofibril
    E. none of the above

*Answers on page 307.

10

NERVOUS SYSTEM

By Jay Angevine

CHAPTER OUTLINE

The Neuron
    Dendrites
    Axon
    Nerve Impulse
    The Synapse
    Myelin Sheath
Peripheral Nerves
Distribution of Neurons
    Cerebral Cortex
    Cerebellar Cortex
    Spinal Cord
Neuroglia
    Astrocytes
    Oligodendrocytes
    Microglia
Autonomic Nervous System
    Sympathetic Division
    Parasympathetic Division
Meninges
    Dura Mater
    Arachnoid
    Pia Mater
Choroidal Plexuses and Cerebrospinal Fluid
Arachnoid Villi
Blood-Brain Barrier

KEY WORDS

Acetylcholine	Myelinated
Action Potential	Neurofibril
Afferent	Neurofilament
Anterograde	Neuroglia
Transport	Neurokeratin
Arachnoid	Neuron
Axolemma	Neurotransmitter
Axon	Nissl Bodies
Axon Hillock	Node of Ranvier
Bipolar Neuron	Norepinephrine
Blood-brain Barrier	Paravertebral
Bouton	Pedicel
Cerebrospinal Fluid	Perineurium
Choroid Plexus	Pia
Craniosacral	Pilomotor
Dendrite	Proprioceptor
Denticulate Ligament	Purkinje Cell
Dorsal Root	Pyramidal Cell
Dura	Resting Potential
Dynein	Retrograde Transport
Efferent	Saltatory Conduction
Endoneurium	Schmidt–Lantermann
Ependymal Cell	Cleft
Epidural Space	Schwann Cell
Epinephrine	Soma (Cell Body)
Epineurium	Stellate Cell
Ganglia	Sudomotor
Gray Matter	Synapse
Horizontal Cell	Synaptic Cleft
Interneuron	Terminal Arborization
Kinesin	Thorn (Spine)
Lipofuchsin	Unipolar Neuron
Melanin	Vasomotor
Mesaxon	Ventral Root
Multipolar Neuron	Ventricle
Myelin Sheath	White Matter

The **nervous system** has two major divisions: the **central nervous system (CNS),** consisting of the brain and spinal cord, and the **peripheral nervous system (PNS)** made up of **nerves** emerging from the CNS and small encapsulated aggregations of nerve cell bodies called **ganglia.** The indispensible functions of the CNS are to receive sensory stimuli from various parts of the body, to analyze this information, and to respond by generating signals that are transmitted over peripheral nerves to initiate and integrate muscular, secretory, and other activities of the body. However, the CNS is not limited to integrating information from the periphery but also has less well-understood endogenous neural activity that underlies reasoning, conscious experience, and regulation of behavior.

THE NEURON

The nervous system is made up of billions of cells, called **neurons,** that are specialized to respond to stimuli and to transmit a signal to activate other cells. It also contains a host of nonexcitable supporting cells constituting the **neuroglia.** The typical neuron consists of a **cell body (soma)** which has many radiating processes called **dendrites,** which are specialized to receive signals from other neurons, and a single long process, the **axon,** which is capable of generating a **nerve impulse** and conducting it over a long distance to stimulate other neurons in the CNS or muscular or secretory cells elsewhere in the body (Fig. 10-1A). As it approaches its end, the axon branches repeatedly in a **terminal arborization.** Each branch of this arborization ends in a small expansion called an **endbulb** or **terminal bouton** that makes contact with another cell to form a **synapse,** where chemical or electrical signals pass from the neuron to another cell, the **effector cell.** At these contacts, the communicative function of the neuron depends on compounds that they synthesize and release to activate the effector cell. These include various **neurotransmitters** that act rapidly and locally to activate their target cells and **neuromodulators** that regulate these events in various ways and that exert slower effects by diffusion through the extracellular fluid or by transport in the blood.

The size and shape of neurons, as well as the mode of branching of their cell processes, are highly variable. Neurons are therefore classified according to the geometry of their processes (Fig. 10-1B). **Unipolar neurons** have an axon but no dendrites. These are rare. Somewhat more common are **pseudounipolar neurons,** in sensory ganglia, which have a short process (an axon) with a T-shaped branching, one member of which leads to the CNS and the other goes to an ending in the periphery. **Bipolar neurons** are similar, but have two processes (both axons) emerging directly and oppositely from the cell body. **Multipolar neurons,** in contrast, have one axon and many dozens of

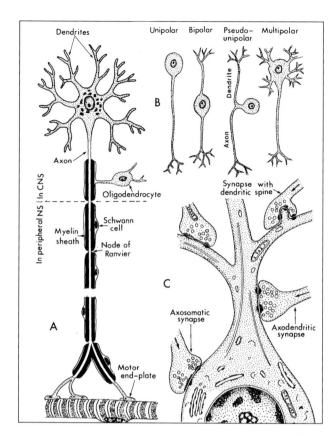

Fig. 10-1 (A) Drawing of the components of a typical neuron. (B) Types of neurons according to their polarity. (C) Types and terminology of the synapses occurring on the cell body or dendrites. (B adapted from A.W. Ham, *Histology,* 6th ed., J.P. Lippincott, Philadelphia, 1969; C redrawn after R. Bunge, in *Bailey's Textbook of Histology,* 16th ed. Williams and Wilkins, Baltimore, 1971.)

dendrites. This latter type is very common in the CNS. The number of synapses on a neuron depends, in large measure, on the number and length of its dendrites. In addition to their classification by shape and number of processes, neurons can be assigned to one of three categories based on their function. **Motor neurons** are involved in stimulating muscles or glands in the periphery; **sensory neurons** receive sensory stimuli from the environment or from the tissues and organs of the body; **interneurons** maintain connections between neurons in the CNS.

A typical neuron has a pale-staining nucleus with a conspicuous nucleolus and relatively little heterochromatin (Fig. 10-2 [see Plate 12]). The cytoplasm is crowded with organelles and filamentous cytoskeletal elements arranged more or less concentrically around the nucleus. This central region of the cytoplasm is often referred to as the **perikaryon.** In sections stained with basic dyes, the most conspicuous components of the perikaryon are large clumps of basophilic material (**Nissl bodies),** once thought to be unique to neurons. In electron micrographs, each of these is found to be an aggregation of many parallel cisternae of the rough endoplasmic reticulum (RER) (Fig. 10-3). RER is also found in the dendrites, but there, it takes the

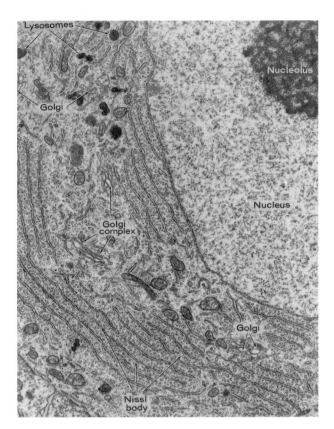

Fig. 10-3 Electron micrograph of a portion of the perikaryon of a typical neuron, illustrating its principal organelles. (Micrograph courtesy of S. Palay.)

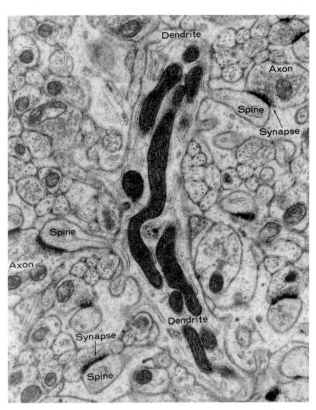

Fig. 10-4 Electron micrograph of a small area of the cerebellum. A small branch of the dendritic tree of a Purkinje cell runs vertically through the field and contains several mitochondia. Projecting laterally from the dendrite are "spines" or "thorns" with bulbous tips and narrow stalks. On these are synapses of granule cells. (From S.L. Palay and V.C. Palay, Cerebellar Cortex, Springer-Verlag, 1974.)

form of tubules or smaller arrays of cisternae. Smooth endoplasmic reticulum forms a loose network of tubules throughout the perikaryon and continues into the dendrites and axon. In certain neurons, it may form flat cisternae adjacent to the plasmalemma. The Golgi complex is prominent in all neurons and appears, in electron micrographs, as multiple small arciform stacks of cisternae slightly expanded at their ends. The cistern at the concave surface of each stack is fenestrated and is continuous with a trans-Golgi network of tubules. The function of the Golgi in these cells is much the same as in other cells. It is involved in the concentration of products synthesized in the endoplasmic reticulum. Some of the numerous small vesicles around it contain the neurotransmitter that will be transported along the axon for release at its endings. After severance of a nerve axon, the Golgi complex in the perikaryon regresses to such an extent that it may no longer be detectable with the light microscope. Finally, throughout the perikaryon and the dendrites, there are many slender mitochondria. They also occur along the axon and are especially numerous in the axon terminals. Lysosomes are present in small numbers in the perikaryon.

Cytoplasmic inclusions are uncommon in neurons and largely limited to irregularly shaped granules of lipofuscin pigment which represents accumulated end products of

lysosomal activity. In old age, lipofuscin may accumulate to such an extent as to displace the nucleus and organelles to one side of the cell. In the neurons of a few regions of the brain, coarse granules of the pigment **melanin** are also be found in the neurons. Its physiological significance in these sites is unknown.

In specimens prepared for light microscopy by traditional silver-impregnation methods, a network of **neurofibrils** could be seen in the perikaryon, weaving among the organelles and extending into the dendrites and the axon. With the electron microscope, three kinds of filamentous structures are found: **neurofilaments,** 10 nm in diameter, **microfilaments,** 3–4 nm in diameter, and **microtubules,** 20–28 nm in diameter. The neurofilaments correspond to the intermediate filaments of other cell types. Bundles of neurofilaments probably make up the neurofibrils visible with the light microscope. The microfilaments are filaments of actin that occur in the cytoplasm of cells in general. The microtubules are similar to those of other cells, but there are slight regional differences in the microtubule-associated proteins that regulate their stability and promote their assembly. Microtubules in the cell body are constantly turning over, and their depolymerization and repolymerization in changing orientation affect cell shape. The microtubules of the axon are of greater functional significance, in that they serve as conveyor lines along which vesicles are transported from the Golgi bodies to the nerve endings.

*One of the most common of the degenerative diseases of the CNS in the aging population is **Alzheimer's disease.** Neurons in the cerebral cortex accumulate tangled masses of filaments in their cytoplasm and ultimately degenerate. There is little or no involvement of the motor system. It begins with loss of memory and progresses to loss of intellectual capacity (dementia). Its cause is unknown.*

Dendrites

The ability of nerve cells to receive and integrate signals depends, in large measure, on their dendrites. Their extensive branching greatly increases the cell surface available for receiving signals from other neurons. Their branching pattern typifies each type of neuron. The dendritic tree of spinal motor neurons may receive up to 10,000 synapses, and the exceptionally elaborate dendritic arborization of cerebellar **Purkinje cells** may have up to 250,000 synapses with axons of other neurons. The main branches of dendrites tend to be smooth-surfaced, but their lateral branches are often quite irregular due to the presence of numerous small lateral projects called **thorns** or

spines. These are preferential sites of synaptic contact and they occupy concavities in the end-bulbs of axons terminating upon the neuron (Figs. 10-1 and 10-4). The capacity of the neuron to integrate input from many different sources is directly related to the degree of branching of their dendrites and the number of their spines.

In the tapering initial reaches of the dendrites, the organelles resemble those of the perikaryon except for the absence of Golgi bodies. With increasing distance from the cell body (soma), smooth endoplasmic reticulum and neurofilaments are reduced, but longitudinal microtubules are prominent and mitochondria are aligned parallel to them.

Axon

The axon arises from a conical extension of the cell body, the **axon hillock.** The axon is more slender and usually very much longer that the dendrites of the same cell. Unlike the dendrites which diminish in diameter as they branch, the axon has essentially the same caliber throughout its length. In spinal motor neurons supplying muscles in the feet, the axon may be as much as 40 in. in length. Its content, the **axoplasm,** lacks Nissl bodies (RER) but contains short segments of smooth endoplasmic reticulum and long, slender mitochondria. In cross section, the neurofilaments are spaced a uniform distance apart throughout the axoplasm (Fig. 10-5). Microtubules are also numerous but less uniformly distributed than the neurofilaments.

In addition to its episodic conduction of a nerve impulse along its membrane, the axon is continually

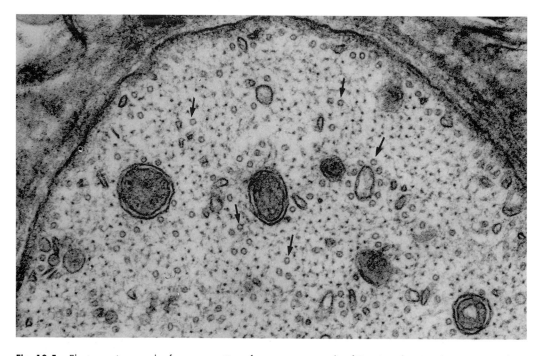

Fig. 10-5 Electron micrograph of a cross section of an axon at a node of Ranvier, showing the very even distribution of the neurofilaments and a less even distribution of the microtubules (at arrows) that are essential for axonal transport (Courtesy of R.L. Price.)

engaged in **axonal transport.** Transport is bidirectional: **anterograde transport** from the perikaryon to the axon terminal, and **retrograde transport** from the axon terminal to the cell body. Fast and slow components have been recognized in anterograde transport. Organelles and small vesicles are moved down the axon by fast transport, at a rate of 20–400 mm/day. Movement of enzymes and protein components of the microtubules and neurofilaments proceeds by slow transport at a rate of 0.2–0.4 mm/day. Anterograde transport is especially important for delivery of the small vesicles containing neurotransmitter to the nerve ending. Its mechanism has been thoroughly studied. The microtubules of the axon are polarized, with their "plus end" toward the axon terminal, and their "minus end" toward the cell body. The protein called **kinesin** is the motor for movement of the vesicles. One end of the molecule attaches to the vesicle and the other end undergoes cyclic interaction with binding sites on the microtubule, resulting in movement of the vesicle from the perikaryon toward the plus end at about 3 μm/s. Some neuropeptide granules synthesized in the perikaryon can be observed in movement along the axon of living neurons in vitro. It was formerly thought that all neurotransmitters reached the nerve endings in vesicles transported in this way. It is now believed that this mechanism may be less important than synthesis of the neurotransmitter at the nerve ending. Retrograde transport depends on another protein, **dynein,** that moves vesicles along the microtubules toward the cell body.

In the peripheral nervous system (PNS), the axons are enveloped in a thin sheath of **Schwann cells** that are closely applied to the **axolemma,** the limiting membrane of the axon. In the CNS, the axons are ensheathed by **oligodendroglial cells.**

Nerve Impulse

The ability of neurons to transmit signals depends on transient electrochemical changes that travel along their axons. The limiting membrane of the axon, the **axolemma,** is able to pump sodium out of the **axoplasm** to maintain, in its interior, a sodium ion (Na+) concentration that is only about a tenth of that in the extracellular fluid, whereas the intracellular potassium (K+) concentration is maintained at a level many times greater than that prevailing in the extracellular environment. This results in a potential difference across the axolemma of about −90 mV, with the inside negative to the outside. This is referred to as the **resting membrane potential.** Under these circumstances, the ion channels in the cell membrane are inactive. When a neuron is stimulated, the ion channels open, and there is a sudden influx of extracellular sodium ions lowering the resting potential. This is followed by a restoration of the potential, by outflow of potassium ions. These changes, creating an **action potential,** occupy only about 5 ms. However, dif-

fusion of the sodium from that initial site toward the axon ending depolarizes the neighboring region of the membrane, generating an action potential there, and this process continues. Thus, an action potential, initiated in the initial segment of the axon, is propagated along its entire length. Upon arriving at the nerve ending, it initiates discharge of stored neurotransmitter that stimulates another nerve cell or a non-neural effector cell.

The Synapse

See also p. 102

The specialized region of contact where neurotransmitter is released from an axon to stimulate another cell is called a **synapse.** In the CNS, such contacts are usually with the dendrites of other neurons **(axodendritic synapses),** but they may be with the cell body **(axosomatic synapses),** and less frequently with the axon **(axoaxonic synapses).** The numbers of synapses in the CNS is astronomical, being estimated at 10^{14}.

In the PNS, the synaptic contact of motor nerves is usually with muscle or glandular epithelial cells. A common neurotransmitter is **acetylcholine,** but a growing number of other compounds serving this function have been identified to date, including certain monoamines, the catecholamines **noradrenaline** and **dopamine,** the indolamine **serotonin,** and at least one amino acid.

At a synapse, the **presynaptic** and **postsynaptic membranes** are parallel and separated by a **synaptic cleft,** 12–20 nm in width, that contains a moderately dense material that may contribute to their cohesion. The cytoplasm of the nerve ending contains a few mitochondria and occasional tubules of smooth endoplasmic reticulum, but its most conspicuous constituents are numerous, small **synaptic vesicles,** 20–40 nm in diameter, clustered near the presynaptic membrane (Fig. 10-6). This membrane is decorated on its inner surface with small conical densities of unknown chemical nature. The region of presynaptic membrane bearing these densities and the associated synaptic vesicles are referred to as the **active zone** of the synapse. When an action potential traveling down the axon reaches its terminal, voltage-gated channels are opened, permitting Ca2+ ions to enter. This triggers release of neurotransmitter into the synaptic cleft by exocytosis of synaptic vesicles docked in the active zone. The neurotransmitter binds to specific **receptors** in the postsynaptic membrane. This results in a conformational change in the receptors in that membrane, opening ion channels. Entry of ions into the postsynaptic cytoplasm causes depolarization of the membrane and excitation of the target cell. Membrane added to the active zone in exocytosis of synaptic vesicles moves laterally from the release site and is retrieved by endocytosis in clathrin-coated vesicles. These lose their coat and fuse with tubules of smooth endoplasmic reticulum in the ending. New vesicles are believed to be formed and charged with neurotransmitter in this organelle.

See Cormack 2nd Ed. p. 214

Sodium ions (p. 102

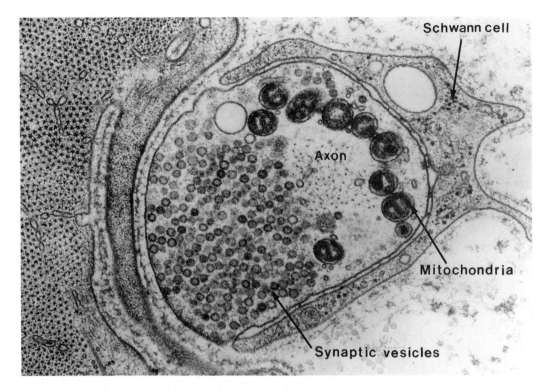

Fig. 10-6   Nerve ending on muscle, showing a large accumulation of synaptic vesicles. The components of synapses in the central nervous system are similar to those shown here. (Micrograph courtesy of T. Reese.)

Synapses may be **excitatory** or **inhibitory,** depending on whether the transmitter depolarizes or hyperpolarizes the postsynaptic membrane. Which of these effects occurs depends on the chemical nature of the neurotransmitter and the type of receptors in the postsynaptic membrane.

Myelin Sheath

The axons of many peripheral nerves are invested by a highly refractile layer called the **myelin sheath** (Fig. 10-7 [see Plate 13]). The lipids that make up the bulk of this layer (cholesterol, phospholipid, and glycolipids) are extracted in specimen preparation for light microscopy, leaving behind a delicate network of material called **neurokeratin** (Fig. 10-7A [see Plate 13]). Myelin is better preserved by osmium fixation and appears as a dense layer of varying thickness, made up of concentric dense and less-dense lines (Figs. 10-7B [see Plate 13] and 10-8).

The myelin sheath is an integral part of the investing layer of **Schwann cells** that are arranged end-to-end, with each completely surrounding the axon. The nature of the myelin sheath is best understood from a study of its formation. The axon initially occupies a deep recess in the surface of the Schwann cell. The borders of the processes surrounding it come into contact and the apposed membranes are described as the **mesaxon** (Figs. 10-9A and 10-10). In the subsequent development of the myelin sheath, formation of additional membrane results in

lengthening of the mesaxon, which becomes spirally wound around the axon (Fig. 10-9B). As the spiral tightens, cytoplasm between successive turns is completely excluded and the inner surfaces of the plasmalemma of successive turns of the spiral come into contact and appear to fuse. Thus, the myelin sheath is made up of a coil of Schwann cell membrane around the axon. In cross sections of the sheath, viewed with the electron microscope, the fused cytoplasmic leaflets of the plasmalemma form a **major dense line,** about 3 nm thick, spiraling around the axon. Alternating with the major dense line is a thinner, less dense, **intraperiod line** formed by the close apposition of the external surfaces of the membrane in successive turns of the spiral. In micrographs of very high resolution, a narrow space (0.2 nm) is visible between these apposed outer surfaces of the membrane. This so-called **intraperiod gap** is continuous through the spiral from the endoneurial to the periaxonal extracellular space.

At intervals along the axon, there are short gaps in the myelin sheath, called the **nodes of Ranvier** (Figs. 10-1A and 10-11A). These are spaces between the successive Schwann cells of the sheath. Small processes of the neighboring Schwann cells interdigite in these spaces but do not completely seal off the axolemma from the extracellular fluid around the nerve. The segment of the sheath between successive nodes, called an **internode,** is the length of one Schwann cell, approximately 1–2 mm.

In longitudinal histological sections, one or more narrow paler areas can be seen crossing the sheath obliquely. These

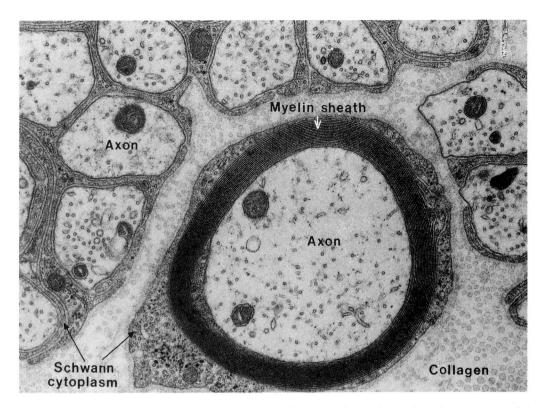

Fig. 10-8   Electron micrograph of a myelinated nerve and the axons of several unmyelinated nerves surrounded by the cytoplasm of Schwann cells.

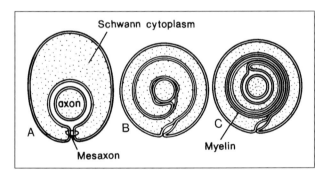

Fig. 10-9   Diagram illustrating stages in development of the myelin sheath of a nerve. (A) Axon enveloped by the process of a Schwann cell. (B) Intermediate stage: Unit membranes of the mesaxon and, to some extent, of the axon have come together, with the line of contact representing the future intraperiod lines of the myelin sheath. (C) Later stage: A few layers of compact myelin have formed by contact and fusion of the cytoplasmic surfaces of the spiraling mesaxon loops. This line of fusion creates the major dense lines of the sheath. (Redrawn from J.D. Robertson, Progress in Biophysics 10:349, 1960.)

have traditionally been called **Schmidt–Lantermann clefts.** It is apparent in electron micrographs that these are not clefts but are sites in which a small amount of cytoplasm persists between the two leaves of the major dense line (Fig. 10-11B). Thus, these oblique lines represent thin threads of Schwann cell cytoplasm that pursue a spiral course from the cell body nearly to the axon. Their func-

tional significance is not clear. They may provide a path through which metabolites can diffuse into the depths of the myelin or may simply represent failure to express all of the cytoplasm in the tightening of the spiral during formation of the sheath. The myelin sheath of peripheral nerves begins a short distance from the cell body. The part of the axon between the axon hillock and the beginning of the sheath is called its **initial segment.**

The presence of a myelin sheath greatly influences the ability of an axon to conduct an impulse. It acts as an insulator with the axon exposed to the extracellular space only at the nodes of Ranvier. The internodal segments of the myelin sheath prevent the interchange of ions necessary to generate an action potential. However, the action potential is regenerated at each node of Ranvier. This is called **saltatory conduction** and is very much faster (10–100 times) than conduction in axons lacking a myelin sheath. The speed of conduction varies directly with the diameter of the axon and the number of layers in the myelin sheath.

Myelin also occurs in major tracts that represent long-distance connections in the CNS. The axons are large and have thick myelin sheaths, and hence, high conduction velocity. Myelin of the CNS is not made by Schwann cells but by **oligodendrocytes,** one of the several types of neuroglial cells (see below). It is the myelin sheaths of nerve tracts that are responsible for the glistening light color of the white matter of the brain.

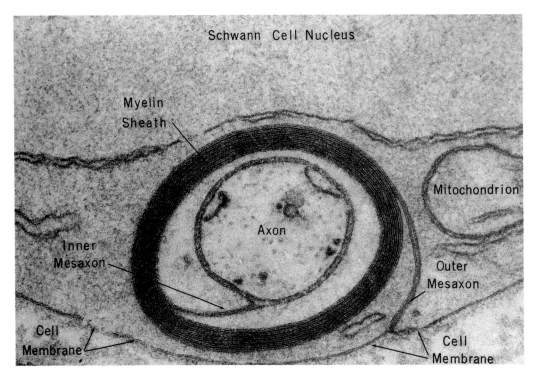

Fig. 10-10 Electron micrograph of a small myelinated nerve showing the internal and external mesaxons.

*The central nervous system is subject to several diseases in which the dominant feature is a destruction of the myelin sheaths. Among these is **multiple sclerosis**. The loss of function depends on where in the CNS the focal areas of demyelinization occur. Weakness, loss of position sense, and paralysis of one or more limbs are common sequelae. The cause of the disorder is unknown.*

In the PNS, Schwann cells also ensheath **unmyelinated axons.** They harbor individual axons, or more often, several axons (Figs. 10-12). The successive Schwann cells along the axons are in close contact with no gaps corresponding to nodes of Ranvier. Unmyelinated axons therefore conduct much more slowly than myelinated axons.

PERIPHERAL NERVES

The nerves of the PNS consist of varying numbers of myelinated and unmyelinated axons originating from neurons located in the brain, spinal cord, or ganglia. They are enclosed in three layers of differing character. The outermost, the **epineurium,** consists of dense irregular connective tissue with the majority of its collagen fibers oriented longitudinally to limit the extent to which the nerve can be stretched. Its cellular elements are fibroblasts, mast cells, and limited numbers of adipose cells. Thinner extensions

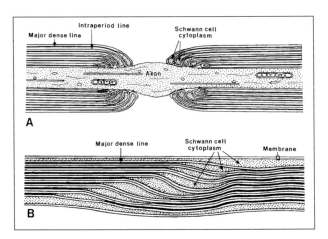

Fig. 10-11 (A) Drawing of a node of Ranvier of a myelinated nerve showing the major dense lines and interperiod lines of the myelin sheath. (B) Drawing of a longitudinal section of the myelin sheath showing the oblique alignment of small fusiform areas of cytoplasm in dilatations of the lamellae. These are recognized with the light microscope as the clefts of Schmidt–Lantermann.

of this layer penetrate into the nerve as the **perineurium,** a thin sleeve of flattened cells surrounding small bundles of nerve axons. The cells of this layer are joined by tight junctions, making the perineurium an effective barrier to penetration of macromolecules. Within each bundle of nerve fibers there is an **endoneurium** consisting of a delicate network of reticular fibers surrounding each Schwann cell–axon complex.

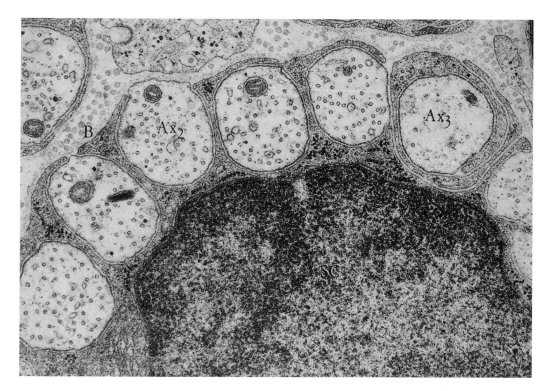

Fig. 10-12 Electron micrograph of a Schwann cell in a peripheral nerve, showing several unmyelinated axons occupying deep recesses in its surface. Most are completely surrounded by Schwann cell cytoplasm, but one (Ax 2) is only partially enclosed and covered only by the basal lamina. (From A. Peters, S.L. Palay, and H. deF. Webster, The Fine Structure of the Nervous System, 3rd ed., Oxford University Press, New York, 1991.)

Nerves are the pathways of communication between centers in the brain and spinal cord and the rest of the body. They contain **afferent fibers,** which carry information from the surface or the interior of the body to the CNS, and **efferent fibers,** which carry nerve impulses from the CNS to tissues and organs in the periphery. Afferent nerves from end organs sensing heat, cold, touch, or pain are called **sensory nerves.** Efferent nerves to muscles, stimulating their contraction, are called **motor nerves,** and the tissues responding to motor nerves are referred to as **effectors.** Many of the peripheral nerves contain both sensory and motor fibers and are, thus, termed **mixed nerves.**

DISTRIBUTION OF NEURONS

Different regions of the CNS are distinguishable with the naked eye by slight differences in color and texture. The **gray matter** contains the cell bodies of neurons, their dendrites, and the terminations of axons arriving from other regions. The **white matter** is largely devoid of neuronal cell bodies and consists mainly of myelinated axons, the cell bodies of which are in the gray matter or the dorsal root ganglia. Neuroglial cells and their processes are present in great numbers and variety in both gray and white matter, but they may be distinguished only with special metallic impregnation methods, or with electron microscopy (see below).

Cerebral Cortex

The **cerebral cortex** is an outer zone of gray matter over the hemispheres of the brain. It receives and analyzes sensory information from the body and responds by voluntary initiation of motor activity. It is also involved in learning and memory. The cerebral cortex contains over 2600 million neurons of many types. It is beyond the province of histology to consider in detail their form and functional connections, but a few cell types will be described. The cells are arranged in six major layers. Its most characteristic type is the **pyramidal cell** (Fig. 10-13). Its soma is roughly triangular in section with a large vesicular nucleus and abundant Nissl bodies in the perikaryon. A long apical dendrite extends toward the surface of the brain with many branches that are sites of axodendritic synapses. An axon arises from its base and descends through the deeper layers of the cortex. The pyramidal cells in the various layers of the cortex vary in size and in the pattern of their dendritic and axonal branching. The dendritic arborization of the smallest is about 10 μm wide, whereas the largest, in the region generating motor activity, is 30–60 μm in width and up to 120 μm in height. Another major cell type is the **stellate** or **granule cell.** These are relatively small, 6–10 μm in diameter, with numerous highly branched dendrites radiating from the cell body and a single relatively short axon. **Horizontal cells,** largely confined to one layer of the cortex, are fusiform, with radiating dendrites and a short axon that divides near the cell body, with the branches running in opposite directions.

> ***Amyotrophic lateral sclerosis** is a progressive loss of motor neurons in the cerebral cortex and spinal cord, resulting in atrophy of the muscles innervated by the neurons affected. The sensory system is unaffected. There is tremor, unsteady gait, and paralysis of muscles of mastication and facial expression. Involvement of the respiratory muscles may lead to death. The cause of this disease is unknown.*

Cerebellar Cortex

The **cerebellar cortex** (Fig. 10-14) receives informational input from the eyes, ears, and stretch receptors in the muscles. It does not initiate muscular activity but has an important role in its coordination and in the maintenance of balance and normal posture. Three layers are recognizable. The outer, so-called **molecular layer** contains relatively few small neurons and many unmyelinated nerve fibers. The middle layer consists of a single layer of large **Purkinje cells** (Fig. 10-15 [see Plate 13]). These have an

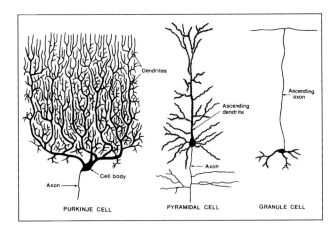

Fig. 10-13 Form of some of the neuron types in the central nervous system. The Purkinje cells of the cerebellum have a remarkably elaborate arborization of dendrites. The small granule cells of the cerebellum send an axon outward to synapse with dendrites of the Purkinje cells. Pyramidal cells of the cerebral cortex have fewer dendrites and these are covered with very large numbers of spines.

apical dendrite that ascends into the molecular layer where it undergoes remarkably elaborate branching in a single plane (Fig. 10-13). The axon extends downward through the underlying granular layer. The **granule cell** layer consists of closely packed small cells with short dendrites and an axon that courses upward to the molecular layer to form parallel fibers synapsing with the Purkinje cells.

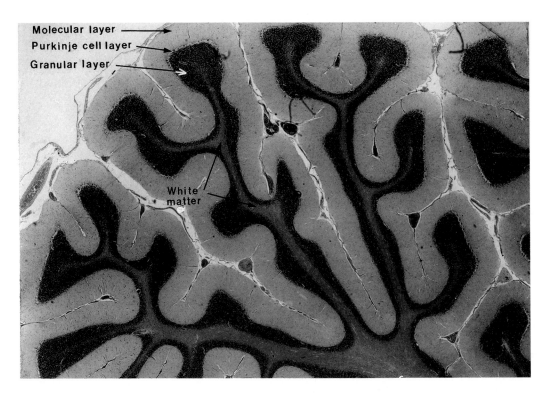

Fig. 10-14 Photomicrograph of a portion of the cerebellum. Each lobule of the highly convoluted organ contains a core of white matter surrounded by gray matter consisting of layers of granular cells, Purkinje cells, and a molecular layer containing the dendritic processes of the Purkinje cells and recurrent branches of cells of the granular layer.

Spinal Cord

The **spinal cord** receives **motor** commands from the brain and relays them over **spinal nerves** emerging at each segment of the vertebral column, to innervate the muscles and other effectors in the periphery. It receives **sensory** input from the body and relays this information to the brain. Nerve fibers enter and leave the spinal cord at regular intervals via **dorsal** and **ventral roots** projecting laterally from both sides of the cord (Fig. 10-16 [see Plate 14]). There are 31 pairs of roots along its length. Sensory fibers enter the cord through the dorsal roots and motor fibers leave through the ventral roots. A short distance from the cord, the dorsal and ventral roots join to form a sizable **spinal nerve,** containing both motor and sensory fibers that are widely distributed in the segment of the body served by that spinal nerve.

In a cross section of the spinal cord, there is a central H-shaped area of **gray matter** containing nerve cell bodies and their dendrites (Fig. 10-17 [see Plate 14]). Around the gray matter are **dorsal, lateral,** and **ventral columns** of **white matter** made up of ascending and descending myelinated nerve fibers communicating with other levels in the spinal cord and with nerve centers in the brain.

The cell bodies of sensory neurons entering the cord are located in a fusiform expansion of each dorsal root, called the **dorsal root ganglion.** These are pseudounipolar neurons with a short axonal process that divides into two myelinated branches; a long **peripheral fiber** that courses to distant sensory endings and a shorter **central fiber** that enters the spinal cord and synapses with neurons in the dorsal horn of its gray matter. The axons of these latter neurons enter the white matter and form ascending and descending tracts in the dorsal column of the spinal cord.

NEUROGLIA

The supporting cells of the central nervous system are collectively called the **neuroglia** ("nerve glue"). In addition to providing mechanical support, they maintain a microenvironment conducive to optimal functioning of the neurons. Although they outnumber the neurons 5–10-fold, they have been less thoroughly studied, for in routine histological sections little more than their nuclei can be identified. Our knowledge of their shape has depended on the use of special techniques involving their impregnation with silver or gold. In the elaborate intermingling of cell processes in the brain, their spatial, and especially their functional, relationships to each other and to the neurons have not been entirely clarified by electron microscopy. However, it is clear that wherever a neuron or a neuronal process is not in synaptic contact with another neuron, it is enveloped by the cell bodies or processes of neuroglial

cells. It is evident that the neuroglia prevent contact between neurons at sites other than those appropriate to their specific function. By providing this isolation, as well as parcellation of inputs these cells seem to play an important ancillary role in the communication function of the nervous system. The principal types of neuroglial cells of the CNS are the **astrocytes, oligodendrocytes, microglia,** and the **ependymal cells.** Within these major types, a rich variety of shapes and sizes is to be found.

Astrocytes

Astrocytes occur in several forms. **Protoplasmic astrocytes,** found mainly in the gray matter of the brain, have a stellate form with multiple radiating processes (Fig. 10-18A). They have abundant cytoplasm and a spherical nucleus that is larger and paler-staining than that of other neuroglial cells. Some of their many processes end with expansions, called **vascular feet** or **pedicels,** applied to the wall of blood vessels. The intimate relation of these processes to the blood vessels suggests that they may have some role in nutrition of the neurons, but as yet there is little supporting evidence. A smaller type of astrocyte is situated close to the cell bodies of neurons as a form of satellite cell. Another subtype, called **velate astrocytes,** have thin veil-like processes that extend between neurons or surround bundles of axons.

Fibrous astrocytes are common in the white matter but also occur in some regions of the periventricular gray matter (Fig. 10-18B). They have an ovoid euchromatic nucleus, pale-staining cytoplasm, and long, thin processes that branch less frequently than those of protoplasmic astrocytes. In electron micrographs, the cytoplasm of both types of astrocyte contains relatively few organelles, but there are conspicuous bundles of filaments that are small-

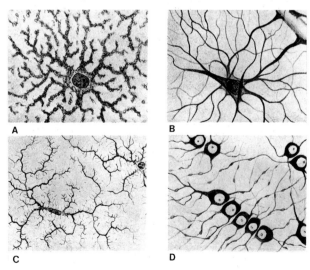

Fig. 10-18 Neuroglial cells of the central nervous system. (A) Protoplasmic astrocytes; (B) fibrous astrocyte; (C) microglia; (D) oligodendroglia.

er (8 nm) and more closely aggregated than the intermediate filaments of somatic cells. The filaments are also chemically distinct, consisting of **glial fibrillar acidic protein.**

Astrocytes are believed to clear the extracellular spaces of potassium ions, glutamate, and γ–aminobutyric acid that accumulate as by-products of neuronal activity. They are also cells containing reserves of glycogen from which glucose can be liberated through glycogenolysis induced by certain neurotransmitters. Therefore, they probably make a significant contribution to the energy metabolism of the cerebral cortex.

Oligodendrocytes

Oligodendrocytes are smaller than astrocytes and have fewer processes. The processes are not highly branched (Fig. 10-18D). Their small, round, heterochromatic nucleus is deeply staining. In electron micrographs, the cytoplasm is relatively dense, is rich in rough endoplasmic reticulum, and has many mitochondria. Microtubules are prominent in the cell body and in the cell processes. These cells are found close to the perikarya of neurons in the gray matter. In the white matter, they are localized in rows or columns between bundles of axons. These so-called **interfascicular oligodendrocytes** of the CNS are analogous to the Schwann cells in the PNS. Each internodal segment of the myelin sheath of CNS axons is formed of apposed membranes of an oligodendroglial cell process, wrapped spirally around an axon. Unlike Schwann cells, which ensheath only one myelinated axon, an oligodendrocyte may form segments of the myelin sheath of several parallel axons, perhaps as many as 50 or more.

The **satellite oligodendrocytes** of the gray matter are closely associated with the somata of neurons. Their smooth unspecialized area of apposition gives no hint of interaction between the cells, but in vitro experiments on isolated neurons and their satellite cells indicate some metabolic interdependency.

Throughout life, neuroglia retain the ability to divide, and they are active in repair of the CNS after injury, proliferating and filling the defects left by degeneration of neurons. Astrocytes are especially active in the repair process.

Microglia

The **microglia** comprises small phagocytic cells widely distributed throughout the CNS. They have a dense oval or elongate nucleus, scant cytoplasm, and short tortuous processes decorated with small spinelike projections (Fig. 10-18C). They are believed to represent the mononuclear phagocyte system of the CNS. In areas of injury, they proliferate, lose their spiney appearance, assuming a swollen

form, and become actively phagocytic in clearing cellular debris and ingesting damaged myelin.

AUTONOMIC NERVOUS SYSTEM

The part of the nervous system concerned with reception of sensory impulses and the voluntary generation of motor responses is known as the **somatic nervous system.** Other activities, such as heartbeat, smooth-muscle contraction, and secretion of exocrine glands are regulated automatically and are not subject to voluntary control. These activities are controlled by the **autonomic nervous system (ANS).** As the name implies, its actions are largely independent, but they are influenced to no small degree by conscious processes of the brain, and vice versa. The system has two divisions, the **sympathetic** and the **parasympathetic** divisions. In the somatic nervous system, a motor neuron acts directly on its effector organ, but in the ANS, two motor neurones in series are involved. The first is located in a center in the brain stem or spinal gray matter, whereas the second is in a ganglion outside of the CNS.

Sympathetic Division

The **sympathetic (thoracolumbar) division** of the ANS includes a chain of interconnected ganglia on either side of the vertebral column. As explained earlier, a **ganglion** is an encapsulated collection of nerve cell bodies outside of the CNS. The cell bodies of the preganglionic neurons are situated in the gray matter of the **thoracic** and **lumbar** regions of the spinal cord. Their axons exit the cord through the ventral roots, but soon leave them to enter one of the **paravertebral ganglia** that are interconnected in a chain running parallel to the vertebral column near the junctions of the dorsal and ventral roots (Fig. 10-16 [see Plate 14]). Each preganglionic neuron synapses with multiple postganglionic neurons in the ganglion of the same segment or in ganglia of neighboring segments. The axons of the postganglionic neurons return to spinal nerves and are distributed in peripheral nerves to blood vessels (**vasomotor fibers**), sweat glands (**sudomotor fibers**), hair follicles (**pilomotor fibers**), salivary glands, heart, and lungs. Some preganglionic fibers pass through the paravertebral ganglia without synapsing and travel in **splanchnic nerves** to synapse on nerve cell bodies in the **celiac ganglion** and **mesenteric ganglia** in the abdominal cavity. Postganglionic fibers from these ganglia innervate the gastrointestinal tract, kidneys, pancreas, liver, bladder, and external genitalia. Thus, sympathetic trunks and their ganglia are the avenues of outflow of impulses from the spinal cord to the viscera. The principal neurotransmitter of the sympathetic system is **norepinephrine.**

Parasympathetic Division

In the **parasympathetic (craniosacral) division** of the autonomic nervous system, the cell bodies of the preganglionic neurons are located in the brain stem and in several sacral segments of the spinal cord. Their axons do not synapse in the paravertebral ganglia, but extend for long distances to synapse with postganglionic neurons in small ganglia near, or within, their visceral targets. The preganglionic fibers of the cranial component of this division emerge from the CNS in the oculomotor, facial, glossopharyngeal, and vagus nerves and synapse with postganglionic neurons in the **ciliary, pterygopalatine, submandibular, and otic ganglia.** Those of the sacral component derive from the second to the fourth sacral segments, leaving via the ventral roots and sacral nerves, and synapse with postganglionic neurons in ganglia associated with the pelvic viscera. In the enteric component that controls the activity of the gastrointestinal tract, pancreas, and gall bladder, the neurons are located in complex networks of ganglia and interconnecting nerves in the walls of these target organs (Fig. 10-19 [see Plate 15]). The two major networks are the **myenteric plexus,** between the longitudinal and circular layers of smooth muscle in the gut, and the **submucosal plexus** between the mucosa and the circular muscle layer. The chemical mediator of the parasympathetic division of the autonomic nervous system is **acetylcholine.**

MENINGES

The **meninges** are three layers of connective tissue covering the brain and spinal cord. The outermost is the **dura mater,** the innermost is the **pia mater,** and an intermediate layer between these is the **arachnoid.**

Dura Mater

The **dura mater** covering the brain consists of dense connective tissue adhering rather loosely to the inner aspect of the skull. It was long thought that there was a "subdural space" between the dura and the underlying arachnoid, but in well-preserved specimens examined with an electron microscope, the two are in contact. At their junction, the inner layer of the dura is evidently a rather weak plane of cleavage in the meninges and extravasation of blood can create a space where none normally exists. Therefore, the "subdural hematoma" that often follows head injuries is not beneath the dura, as the name applies, but is an accumulation of blood within a cleft in the dura.

The dura enclosing the spinal cord is separated from the surrounding periosteum by an **epidural space** that contains very loose connective tissue, a plexus of thin-walled veins, and some adipose cells. The internal and external surfaces of the spinal dura are covered by simple squamous epithe-lium. The inner epithelium is connected to the sides of the spinal cord by a series of slender **denticulate ligaments.** These attachments help to support the spinal cord.

Arachnoid

The **arachnoid** component of the meninges consists of an outer layer of closely apposed cells in contact with the dura and an inner region of long arachnoid trabecular cells that traverse a **subarachnoid space** to connect the arachnoid to the underlying pia mater (Fig. 10-20). This space contains cerebrospinal fluid.

Pia Mater

The **pia mater** is a layer of very loose connective tissue covered, on the side toward the arachnoid, by squamous cells of mesenchymal origin (Fig. 10-20). These cells usually form a thin, single layer. Fine collagenous and elastic fibers are interposed between the layer of squamous pial cells and the underlying neural tissue. The pia mater closely conforms to the surface contours of the brain and spinal cord and is so intimately associated with the arachnoid that they are often considered to be a single layer, the **pia–arachnoid.** Macrophages are common among the pial cells and in the walls of its many blood vessels. In the human, they often contain large amounts of a yellow pigment that reacts positively for iron. Scattered mast cells and small groups of lymphocytes may also be found along the pial blood vessels.

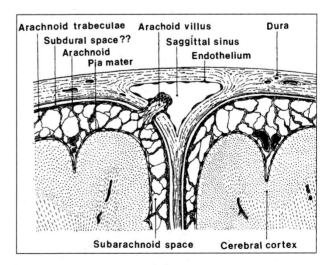

Fig. 10-20 Diagram of the organization of the connective tissue sheaths of the brain. Cerebrospinal fluid, formed in the choroid plexus, circulates in the subarachnoid space and is absorbed into the venous sinuses through the arachnoid villi, one of which is shown projecting into the saggital sinus. The subdural space shown here is now thought to be an artifact. (From L.H. Weed, American Journal of Anatomy 31:191, 1922.)

CHOROID PLEXUSES AND CEREBROSPINAL FLUID

The CNS develops from the embryonic neural tube and is still a hollow organ in the adult. There are two cavities in the end-brain (telencephalon):—the **lateral ventricles,** one in each cerebral hemisphere; a **third ventricle** in the roof of the between-brain (diencephalon); and a **fourth ventricle** in the roof of the hind-brain (pontine region and medulla oblongata). The ventricles are lined by the **ependyma,** a cuboidal epithelium. Its cells have numerous mitochondria, a small Golgi, and some rough endoplasmic reticulum. Some bear motile cilia. A zonula adherens and occasional gap junctions are present on their lateral surfaces, but a zonula occludens is said to be absent. The base of some cells taper into a long process that extends down into the underlying neural tissue.

On the medial wall of the lateral ventricles is an area where neural tissue is lacking, and the highly vascular pia mater over the medial side of the cerebral hemisphere comes into contact with the ependyma. These two layers form elaborate folds that project into the ventricle, forming the **choroid plexus.** The folds, in turn, bear numerous villi, which are diverticuli of the subarachnoid space. Each is capped by modified ependymal epithelium overlying pial blood vessels. The epithelial cells have an atypical brush-border in which the microvilli are expanded at their ends. The choroid plexuses have a surface area estimated to be in excess of 200 cm². Their function is to produce the **cerebrospinal fluid (CSF)** which fills the ventricles and passes out into the subarachnoid space, bathing the entire outer surface of the brain. The fluid is of low density, contains little protein, and has an ionic composition similar to that of blood plasma.

The choroid plexuses in the lateral ventricles maintain the constancy of the fluid environment of the CNS by producing fluid at the rate of 14–36 ml/h. The total volume of CSF (about 150 ml) is replaced four or five times a day. An osmotic gradient across the epithelium results in diffusion of water from the blood into the ventricles. Although water makes up 90% of the fluid, its ionic composition is carefully regulated. Molecules, such as glucose and amino acids needed by the brain, move by facilitated diffusion down the concentration gradient. Other molecules are believed to be actively secreted.

Arachnoid Villi

A thin process of the dura, the **falx cerebri,** extends inward between the two hemispheres of the brain. Situated at its base is the **sagittal venous sinus.** The dura around the sinus is penetrated by many small protrusions of the arachnoid, the **arachnoid villi,** which extend a short distance into the lumen of the sinus (Fig. 10-20). The interior of each villus communicates at its base with the subarachnoid space containing CSF. The fluid in the core of the villus is separated from the blood only by a thin cap of the endothelium of the sinus. In the continual turnover of CSF, the arachnoid villi act as one-way valves permitting flow from the subarachnoid space to the blood. Just how this flow is maintained is debated. Dyes injected into the subarachnoid space are detectable in the blood in from 10 to 30 s.

BLOOD-BRAIN BARRIER

Between the blood and the brain there is an effective **blood-brain barrier.** The barrier depends on special properties of the endothelium of cerebral capillaries. Capillaries elsewhere in the body have fenestrated endothelium or have intercellular junctions that offer little resistance to passage of ions or small molecules. Those of the CNS are not fenestrated and have intercellular tight junctions between endothelial cells that are highly resistant to passage of ions or small molecules. Moreover, these capillaries do not exhibit transendothelial transport in small vesicles. It is speculated that the neuroglial cell processes that surround the capillaries may somehow influence them to express these unique properties. When a dye such as Trypan Blue is injected into the blood, it diffuses through capillary walls and stains most tissues of the body, but the brain remains unstained because of the blood–brain barrier. This barrier serves to protect the brain against abrupt changes in concentration of ions in the extracellular fluid and against molecules in the circulation that might interfere with normal neural function. Nutrients such as glucose and amino acids needed by the neural tissue reach it by facilitated diffusion or active transport across the endothelium.

QUESTIONS*

1. The principal metabolic center of a neuron is its

   A. axon hillock
   B. dendritic tree
   C. axonal arborization
   D. cell body
   E. synaptic vesicles

2. Along its extent from the cell body of origin in the spinal cord to its muscle target in the periphery, the myelin associated with a motor neuron axon is contributed by

   A. oligodendrocytes
   B. Schwann cells
   C. First A then B
   D. First B then A
   E. Neither A nor B

3. The fact that most synaptic transmission is indirect and involves extracellular diffusion of neurotransmitters is best exemplified by the existence of

   A. presynaptic membranes
   B. postsynaptic membranes
   C. gap junctions
   D. axonal transport
   E. synaptic clefts

4. Within the CNS, phagocytosis of cellular debris is carried out by

   A. microglia
   B. protoplasmic astrocytes
   C. fibrous astrocytes
   D. ependymal cells
   E. none of the above

5. In a peripheral nerve, which of the following layers is composed of dense connective tissue?

   A. perineurium
   B. epineurium
   C. endoneurium
   D. all of the above
   E. none of the above

6. The layer of the meningeal covering of the brain which is most like the epineurium of nerves is the

   A. pia
   B. arachnoid
   C. dura
   D. subarachnoid space
   E. venous sinuses

7. The space between two independent segments of the myelin sheath along an axon is known as the

   A. major dense line
   B. intraperiod line
   C. node of Ranvier
   D. Schmidt–Lantermann cleft
   E. mesaxon

8. Within the CNS, myelin is produced by

   A. microglia
   B. fibrous astrocytes
   C. protoplasmic astrocytes
   D. oligodendrocytes
   E. Schwann cells

9. Which of the following cellular structures is found in neuronal cell bodies but not in axons?

   A. rough endoplasmic reticulum
   B. microtubules
   C. mitochondria
   D. membrane vesicles
   E. neurofilaments

10. The term multipolar neuron best refers to a nerve cell which

    A. has multiple axons
    B. has multiple dendrites
    C. synthesizes more than one type of neurotransmitter
    D. is binucleated
    E. is implicated in schizophrenia

11. Choroid plexus is formed where which of the following come into contact?

    A. pia and ependyma
    B. pia and arachnoid
    C. dura and arachnoid
    D. arachnoid and ependyma
    E. dura and ependyma

12. The proper order of the meningeal layers, from most superficial to deepest, is

    A. pia, arachnoid, dura
    B. arachnoid, pia, dura
    C. arachnoid, dura, pia
    D. dura, pia, arachnoid
    E. dura, arachnoid, pia

*Answers on page 307.

11

CIRCULATORY SYSTEM

CHAPTER OUTLINE

Heart
   The Conducting System
Arteries
   Elastic Arteries
   Muscular Arteries
   Arterioles
   Physiology of Arterioles
   Age Changes in Arteries
Capillaries
   Physiology
Veins
Arteriovenous Anastomoses
Carotid Bodies
Carotid Sinus
Lymphatics

KEY WORDS

Annuli Fibrosi	Pericyte
Aorta	Pulmonary
Atrioventricular	Purkinje Fibers
Canal	Membranaceum
Atrioventricular Node	Sheath Cell
Atrium	Sinoatrial Node
Bicuspid Valve	Systole
Bundle of His	Thoracic Duct
Carotid Sinus	Transcytosis
Diastole	Tricuspid Valve
Endocardium	Tunica Adventitia
Epicardium	Tunica Intima
External Elastic	Tunica Media
Lamina	Valves
Glomus Cell	Vasa Vasorum
Internal Elastic	Vasoconstrictor
Lamina	Vasodilator
Interventricular	Vasomotor Center
Septum	Vena Cava
Lactic Acid	Ventricle
Metarterioles	von Willebrandt
Myocardium	Factor
Pacemaker	Weibel–Palade
Pericardium	Bodies

The **circulatory system** (vascular system) distributes oxygen to the tissues of the body and collects carbon dioxide and other waste products of metabolism from them, for elimination by the lungs and kidneys. It consists of a muscular pump, the **heart,** and two systems of blood vessels—the **pulmonary circulation,** carrying blood to and from the lungs, and the **systemic circulation,** distributing blood to all of the other tissues and organs of the body. In both, the blood pumped from the heart passes through **arteries** of diminishing caliber to networks of thin-walled **capillaries,** and then back to the heart through **veins** of increasing caliber.

The initial velocity of blood flowing from the heart into the **aorta** and **pulmonary artery** is about 33 cm/s, but the rate of flow gradually decreases as the total cross-sectional area of the vascular system is increased by repeated branching of the arteries. A further increase in the cross-sectional area of the system occurs rather abruptly at the level of the arterioles and capillaries, resulting in a decrease in rate of flow to about 0.3 cm/s. This slow flow provides ample time for the exchange of metabolites between the blood and the tissues. The extensive networks of capillaries present a total surface area of about 700 m² for this exchange. At any given moment, only about 5% of the blood volume is in the capillaries and 95% is on its way to or from them.

HEART

The heart is the pump of the circulatory system. It consists of four chambers: the **left atrium** discharging its content into the **left ventricle,** and **right atrium** emptying into the **right ventricle.** The right atrium receives venous blood returning from the body and expels it into the right ventricle, which pumps it to the lungs through blood vessels of the **pulmonary circulation.** The left atrium receives oxygenated blood returning from the lungs and expels it into the left ventricle, which pumps it through blood vessels throughout the **systemic circulation** (Fig. 11-1A). Backflow from the aorta and pulmonary artery between beats (diastole) is prevented by cup-shaped tricuspid valves at their base. Similarly, backflow of blood from the ventricles into the atria is prevented by a **tricuspid valve** in the right atrioventricular canal and a **bicuspid valve** in the left atrioventricular canal. The valve leaflets are thin sheets of dense connective tissue covered by squamous endothelium.

The wall of the heart is made up of three layers: the **endocardium,** the **myocardium,** and the **epicardium.** The endocardium is a lining layer of squamous endothelium, underlain by a thin layer of loose connective tissue. Its denser deep portion is continuous with connective tissue that surrounds bundles of cardiac-muscle fibers in the wall of the heart. The myocardium is made up of several layers of cardiac-muscle cells of differing orientation. The fibers of the atria converge upon rings of dense connective tissue around the origins of the aorta and the pulmonary artery. Those of the ventricles insert into similar rings of connective tissue encircling the two atrioventricular orifices. These four rings, called the **annuli fibrosi,** together with the **septum membranaceum** in the upper part of the interventricular septum, constitute the **cardiac skeleton.**

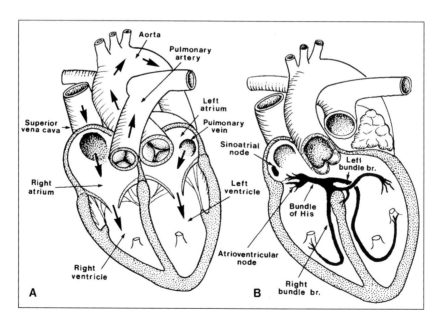

Fig. 11-1 (A) Diagram of the posterior half of the heart showing the path of blood through the chambers and great vessels. (B) Diagram of the impulse generating and conducting system. (Redrawn from L.C. Junquiera, J. Carniero and R.O. Kelly, Basic Histology, Appleton and Lange, 1992.)

*A common cause of heart disease is **rheumatic fever**, an inflammation of connective tissues of the heart and joints following a pharyngeal infection with group A streptococci. Involvement of the endocardium (endocarditis) often leads to thickening and adherence of cusps of the mitral and aortic valves. These lesions may result in narrowing of the atrioventricular orifice (mitral stenosis) and/or backflow of blood from the aorta between beats (aortic regurgitation). Serious impairment of cardiac output may require surgery for valve replacement.*

The Conducting System

For the heart to pump efficiently, the right and left ventricles of the heart must act synchronously, and the contraction of the atria and ventricles must occur sequentially to expel the blood in the atria into the ventricles before their contraction. Coordination of these events of the cardiac cycle depends on an impulse-conducting system made up of modified cardiac-muscle cells that are specialized for generating and conducting impulses throughout the heart. The **pacemaker** of the heart is the **sinoatrial node**, located near the junction of the superior vena cava with the right atrium (Fig. 11-1B). It consists of specialized cardiac-muscle fibers that are more slender than the working atrial-muscle fibers and contain few myofibrils. The fibers of the node undergo spontaneous rhythmic depolarization of their membrane, generating impulses that travel through the myocardium activating the working muscle cells. The node is enclosed in connective tissue and innervated by both divisions of the autonomic nervous system. The heartbeat can be accelerated by nerves of the sympathetic nervous system or slowed by the parasympathetic nerves. The electrical depolarization of fibers in the sinoatrial node spreads over **internodal tracts** of conducting Purkinje fibers to the **atrioventricular node**, located beneath the endocardium of the interatrial septum. The microscopic structure of this node is similar to that of the sinoatrial node. From there, the wave of depolarization is conducted along a tract known as the **atrioventricular bundle of His**, which penetrates the ring of fibrous tissue around the atrioventricular orifice and divides into **right** and **left bundle branches** that course down either side of the interventricular septum beneath the endocardium. The conducting fibers are larger than ventricular muscle fibers and have a few myofibrils around a core of cytoplasm containing the nucleus and a large amount of glycogen. At the apex of the heart, the bundle branches turn back onto the lateral wall of the ventricles and communicate with many working cardiac-muscle cells via gap junctions. This deployment of conducting fibers ensures that the apex of the ventricles begin to contract before their base,

and this facilitates the ejection of blood from the ventricles into the aorta and pulmonary artery.

*The disorder called **heart block** may result from an occlusion of the coronary artery that results in damage to the atrioventricular bundle of His. Coordination of the contractions of the atrium and ventricles is lost and the two chambers beat independently and inefficiently.*

ARTERIES

The walls of the larger blood vessels are made up of three layers: (1) The innermost layer, the **tunica intima**, consists of an endothelium of squamous cells with their long axes oriented longitudinally and supported by a thin underlying layer of areolar connective tissue; (2) an intermediate layer, the **tunica media**, composed of circumferentially oriented smooth-muscle cells; and (3) an outer layer, the **tunica adventitia** consisting of longitudinally oriented fibroblasts and associated collagen fibers (Figs. 11-2 and 11-3). The thickness of the media and adventitia varies greatly in vessels of different size.

In arteries, there is a fenestrated sheet of elastin called the **internal elastic lamina (elastica interna)**, at the boundary between the intima and media. This is especially prominent in arteries of medium caliber (Fig. 11-4). A thinner **external elastic lamina (elastica externa)** is also identifiable between the media and the adventitia of many arteries. From the largest arteries down to the smallest, there is a continuous gradation in the character of their wall. Arteries are classified as (1) **elastic arteries** (conducting arteries), (2) **muscular arteries** (distributing arteries), and (3) **arterioles**, on the basis of their diameter, and

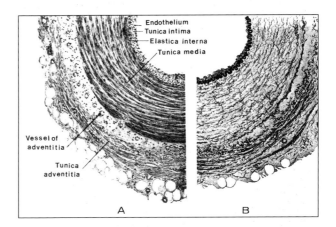

Fig. 11-2 (A) Drawing of the wall of a medium-sized artery, in cross section, showing the tunica intima, media, and adventitia, stained with hemotoxylin and eosin; (B) the same, stained with orcein to reveal the elastin component of the wall.

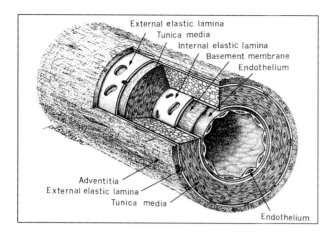

Fig. 11-3 *Schematic representation of the structural components of a medium-sized artery. (Redrawn from Williams and Warwick, in Gray's anatomy. 38th British ed., W.B. Saunders Co., Philadelphia, 1980.)*

the thickness and dominant component of their tunica media. Although this classification is useful for descriptive purposes, there is actually a continuous gradient in the character of the arterial wall from the largest down to the smallest, and it is not always easy to assign a given artery to one of these categories.

Elastic Arteries

The large **elastic arteries** include the pulmonary artery emerging from the right ventricle, the aorta from the left ventricle, and their major branches. Their tunica intima consists of endothelium separated from the elastica interna by a relatively thick layer of connective tissue containing fibroblasts and thin, longitudinally oriented collagen fibers. In electron micrographs, the endothelial cells are unusual in that they contain rodlike cytoplasmic inclusions called **Weibel–Palade bodies** that are sites of storage of the **von Willebrandt factor**, a glycoprotein synthesized and secreted into the blood by all endothelial cells but stored in visible inclusions only in the large elastic arteries. This factor participates in blood clotting.

The tunica media of elastic arteries consists of 20–50 concentric, fenestrated lamellae of elastin, alternating with thin layers of circularly oriented smooth-muscle cells, reticular fibers, and elastin fibrils in a proteoglycan-rich extracellular matrix (Fig. 11-4). In histological sections, internal and external elastic laminae are not distinguishable from the numerous other elastic lamellae of the media. Due to the abundance of these lamellae, smooth muscle makes up a smaller fraction of the media of these large arteries than it does in medium-sized arteries. The adventitia is relatively thin but contains many longitudinal collagen fibers.

In these large elastic arteries, diffusion of metabolites from the lumen is inadequate to meet the needs of the very

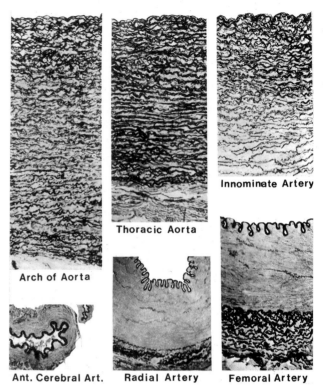

Innominate Artery

Thoracic Aorta

Arch of Aorta

Ant. Cerebral Art.   **Radial Artery**   **Femoral Artery**

Fig. 11-4 *Photomicrographs of the wall of elastic arteries (above) and large muscular arteries (below) showing the differences in thickness of their wall and in the amount of elastin, which appears black. (From E.V. Cowdry, Textbook of Histology, Lea and Febiger, Philadelphia, 1950.)*

thick media, and their adventitia contains small blood vessels, called **vasa vasorum**, that send capillary branches a short distance into the media.

Muscular Arteries

These vessels, of smaller diameter than the elastic arteries, make up the great majority of the arteries in body. Their intima consists of the endothelium and a thin subendothelial layer of areolar connective tissue. The internal elastic lamina is prominent and, in vessels that have contracted upon immersion in fixative it has a scalloped or folded appearance (Figs.11-5[see Plate 15] and 11-6). The tunica media consists of a conspicuous layer of circumferentially oriented smooth-muscle fibers and associated reticular fibers (Fig. 11-7). There are no elastic laminae in the media, but there are varying numbers of slender elastic fibers. The elastin and collagen are produced by the smooth-muscle cells. An external elastic lamina is present only in the largest muscular arteries. The tunica adventitia consists of scattered fibroblasts and longitudinally oriented collagen fibers that merge with those of the surrounding connective tissue.

The thickness of the media in muscular varies according to the blood pressure in the system at that level. For

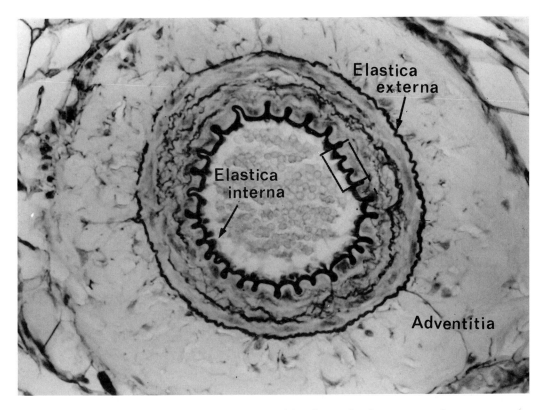

Fig. 11-6 Photomicrograph of a muscular artery stained for elastin. The elastin interna, elastica externa, the media and an unusually thick adventitia are easily distinguished.

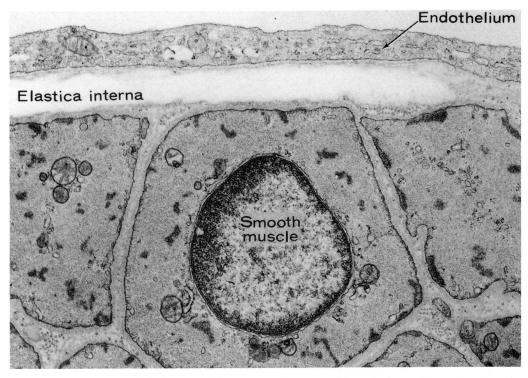

Fig. 11-7 Electron micrograph of a longitudinal section of a portion of the wall of a small muscular artery. The elastica interna is unstained and appears as a clear area between the endothelium (above) and the smooth muscle of the tunica media (below).

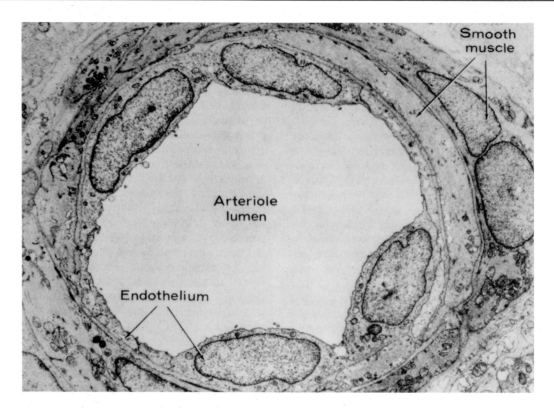

Fig. 11-8 Electron micrograph of a small arteriole. Note the single layer of smooth-muscle cells around the endothelium.

example, the coronary arteries of the heart, which are subjected to relatively high pressure, have thicker media than other muscular arteries. On the other hand, blood pressure in the pulmonary circulation is considerably lower and the tunica media of arteries in the lung is relatively thin.

Arterioles

The small muscular arteries and the **arterioles** are physiologically important elements of the circulatory system, for they are the major component of the peripheral resistance to blood flow that regulates the blood pressure. Arterioles range in diameter from 200 μm down to 40 μm. The tunica intima includes the endothelium and a very thin subendothelial layer of reticular fibers. A very thin, fenestrated elastica interna is present in the larger arterioles but absent in the terminal arterioles. In the larger arterioles, the tunica media consists of one or two layers of circular smooth-muscle cells. In the smallest arterioles, there may be a single layer in which the individual smooth muscle cells are long enough to completely encircle the tube of endothelium (Fig. 11-8). Collagen fibers and occasional fibroblasts form a thin adventitia. In the transition from **terminal arterioles** to capillaries, the smooth-muscle layer becomes discontinuous. Individual smooth-muscle cells, spaced a short distance apart, completely encircle the tube of endothelium. Such vessels are sometimes called

metarterioles. Where they are continuous with capillaries, the circular smooth-muscle cells act as a **precapillary sphincter**. Their contraction slows or stops flow through a region of the capillary network. Blood may flow, instead, directly to venules through lateral branches, somewhat larger than capillaries, that bypass the capillary bed. Whether these remain open or closed depends on the metabolic needs of the local tissues.

Physiology of Arteries

The intermittent contraction of the heart results in a pulsatile flow of blood in the large **elastic arteries**. The abundant elastic tissue in their walls enables them to expand slightly during contraction of the heart (systole), storing some of the force of the heartbeat. The potential energy so accumulated is dissipated in the elastic recoil of their wall in the interval between heartbeats (diastole). Their recoil thus serves as an auxiliary pump, forcing the blood onward when no force is being exerted by the heart. This ensures a continuous flow through the capillaries despite the intermittent contraction of the heart.

Impulses continuously generated in the **vasomotor center** of the brain travel via the spinal cord to the sympathetic chain of ganglia and then over **vasomotor nerves** to the arteries. As a result of these nerve impulses, smooth muscle in the media of medium-sized and small arteries is maintained in a state of partial contraction called **vasomotor tone**. The nerves to the blood vessel walls include both **vasoconstrictor** and **vasodilator fibers**, providing for decrease or increase in the caliber of the vessels. Because the arteries offer the principal resistance to blood flow, a generalized vasoconstriction results in a marked rise in the blood pressure. A change in the caliber of a single distributing artery increases or decreases the flow to the tissue or organ served by that vessel (Fig. 11-9).

Products of tissue injury may cause local vasoconstriction, an effect that limits blood loss from the site. Conversely, oxygen deprivation and accumulation of lactic acid in an area of tissue causes relaxation of smooth muscle in the arteries and consequent vasodilatation. This so-called **reactive hyperemia** is independent of the nervous system. It serves to correct any local deficit of oxygen or other metabolites.

Age Changes in Arteries

The walls of large arteries normally continue to undergo developmental changes from birth to age 25. There is progressive thickening of the wall of elastic arteries with development of increasing numbers of elastic lamellae. In muscular arteries, there is an increase in the thickness of the media. From middle age onward, there is a continuous slow thickening of the intima of the arteries, with an increase in collagen and a migration of some smooth-muscle cells from the media into the intima. These tend to accumulate lipid droplets rich in cholesterol esters. These diffuse normal changes with aging are described as **arteriosclerosis**. They are not to be confused with the pathological process of **atherosclerosis**. This consists of patchy accumulation of lipid-filled smooth-muscle cells, macrophages, and fibrous tissue

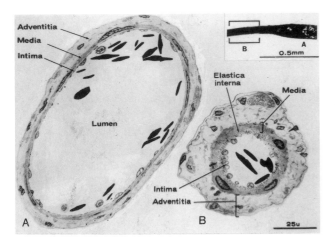

Fig. 11-9 A dramatic example of vasoconstriction. A microdroplet of norepinephrine was applied to a living vessel, causing vasoconstriction of the area indicated by brackets in the inset. The vessel was then fixed and sectioned. Cross sections less than 2 mm apart are shown at A and B. (From P.C. Phelps, and J.H. Luft, American Journal of Anatomy 125:399, 1969.)

that form elevated plaques in the intima. Platelets may adhere to their rough surface, initiating the formation of a blood clot that occludes the lumen. When this occurs in a coronary artery, it causes a "heart attack" (**myocardial infarction**). When it occurs in an artery in the brain, it causes a "stroke" (**cerebral thrombosis**).

CAPILLARIES

Capillaries are thin-walled endothelium-lined tubes of uniform diameter that branch repeatedly to form extensive networks throughout the tissues of the body (Figs. 11-10 [see Plate 16] and 11-11). Their diameter of 8–11 μm is just large enough to permit unimpeded passage of blood cells. A capillary forming one mesh of the network is only 0.25–1 μm in length, but the total length of the capillaries in the body is estimated to be 40,000 miles or more. The capillary wall is an extremely thin endothelium with a basal lamina supported by a loose network of reticular fibers (Fig. 11-11). There is no media or adventitia. The endothelial cells are elongated in the direction of blood flow and the cell nucleus is flattened and thus appears elliptical in cross sections. The thicker perinuclear region of the cytoplasm bulges slightly into the lumen, but the attenuated peripheral portion of the cell is so thin that the adlumenal and ablumenal membranes are separated by a layer of cytoplasm only 0.2–0.4 μm in thickness. The cells have few organelles. The lumenal surface of the endothelium is smooth, but the thin margins of adjacent cells may overlap, with the free edge of the uppermost cell projecting a short distance into the lumen. Zonulae adherentes and desmosomes are rare or absent, but freeze-fracture preparations reveal a few strands in the opposing membranes that resemble those of the zonula occludens of other epithelia. However, there are discontinuities in these occluding cell junctions through which a small amount of fluid or emigrating leukocytes can pass.

Most capillaries are similar in appearance in histological sections, but with the electron microscope, two principal types can be distinguished. Muscle, brain, connective tissues, and lung have **continuous capillaries** (somatic capillaries) in which the endothelium is uninterrupted (Figs. 11-11 and 11-12A). The pancreas, endocrine glands, intestinal villi, and renal glomeruli have **fenestrated capillaries** (visceral capillaries) in which the thin peripheral portions of the endothelial cells are traversed by minute circular **pores**, 60–70 nm in diameter, each closed by a thin **pore diaphragm** (Figs. 11-12B and 11-13). In certain areas of the cell, the pores are uniformly distributed with a center-to-center spacing of about 130 nm, whereas other areas are unfenestrated.

Spaced at intervals along the outside of capillaries are cells called **pericytes** that have primary processes deployed longitudinally along the capillary wall, and secondary lateral processes extending around the vessel (Figs.

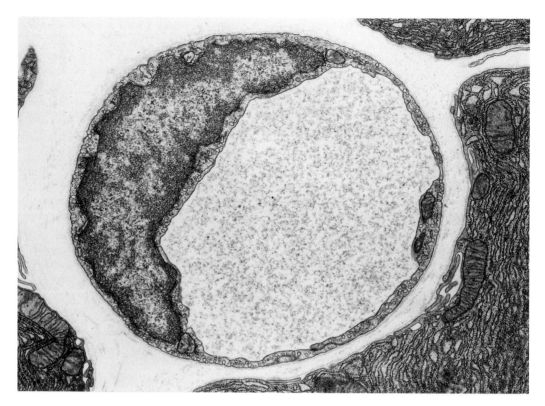

Fig. 11-11 Electron micrograph of a continuous capillary. In this example, the entire circumference of the vessel is made up of a single endothelial cell. (Micrograph courtesy of R. Bolender.)

11-14 and 11-15). The pericytes are covered by a thin external lamina that is continuous with the basal lamina of the endothelium, except at focal gap junctions between pericyte processes and the underlying endothelial cells. Their cytoplasm contains microtubules in the axis of the processes and bundles of filaments in the peripheral cytoplasm that terminate in densities on the inner aspect of the plasmalemma. It was long speculated that the pericytes might be contractile. This has now been verified by the finding that they contain tropomyosin, myosin of smooth-muscle type, and a protein kinase similar to one which is involved in contraction of striated muscle.

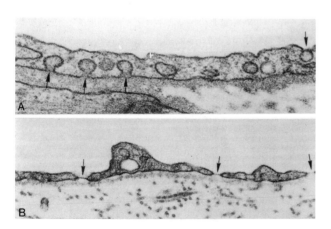

Fig. 11-12 Electron micrographs of short segments of endothelium (A) from a continuous capillary and (B) from a fenestrated capillary. Note the thin diaphragms closing the pores of the fenestrated capillary. (Micrographs courtesy of E. Weihe.)

A third type of capillary is found in the liver, bone marrow, and spleen. These vessels, having a larger diameter (30–40 µm) and a variable cross-sectional shape, are called **sinuses** or **sinusoidal capillaries**. They have multiple discontinuities in their wall that are much larger than the pores of visceral capillaries, and these are not closed by diaphragms. Blood cells easily cross the wall of the sinuses in the bone marrow and spleen. Macrophages are closely associated with the wall of sinuses in the liver and, in some cases, appear to be included in the endothelium.

Physiology

The mechanism of exchange across the capillary wall was long a subject of lively debate. This has been clarified by studies involving intravascular injection of electron-opaque molecules of known dimensions greater than 10 nm. In continuous capillaries, these particles are rapidly taken up in small flask-shaped vesicles (**caveolae**) opening onto the adlumenal surface of the endothelium. These are then closed and ferried across the cytoplasm to discharge their content into the extravascular space by fusion of the vesicles with the ablumenal plasmalemma (Fig. 11-12A). Transient transendothelial channels may be formed by fusion of endocytosis vesicles. The term **transcytosis** has been suggested to distinguish this activity from pinocytosis in other cell types, where such vesicles do not cross the cell but are a mechanism for uptake of substances for use by the cell.

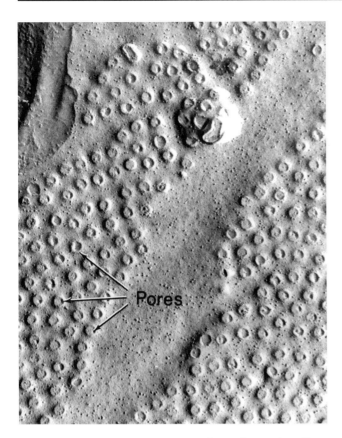

Fig. 11-13 Freeze-fracture preparation of a small area of capillary endothelium showing the numerous uniformly spaced pores.

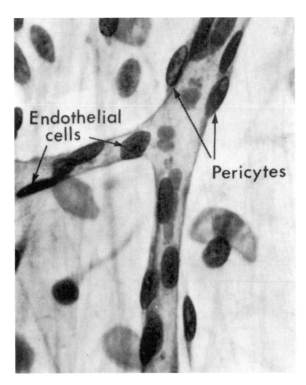

Fig. 11-14 Photomicrograph of an intact capillary in a whole mount of rat mesentery. The nuclei of the endothelial cells lining the capillary can be distinguished from those of the pericytes which bulge outward from the wall.

In fenestrated capillaries, injected macromolecules pass freely through the pores. The capillaries of the renal glomeruli are unique in having an unusually thick basal lamina and pores lacking a diaphragm. Fluid and particulate tracers traverse the wall of these capillaries nearly 100 times more rapidly than in continuous muscle capillaries.

Intravenously injected dyes that readily leave the capillaries of most tissues are retained in the lumen of brain capillaries. The endothelial cells of these capillaries are joined by uninterrupted tight junctions. These are believed to be the basis for the so-called **blood-brain barrier**. A blood-ocular barrier and blood-thymus barrier depend on similar properties of their capillaries.

The function of endothelial cells is not confined to providing a smooth, nonthrombogenic lining for the capillaries. They are able to degrade lipoproteins in the plasma to yield fatty acids that are utilized by the surrounding tissue or are stored in adipose cells. Under certain circumstances, they can secrete molecules that are involved in blood clotting (**platelet-activating factor**). At sites of inflammation, they secrete, onto their surface, adhesion molecules that facilitate the emigration of neutrophilic leukocytes.

VEINS

The capillary networks are drained by **venules**, thin-walled vessels only slightly larger than capillaries. Their

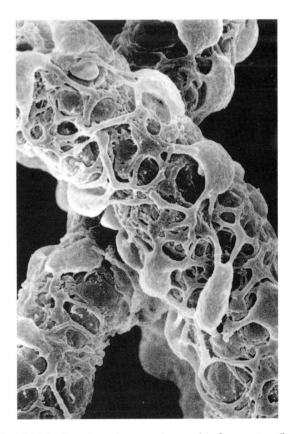

Fig. 11-15 Scanning electron micrograph of a postcapillary venule, showing highly branched pericyte processes forming a lace-like network over the surface of the vessel. (From T. Fujiwara and Y. Uehara, *American Journal of Anatomy* 170:38, 1984.)

wall consists of endothelium and occasional pericytes enclosed within a basal lamina. Exchange of metabolites between the blood and the tissues continues in the smallest venules, and in acute inflammation, these are the principal vessels through which fluid escapes to produce the local swelling (edema). Leukocytes emigrating from the blood to attack the bacteria also pass through the wall of small venules. Slightly larger venules (0.2–1 mm) have a layer of smooth muscle around the endothelium and more collagen fibers.

Small and medium-sized **veins** have an intima of endothelium with little or no subendothelial connective tissue. A thin internal elastic lamina is rarely detectable, and their media consists of one or two layers of circular smooth-muscle with associated reticular and elastic fibers. The media is much thinner and less compact than that of arteries of comparable size (Fig. 11-16 [see Plate 16]). The adventitia consists of longitudinally oriented collagen, elastic fibers, and fibroblasts, and it is thick, relative to the adventitia of arteries of comparable diameter.

A distinctive feature of medium-sized veins is the presence of **valves**. These consist of two semilunar folds of the intima that project into the lumen from opposite sides. Although normally pressed against the lining epithelium by the flow of blood toward the heart, any obstruction of the vessel distal to them causes the free edges of the valve leaflets to come together, preventing the retrograde flow of blood. The space between a closed valve cusp and the vessel wall is called the **sinus** of the valve. Just above the arc of attachment of the valve cusps, the vessel wall is thinner. In distended veins, this thinner region bulges slightly, making it possible to locate the site of valves, with the naked eye, in the intact vessel. Valves are numerous in veins of the legs, where they are needed to prevent backflow due to the force of gravity on the column of blood.

Large veins include the vena cava, portal, splenic, external iliac, and azygos veins. These have a thicker subendothelial layer of connective tissue. In general, the media is poorly developed and contains little circular smooth muscle. The relatively thick adventitia of large veins is rich in elastic fibers and longitudinally oriented collagen fibers. Where the vena cava and pulmonary vein enter the heart, strands of cardiac muscle may extend a short distance into their wall.

The thick adventitia of large veins contains the small nutrient vessels, called **vasa vasorum**. These are needed to maintain viability of the outer portion of the wall, for the distance from the lumen is relatively long and the venous blood carries no oxygen.

ARTERIOVENOUS ANASTOMOSES

In many parts of the body, lateral branches of small arteries are directly connected to veins by **arteriovenous anastomoses**. Three morphologically distinct segments

are recognizable along their length. The initial segment is similar in structure to the small artery of which it is a branch. The terminal segment resembles the small vein with which it is confluent. Between these is a contractile intermediate segment with a wall unusually thick for a vessel of its size. It has a subendothelial layer of longitudinally oriented, modified smooth-muscle cells. When this segment is contracted, blood flows through the capillary bed. When it is relaxed, blood can flow directly from small arteries to small veins bypassing the local capillaries. Arteriovenous anastomoses therefore play an important role in regulating blood flow to a region. They are abundant in the skin, where they enable the body to conserve heat by diverting the blood away from the superficial network of capillaries.

CAROTID BODIES

Although sensory nerves are associated with arteries throughout the vascular system, they are especially abundant in the **carotid bodies** that have an important role in regulating respiration, heart beat, and the vasomotor activities that control blood pressure. These are inconspicuous organs (3×5 mm) at the bifurcation of the common carotid artery. They contain **chemoreceptors** responsive to changes in the oxygen, carbon dioxide, and hydrogen ion concentrations of the blood. The carotid body consists of multiple clusters of pale-staining **type-I cells (glomus cells)** surrounded by **type-II cells (sheath cells)**. These, in turn, are surrounded by connective tissue that contains many fenestrated capillaries. The most distinctive feature of the type-I cells is the presence of numerous dense-cored vesicles (60–200 nm) in their cytoplasm. These contain dopamine and other neurotransmitters. The sheath cells have thin lamellar processes that envelop clusters of two to six type-I cells. The exact location of the chemoreceptor function of the carotid bodies is in dispute, but it is the prevailing view that the membrane of the type-I cells contains a heme protein that binds oxygen. In the presence of adequate partial pressures of oxygen, K+ channels associated with the heme protein are open and Ca channels are closed. In anoxia, the K+ channels close, Ca channels open, and the type-I cells release neurotransmitters that stimulate afferent nerves communicating with regulatory centers in the brain controlling respiration. Similar **aortic bodies**, situated on the arch of the aorta, are assumed to have much the same function as the carotid bodies.

CAROTID SINUS

The **carotid sinus** is a slightly dilated region of the internal carotid artery, where the wall is thinner and contains many sensory nerves. Its nerves are stimulated by stretch and the thinning of the media in this region makes

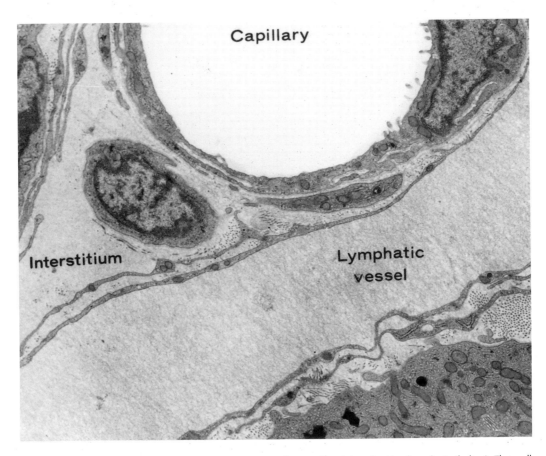

Fig. 11-17 Electron micrograph permitting comparison of a capillary (above) with a lymphatic (below). The wall consists of a very thin endothelium with no associated pericytes.

the wall more distensible. The carotid sinus therefore serves as a **baroceptor** that reacts to changes in blood pressure and initiates afferent impulses to centers in the brain. These, in turn, generate efferent impulses that cause vasodilation or vasoconstriction of peripheral arteries and thus maintain blood pressure within normal limits.

LYMPHATICS

In addition to the blood vascular system, the body has a **lymphatic system** made up of thin-walled vessels that carry excess fluid from the interstitial compartment back to the blood. Fluid collected in **lymphatic capillaries** in the periphery is conducted through vessels of increasing size to empty into the circulatory system by two main ducts: the **thoracic duct** and the **right lymphatic duct**. These join the blood vascular system at the junction of the subclavian and internal jugular veins. The clear fluid transported in the lymphatics is called **lymph**. Occasional lymphocytes and smaller particulates in the lymph are filtered out in **lymph nodes** that are interposed in the system at intervals along the path of lymph flow. (See Chapter 12). The lymphatic system is not a circulation system, it is a drainage system.

Lymphatic capillaries are far more variable in size and in cross-sectional outline than are blood capillaries

(Figs. 11-16 [see Plate 16] and 11-17). The endothelium is very thin and there are no tight junctions between cells. A continuous basal lamina is usually absent, but **lymphatic anchoring filaments** extend into the surrounding tissue from small plaques of basement membrane-like material on the ablumenal side of the endothelial cells. These filaments help to maintain the patency of these thin-walled vessels. The endothelial cells are not fenestrated. Lymphatic vessels larger than capillaries have a somewhat thicker wall, but thinner than small veins of comparable size. Three layers are not discernible in the wall. At close intervals along their length, they have bicuspid valves similar to those of veins. Valves are essential to the function of the lymph vascular system which has no pump comparable to the heart. The flow of lymph from the extremities depends, in large measure, on the massaging effect of contraction of the surrounding muscles. The largest lymphatics have some smooth muscle in their wall, they are innervated, and there is visual and cinematographic evidence of their contractility. This may explain lymph flow in organs where there is no muscle-generated movement around them.

The large **lymphatic ducts** have a structure like that of veins, but the wall is thinner and contains smooth-muscle fibers oriented both circularly and longitudinally. The adventitia is relatively thin.

QUESTIONS*

1. Which description is **incorrect** about muscular arteries?

   A. muscular tunica adventitia
   B. an inner elastic membrane
   C. muscular tunica media
   D. vasa vasorum in tunica adventitia
   E. none of the above

2. The sinoatrial node (pacemaker) is found in

   A. the left atrium
   B. the right atrium
   C. the left ventricle
   D. the right ventricle
   E. none of the above

3. The most abundant tissue in the aorta is

   A. dense irregular connective tissue
   B. smooth muscle
   C. elastic
   D. elastic cartilage
   E. none of the above

4. This component of the wall of vascular tissue contains the vasa vasorum:

   A. tunica intima
   B. tunica media
   C. tunica adventitia
   D. all of the above
   E. none of the above

5. The muscular layer of the blood vessels is known as the

   A. tunica intima
   B. tunica media
   C. tunica adventitia
   D. mesothelium
   E. endothelium

6. Sinusoids are a type of

   A. capillary
   B. artery
   C. vein
   D. lymph vessel
   E. Purkinje fiber

7. The aorta is an example of a/an

   A. elastic artery
   B. muscular artery
   C. arteriole
   D. medium vein
   E. large vein

8. Muscular arteries are characterized by

   A. an inner elastic membrane
   B. an external elastic membrane
   C. decreased elastic material in the tunica media
   D. A and B
   E. all of the above

9. Veins differ from arteries in that they generally

   A. have thinner walls
   B. have larger lumens
   C. contain valves
   D. A and C
   E. A, B, and C

10. The cell type which is sometimes found partially surrounding the capillary endothelial cells and may have a contractile function is called a

    A. myocyte
    B. smooth-muscle cell
    C. pericyte
    D. myoblast
    E. fibroblast

*Answers on page 307.

12

IMMUNE SYSTEM

CHAPTER OUTLINE

KEY WORDS

The **immune system** includes the **lymphocytes** of the blood, the **plasma cells** and **macrophages** of the connective tissues, and the lymphoid organs, **thymus, spleen, lymph nodes,** and the **lymphoid nodules** of the gastrointestinal tract. Collectively, the cells of the system defend the body against microorganisms by generating an **immune response** to the invaders. There are two kinds of immune response: (1) the **humoral immune response,** which depends on B lymphocytes producing **antibodies** that bind to the invader and contribute to its destruction and (2) the **cell-mediated immune response** in which cytotoxic T lymphocytes directly attack and lyse foreign cells.

For these mechanisms to succeed, the cells of the immune system must be able to distinguish the body's own cells (self) from those of an invader (nonself). All of our cells have protein surface molecules, called the **major histocompatability complex (MHC),** that have a structure unique to each individual. These molecules fall into two classes—**MHC-I**, found on all cells of the body, and **MHC-II** that are largely confined to the lymphocytes and macrophages of the immune system.

HUMORAL IMMUNE RESPONSE

The principal agents of the humoral immune response are **B lymphocytes** (Fig. 12-1), but these require the cooperation of macrophages and a class of T lymphocytes called **helper T lymphocytes**. During their differentiation in the blood-forming organs, B lymphocytes synthesize **immunoglobulin** molecules and display them on their surface. These are large Y-shaped protein molecules (Fig. 12-2) that have, in the amino acid chains of their diverging arms, identical amino acid sequences that serve as **recognition sites,** enabling the cell to identify and bind to foreign protein. The gene-encoding immunoglobulin consists of several separate segments (minigenes) in different regions of the chromosomes. Before transcription, these must be assembled into a single complete gene. In this process, the several segments are arranged in different sequences in different B cells, and the enzyme that joins the segments randomly inserts extra coding units between their ends. These events result in very great variability in the chemical structure of the immunoglobulin molecules. Hundreds of thousands of different sequences are represented in the immunoglobulins of cells in the B-lymphocyte population. Thus, for any foreign protein, there will be some lymphocytes with matching sequences, and those cells will bind to that foreign protein and initiate synthesis of **antibody** specific for that protein. An antibody is an immunoglobulin molecule that reacts specifically with a foreign molecule (usually a protein or polypeptide). Any foreign (non-self) molecule that induces the immune system to produce antibodies specific for that molecule is referred to as an **antigen.**

For example, when bacteria enter the body, some of the invaders are ingested by macrophages and digested intracellularly (Fig. 12-3). Small residues, usually polypeptides, of bacterial origin are joined to molecules of the **major histocompatability complex** (MHC-II) and inserted into the membrane of the macrophage. This complex constitutes the **antigen** that initiates a humoral immune response. B lymphocytes are not able to respond directly to bacteria with production of antibodies. The bacteria must first be processed by macrophages and antigen presented at their surface in combination with MHC molecules. Thus, macrophages and certain other cell types with similar properties, are commonly referred to as **antigen-presenting cells**.

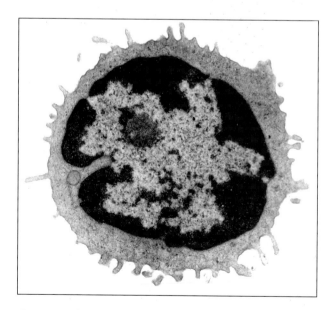

Fig. 12-1 Electron micrograph of a typical small lymphocyte. B lymphocytes cannot be distinguished from T lymphocytes without using labeled antibody to specific surface markers.

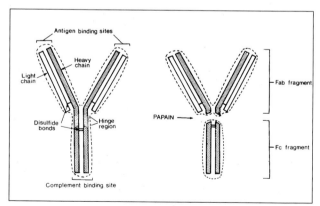

Fig. 12-2 (A) Drawing of the structure of a monomeric immunoglobulin molecule. It is made up of two longer heavy chains and two shorter light chains in a Y-shaped configuration. At the stem end, there is a complement-binding region, and at the ends of the arms, are two antigen-binding regions. (B) Treatment with papain cleaves the molecule into two Fab fragments that bind antibody and one Fc fragment that binds complement.

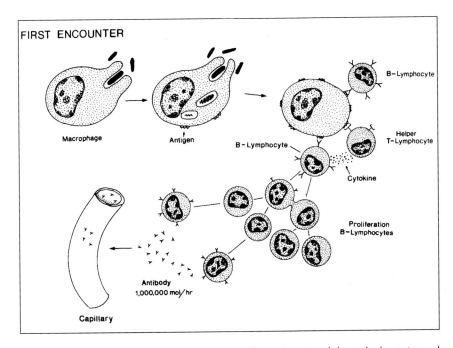

Fig. 12-3 In a primary immune response, macrophages ingest and digest the bacteria, and insert into their membrane a polypeptide of bacterial origin that serves as an antigen. B and helper T lymphocytes bind to the antigen. The helper T lymphocytes release cytokines that activate the B lymphocytes to proliferate, resulting in many more B cells, responding to the antigen. These all produce and release large amounts of specific antibody.

Patrolling B lymphocytes that have surface immunoglobulins that match the antigen presented will bind to it. Binding of the B lymphocytes stimulates them to begin synthesis of **antibody** specific for that antigen. Circulating **helper T lymphocytes** also have variable **antigen receptors** that are not immunoglobulins. Those helper T cells that have receptors matching the antigen presented will bind and secrete diffusable signaling molecules called **cytokines** (lymphokines) that stimulate the B lymphocytes to proliferate, thus producing many more B cells, all of which make antibody specific to that antigen (Figs. 12-3 and 12-4). The activated B lymphocytes each make up to 1 × 10⁶ antibody molecules per hour and these are released into the circulation. Thus, the humoral immune response depends on activation and proliferation of only certain cells of the body's population of B lymphocytes, a process called **clonal selection**.

There are some 8×10^{12} B lymphocytes in the circulation and in the lymphoid organs. Many of these have been programmed in previous immune responses to respond to a host of different antigens. A second exposure to one of these initiates a **secondary immune response**. Upon a second encounter with the same species of bacteria, the diverging arms (*Fab* portion) of the circulating Y-shaped antibody molecules bind to the bacteria (Fig. 12-5). The macrophages have receptors on their surface that bind the other end (*Fc* portion) of the Y-shaped antibody molecules. The antibody thus serves as an **opsonin**, a substance that enhances phagocytosis by binding both to the bacteria and

to the surface of the macrophages. This opsonization of the bacteria greatly accelerates the uptake and processing of the antigen and the rate of development of the immune response. Thus, in a secondary immune response the titer of circulating antibody rapidly rises to 10–100 times the previous level. Many of the B cells remain in, or migrate into, the connective tissues and develop there into **plasma cells** that continue to produce antibody for weeks after the initiation of the secondary response.

Five classes of immunoglobulins are identifiable in the blood and tissue fluids. Of these, **immunoglobulin-G (IgG)** makes up 75% of the antibody produced in humoral immune reactions. A smaller amount is **immunoglobulin-E (IgE)**, formed mainly in response to foreign proteins other than microorganisms. This class binds to receptors on mast cells and basophil leukocytes and causes their release of the histamine that is responsible for many of the discomforts associated with allergies. **Immunoglobulin-A (IgA)** secreted by plasma cells is present in the secretions of the salivary glands, tear glands, intestinal glands, and glands of the respiratory tract, and endows those secretions with protective antibacterial properties.

The random rearrangement of immunoglobulin gene segments in differentiating B lymphocytes inevitably results in some cells bearing immunoglobulins that would react to proteins on the body's own cells. However, the immediate and overwhelming exposure of these **self-reactive B lymphocytes** to the surrounding MHC-I-bearing cells of the bone marrow causes them to undergo apoptosis.

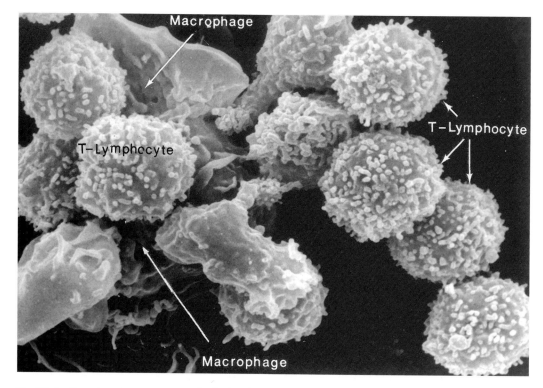

Fig. 12-4 Scanning electron micrograph of T lymphocytes clustered around, and closely associated with, the surface of a macrophage engaged in antigen presentation (Courtesy of M.H. Nielsen and O. Werdelin.)

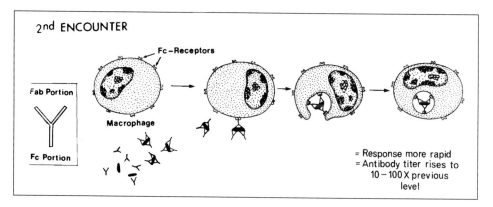

Fig. 12-5 The arms of the antibody molecule (*Fab* portion) bind to antigen. The stem of the Y (*Fc* portion) binds to receptors on the surface of macrophages. In a second encounter with the same bacteria, antibody binds to the bacteria and this complex binds to *Fc* receptors on macrophages. This greatly facilitates uptake and destruction of the bacteria. The secondary immune response is therefore more rapid and efficient, resulting in a 10–100-fold increase in circulating antibody.

Therefore, only B lymphocytes that are not reactive to self are released from the bone marrow into the bloodstream.

CELL-MEDIATED IMMUNE RESPONSE

The cell-mediated immune response is carried out by a subpopulation of lymphocytes, called **cytotoxic T lymphocytes**. These are able to identify, and bind to, infected cells containing viruses or larger parasites that are not accessible to B lymphocytes. MHC molecules synthesized in the endoplasmic reticulum of infected cells serve as transport proteins for antigenic peptides of the virus or parasite. The peptide residing in a groove in the MHC molecule is encorporated in the cell membrane. The presence of the peptide, in association with MHC, informs the T cells that the cell is infected, and they bind to it (Fig. 12-6). Cytotoxic T lymphocytes have small granules in their cytoplasm that contain a chemical called **perforin** and proteases. Binding of T lymphocytes stimulates their release of perforin, which forms holes in the target-cell membrane through which the proteases enter. The cell undergoes lysis

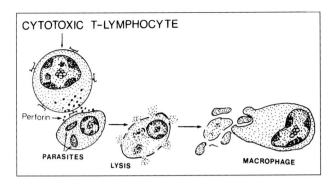

Fig. 12-6 T lymphocytes are able to recognize and bind to cells containing parasites or viruses. Activated by binding, they secrete perforin, a chemical that makes holes in the target cell. This causes the cell to lyse and its fragments are ingested by macrophages.

and macrophages dispose of its remnants (Fig. 12-6).

The cytotoxic T lymphocytes are also the principal agents of the rejection of tissue grafts and transplanted organs. For example, if skin is grafted from one individual to another to cover a severely burned area (Fig. 12-7), patrolling lymphocytes recognize the surrounding skin as "self" and pay no attention to it. However, upon contacting cells of the skin graft, which have on their surface MHC molecules differing from those of the graft recipient, they recognize these as foreign (non-self) and bind to them. This activates the lymphocytes to secrete a cytokine that diffuses to the underlying capillaries where it causes many lymphocytes, circulating in the blood, to adhere to the wall of the blood vessel and migrate through its wall. These migrate up the concentration gradient of the cytokine and attach to the cells of the skin graft (Fig. 12-7). The large number of assembled cytotoxic T lymphocytes secrete perforin, lysing the cells and causing rejection of the skin graft. However, if the skin graft is taken from an identical twin, whose cells would have on their surface MHC molecules identical to those of the graft recipient, the cytotoxic T lymphocytes would recognize them as "self" and would not reject the graft. In the transplantation of organs, which has now become common, the surgery is relatively easy, but the major challenge is in treating the recipient with reagents that block the immune system to prevent rejection of the transplanted organ.

THYMUS

The **thymus** is a lymphoid organ situated in the chest, anterior to the great vessels that emerge from the heart. It is quite large early in life, weighing about 40 g at puberty, but it then slowly regresses to a fraction of this size in older adults. Although its parenchyma is gradually replaced by adipose cells and fibrous tissue, it remains functional. It consists of two lobes, each invested by a thin capsule, from which connective tissue septa extend inward, subdividing each lobe into small lobules (Fig. 12-8). Each lobule has a

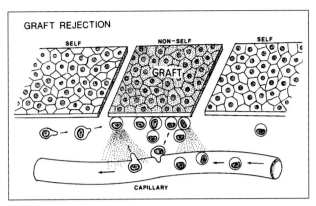

Fig. 12-7 If skin from another individual is grafted to cover a burned area, T lymphocytes wandering through underlying tissue recognize it as nonself and bind to it. They then release a cytokine that diffuses to underlying capillaries where it induces great numbers of lymphocytes to migrate through the vessel wall and up the concentration gradient of the cytokine to join in the attack on the foreign cells. Their combined efforts result in rejection of the graft.

deeply staining peripheral zone, the **cortex**, and a lighter staining central portion, the **medulla** (Fig. 12-9 [see Plate 17]). The principal cell types of the thymus are lymphocytes, macrophages, and reticular cells. Immediately beneath the capsule there is a nearly continuous layer of **epithelial reticular cells**. Deep to this bounding layer, lymphocytes completely fill the interstices of a three-dimensional network of **stellate reticular cells** that have a pale-staining nucleus and acidophilic cytoplasm. Their tapering cell processes are adherent to one another at desmosomes.

In the embryo, the thymus is the first organ to become populated by lymphocytes. It is first seeded with blood-borne lymphoblasts from the yolk sac of the embryo, and later lymphoblasts and prolymphocytes from the liver and bone marrow. In the thymus, these undergo intensive proliferation in the cortex of the lobules, and their progeny differentiate as they slowly move inward toward the medulla. Those in the outer cortex are large and immature and those in the medulla are smaller, mature T lymphocytes. Many of the lymphocytes in the inner cortex and outer medulla have a pycnotic nucleus and appear to be in the process of dying. It is believed that only a small percentage of the thymic T lymphocytes complete their differentiation and leave the organ to populate the other lymphoid organs and the connective tissues of the body. The reason for the death of enormous numbers of lymphocytes in the thymus long puzzled histologists, but recent advances in immunology have provided a possible explanation that will be presented later in the chapter.

In the medulla, lymphocytes are less closely packed than in the cortex, and the reticular cells are more prominent. The reticular cells vary in their appearance and several types have been described. The functional significance of this diversity is not understood. Cells of one type aggregate and become flattened and concentrically arranged to form bodies called **Hassall's corpuscles** (Fig. 12-10 [see

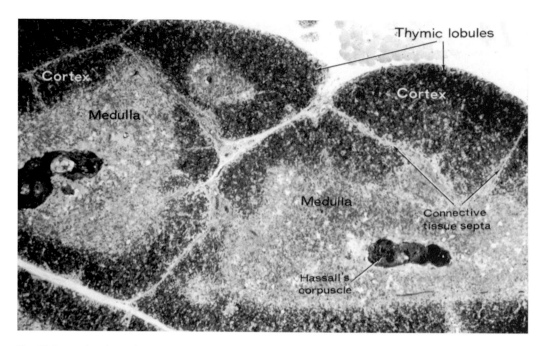

Fig. 12-8 An histological section of the thymus. The thymic lobes are made up of roughly polygonal lobules separated by connective tissue septa. Each lobule has a densely staining peripheral cortex and a paler-staining central region, the medulla. (Courtesy of G.B. Schneider and S. Clark, Jr.)

Plate 16]). The cells in the center of these peculiar bodies lose their nucleus and become filled with keratohyalin granules and keratin filaments. The significance of Hassall's corpuscles is unknown.

Blood Supply

The arteries supplying the thymus ramify in the perilobular connective tissue, and their branches follow the septa inward to enter the parenchyma at the corticomedullary boundary. There, arterioles give off branches that turn inward to the medulla, and capillaries course outward into the cortex. In the outer cortex, these small vessels form branching and anastomosing arcades that turn back toward the medulla. In their recurrent course through the cortex, they join to form somewhat larger capillaries that are confluent with postcapillary venules at the corticomedullary boundary. Joined by venules from the medulla, these leave the thymic parenchyma via the connective tissue septa and join comparable vessels from other lobules to form the interlobular veins.

This unusual vascular pattern, in which the cortex is supplied exclusively by capillaries and the medulla contains arterioles and venules, as well as capillaries, prompted studies with electron-opaque tracers. These showed that there was little movement of macromolecules from the blood to the cortical parenchyma, whereas the medullary capillaries were highly permeable. This suggested that the lymphocytes of the cortex were protected from circulating macromolecules. Ultrastructural studies reveal that the

nonfenestrated capillaries of the cortex have a thick basal lamina (basement membrane) and are surrounded by a sheath of reticular cells that also has a conspicuous external lamina. It has been proposed that the lamina around the perivascular reticular cells and that of the endothelium may constitute a **blood-thymus barrier**, comparable to the blood-brain barrier, and that this may prevent antigens in the blood from reaching the differentiating T lymphocytes in the cortex. For nearly two decades, it has been assumed that lymphocytes mature in the thymus in an antigen-free environment. More recently, studies have cast some doubt on this assumption.

Histophysiology

In recent years, interest in the thymus has centered on its function in the maturation of T lymphocytes. When it is being populated by lymphoblasts and prolymphocytes from the bone marrow, these are induced to emigrate from the blood into the cortex by a chemotactic peptide, **thymotaxin**, that is secreted by the epithelial reticular cells beneath the capsule. Early in their differentiation in the cortex, the lymphocytes synthesize and insert into their membrane certain molecules that make it possible for immunologists to identify different subsets of T lymphocytes by using labeled antibodies to those surface markers. The fate of two of these markers, **CD-4** and **CD-8**, has been thoroughly studied. As they differentiate, the lymphocytes also acquire surface molecules of the **major histocompatability complex** (**MHC**) that enable them to distinguish **self** (the body's own cells) from **non-self** (foreign cells). The acquisition of this ability is thought to require close contact between the reticular cells and the differentiating lymphocytes. Lymphocytes of the CD-8 phenotype bear **class-I MHC** surface molecules that are present on all cells of the body. Lymphocytes of the CD-4 phenotype, that later serve as helper T cells in the humoral immune response, bear **class-II MHC** molecules that are found mainly on cells of the immune system.

> *An essential attribute of the immune system is its ability to distinguish "self" from "non-self." When this ability is compromised, an immune response to self results in an **autoimmune disease**. Cytotoxic T lymphocytes or antibodies may be directed against a single cell type, as in **insulin-dependent diabetes**, where the target is the beta cell of the endocrine pancreas, or they may be directed against an antigen shared by many cell types, as in **systemic lupus erythematosus**.*

In addition to acquiring surface markers in the course of their differentiation, the T lymphocytes synthesize and insert receptors for recognition of antigens into their membrane. These consist of α- and ß-chains that determine both the antigen specificity and MHC specificity of the receptor. In preparation for synthesis of the receptors, the genes for the α- and ß-chains undergo extensive random rearrangements that result in the expression of a great variety of sequences in the antigen receptors of the T-lympho-

cyte population. Those cells that chance to have sequences that would recognize and react to **self-MHC** are now believed to be the ones that degenerate and are eliminated in their transit through the cortex (Fig. 12-11). Only those T lymphocytes capable of reacting to foreign proteins in associations with **class II MHC** complete their differention and enter blood vessels in the medulla of the thymus. This process of degeneration of self-reactive T lymphocytes, called **negative selection**, eliminates about 80% of the lymphocytes that arise from precursors in the cortex. A **positive selection** is accomplished by clonal expansion of those cells bearing receptors for non-self, and it is these T lymphocytes (CD-4) that are released into the blood for distribution to the connective tissues and other lymphoid organs.

The thymic reticular cells also secrete several peptides that are believed to mediate short-range interactions within the thymus. One of these, **thymulin**, is reported to stimulate immature lymphocytes to synthesize their surface markers. Another, the **thymic humoral factor**, is thought to promote differentiation and clonal expansion of the CD-8 T lymphocytes. Another peptide, called **thrombopoietin**, is also thought to promote differentiation. However, it also binds to acetylcholine receptors and, when produced in excess, is somehow involved in the pathogenesis of the serious neuromuscular disorder, **muscular dystrophy**.

The thymus decreases in size and function during adult life, and a number of **autoimmune diseases** are now believed to be due to its failure to eliminate all self-reactive lymphocytes.

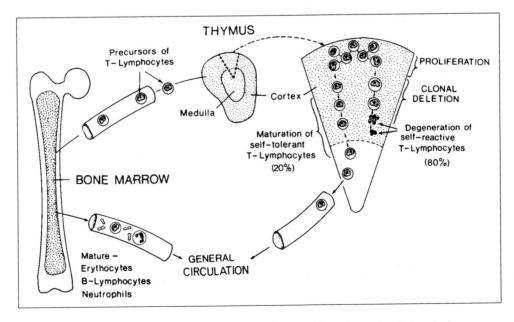

Fig. 12-11 Mature erythrocytes, B lymphocytes, and neutrophils enter the general circulation directly from the bone marrow. Precursors of T lymphocytes are first carried to the thymus. They proliferate in the outer cortex and mature as they slowly move toward the medulla. Those having receptors that would bind to "self" undergo apoptosis and degenerate (clonal deletion). Only those that are self-tolerant are released into the circulation.

*The HIV virus of **acquired immunodeficiency** **syndrome** (AIDS) binds selectively to the CD-4 pro-tein on T lymphocytes and on other cells bearing this marker, including macrophages, and dendritic cells of the thymus. Destruction of these cells accounts for the dysfunction of the immune system of AIDS patients and their consequent vulnerability to bacte-rial, viral, and fungal infections. Victims of AIDS usually succumb to an infection by one or more of these pathogens.*

LYMPH NODES

Lymph nodes are small organs distributed in series along the course of lymphatic vessels. They function as fil-ters for the lymph passing through them. Their principal cell types are **lymphocytes** and **reticular cells**. Lymph nodes are found in groups throughout the prevertebral region, along major blood vessels in the thorax and abdomen, in the mesenteries supporting the intestines, and in the subcutaneous connective tissue of the neck and groin. They are commonly reniform in shape and 5–20 mm in diameter, with a slight indentation on one side, called the **hilus,** where blood vessels enter and lymphatic vessels leave the node.

Microscopic Structure

A lymph node is enclosed in a capsule, from which slender, branching, connective tissue trabeculae extend into its parenchyma (Figs. 12-12 and 12-13 [see Plate 17]). Between trabeculae, the lymphoid tissue is supported by a three-dimensional network of reticular fibers and associat-ed reticular cells. The meshes of this network are filled with closely packed lymphocytes and smaller numbers of macrophages and plasma cells. The afferent lymph enters via lymphatic vessels that pass through the capsule at sev-eral sites on its surface (Fig. 12-12). The efferent lymph leaves through a single lymphatic vessel at the hilum of the node.

At low magnification, a deeper-staining **cortex** can be distinguished from a paler **medulla**. The difference in staining is attributable to the greater concentration of lym-phocytes in the cortex and the greater number and diame-ter of vascular sinuses in the medulla (Fig. 12-12).

Lymph Channels

The **afferent lymph vessels** traversing the capsule are confluent with a **subcapsular sinus** (marginal sinus) that extends around the periphery of the node, between the cap-sule and the cortical parenchyma (Fig. 12-13A [see Plate 17]). At the hilus, the subcortical sinus is continuous with

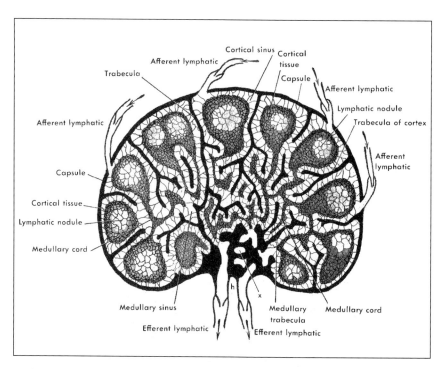

Fig. 12-12 Diagram of a lymph node showing its afferent and efferent lymphatics and their valves. Trabeculae originating from the capsule extend inward, dividing the cortex into sep-arate alcoves. The medullary trabeculae are continuous with those of the cortex. Blood ves-sels are not shown.

the **efferent lymphatic**. Tributary sinuses arising from the subcapsular sinus course into the parenchyma, running along the sides of the connective tissue trabeculae. These continue into the medulla as the **medullary sinuses**, which are larger and more tortuous channels that branch and anastomose repeatedly, subdividing the parenchyma into many **medullary cords** of closely packed lymphocytes. The medullary sinuses are confluent with the subcapsular sinus, at the hilus, where it is continuous with the **efferent lymph vessel** leaving the node.

In scanning electron micrographs, the sinuses are seen to be lined by attenuated squamous cells resembling endothelium. The lumen of the sinus contains a meshwork of reticular fibers and stellate reticular cells that are joined to each other and to the wall of the sinus by slender tapering processes. Also projecting into the lumen, from the wall of the sinus, are numerous macrophages that have thin veil-like processes, sometimes described as undulating membranes. The sinuses also contain lymphocytes that move freely between the lymph and the surrounding parenchyma. The abundant reticular cells and macrophages in the wall of the medullary sinuses make them very well suited to the filtering function of the node. Lymph entering the node from the afferent lymphatics percolates through the sinuses freely exchanging lymphocytes and solutes with the parenchyma. Any bacteria in the afferent lymph are phagocytized by the macrophages.

Parenchyma

The parenchyma of the cortex consists almost entirely of lymphocytes, but local differences in the tightness of their packing and their density of staining make it possible to distinguish **primary lymphoid nodules, secondary lymphoid nodules**, and **diffuse lymphoid tissue**. Primary lymphoid nodules are ovoid areas of homogeneous density where small lymphocytes are more tightly packed than elsewhere. Secondary nodules are of similar character but have a paler-staining central area called the **germinal center**, which is rich in larger lymphocytes. The germinal center is believed to be made up of activated B lymphocytes engaged in antibody synthesis (Fig. 12-14). A few T lymphocytes may also be present. Development of plasma cells from B lymphocytes is initiated in the germinal centers, but they move into the medulla to complete their differentiation. An especially dark-staining zone of closely aggregated small lymphocytes that form a cap on the capsular side of the secondary lymphoid nodule is referred to as the **crescent** when it is confined to the outer aspect of the nodule, or as the **mantle** when it surrounds the nodule.

The primary and secondary nodules at the periphery of the lymph node make up the bulk of the outer cortex. The internodal cortex and the deep cortex consist of diffuse lymphoid tissue, in which the lymphocytes are not as closely packed. There is no distinct boundary between the outer and inner cortex, and the latter grades into the medulla without a clearly defined boundary. These regional terms are useful, however, because the composition of the lymphocyte population differs from region to region. B lymphocytes are concentrated in the primary and secondary nodules, and T lymphocytes make up most of the diffuse lymphoid tissue in the medulla. The deep cortex is populated with lymphocytes of the **recirculating pool** that are involved in immunological surveillance throughout the body. In this region of the cortex, there are distinctive postcapillary venules that have tall endothelial cells. Although many lymphocytes reach the parenchyma via the afferent lymph, these **high-endothelial venules** are the portal of entry for the blood-borne lymphocytes that migrate through their wall into the deep cortex.

The **medullary cords** are aggregations of lymphoid tissue around small blood vessels. They occupy the space between the dilated **medullary sinuses** and are made up of small lymphocytes, macrophages, and plasma cells in a network of reticular cells and reticular fibers.

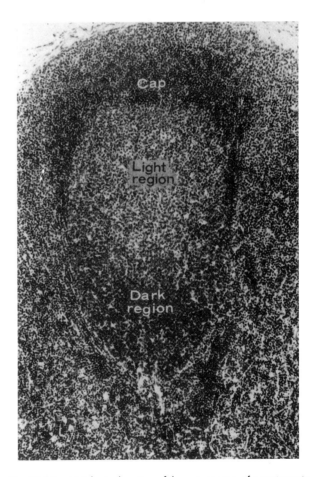

Fig. 12-14 Histological section of the outer cortex of a mesenteric lymph node. Note the cap, or crescent, at the peripheral end of the germinal center.

Blood Vessels

The blood vessels to the lymph node enter through the hilus. Main branches of the artery run in the trabeculae with lateral branches supplying the capillary network of the medullary cords. Smaller arteries continue into the cortex, where they ramify into the capillary networks of the diffuse lymphoid tissue and those that surround, but do not enter, the primary and secondary lymphoid nodules. Postcapillary venules arising from these capillary plexuses have a low endothelial lining and drain into larger venous channels in the trabeculae. The specialized high endothelial postcapillary venules of the deep cortex have no muscular coat. Because the emigration of recirculating lymphocytes from the blood occurs only in these vessels, it is assumed that lymphocytes have receptors that recognize, and bind to, the high endothelial cells. A surface glycoprotein has recently been identified on lymphocytes that seems to be involved in this recognition.

Histophysiology

An important function of lymph nodes is to limit the spread of infection by filtering out and destroying bacteria in the lymph draining the site of their entry. Experiments involving perfusion of a single lymph node with a known number of bacteria, followed by counting the number appearing in the efferent lymph, have shown that the filtering efficiency of a single node is greater than 95%. In the intact organism, those not removed by phagocytes of the first node would likely be eliminated by the next node in the chain. Cells entering the lymph from a cancer are also filtered out in the regional lymph nodes, but unlike bacteria, they survive and proliferate there. Ultimately, some cancer cells invading the sinus are carried away in the efferent lymph and colonize the next node in the path of lymphatic drainage. For this reason, surgeons excising a malignant tumor try to remove all of the regional lymph nodes to prevent further spread (metastasis) of the cancer.

Even if the intact bacteria do not reach a lymph node downstream from a site of infection, antigenic products of their digestion by macrophages in the area of inflammation will reach a node and stimulate its lymphocytes to initiate a humoral immune response. In a lymph node responding to infection, the preexisting germinal centers usually dis-

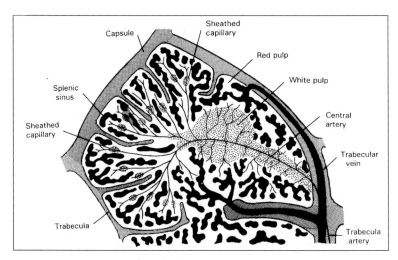

Fig. 12-16 Diagram of the vascular system of a portion of the spleen. The periarterial lymphoid sheaths of the white pulp are the stippled areas around the central arteries leaving the trabeculae. An open circulation is depicted here, with the capillaries not communicating with the sinuses, shown here as irregularly shaped black structures.

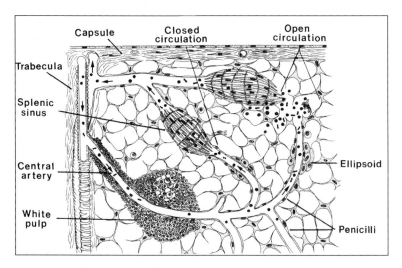

Fig. 12-17 Schematic representation of a small area of the splenic parenchyma, showing the meshwork of reticular cells of the red pulp, the perivascular aggregations of lymphocytes that comprise the white pulp, and the specialized splenic sinuses. The alternative interpretations of an open or a closed circulation are also depicted.

appear, and many large lymphocytes and plasma cells appear in nodules in a greatly enlarged deep cortex and, there, they begin to produce antibodies. Within a day or two, antibody can be detected in the efferent lymph and in the blood. Dense aggregations of lymphocytes then appear in the outer cortex, representing early stages in the development of new secondary lymph nodules. By the end of the first week, the lymph node has usually reverted to its normal architecture with numerous newly formed germinal centers in its cortex. Meanwhile, activated lymphocytes in the efferent lymph have colonized other downstream lymph nodes in the chain, initiating antibody production in them.

SPLEEN

The **spleen** is an elongated organ, weighing about 150 g, located in the abdominal cavity between the fundus of the stomach and the diaphragm. It contains a large volume of lymphoid tissue that participates in immune responses. It also serves as an efficient filter interposed in the circulation to clear the blood of damaged or senescent erythrocytes. It sequesters circulating monocytes, and these differentiate into splenic macrophages that ingest and destroy effete erythrocytes. The spleen also stores as many as a third of the body's platelets and holds them in ready reserve until needed. In some species, the spleen acts as a reservoir of mature erythrocytes that can be added to the blood in response to unusual demands. This function is less evident in man.

Microscopic Structure

The spleen has a collagenous **capsule** that is thickened at the **hilus**. Closely adherent to the capsule is an investment of **peritoneum**, the thin layer of squamous epithelium that lines the interior of the abdominal cavity and covers its viscera. This is continuous with the lienorenal ligament, a fold of peritoneum through which the blood vessels, nerves, and lymphatics enter and leave the spleen. From the capsule, connective-tissue **trabeculae** extend into the parenchyma.

Visual examination of the cut surface of a hemisected spleen reveals many rounded gray areas 0.2–0.7 mm in diameter. Collectively, these relatively light areas are referred to as the **white pulp** of the spleen (Fig. 12-15 [see Plate 18]). They are scattered through a mass of dark-red tissue that constitutes the **red pulp**. Upon microscopic examination, the areas of white pulp (formerly called Malpighian bodies) consist of diffuse and nodular lymphoid tissue resembling the cortex of a lymph node. The red pulp contains many thin-walled vessels of large caliber, the **splenic sinuses**, and between these are highly cellular areas, the **splenic cords** (cords of Billroth). The color of the red pulp is due to the abundance of erythrocytes in the lumen of the sinuses infiltrating the spaces within a loose network of stellate reticular cells.

Blood Vessels

Several branches of the **splenic artery** enter the hilus and ramify in the connective-tissue trabeculae of the parenchyma, as **trabecular arteries**. When their ramification has produced branches about 0.2 mm in diameter, these leave the trabeculae as **central arteries** surrounded by a wide **periarterial sheath** of diffuse and nodular lymphoid tissue that extends for some distance along the artery (Fig. 12-16). Collectively, the many periarterial sheaths of lymphoid tissue make up the white pulp of the spleen.

Upon emerging from the distal end of the periarterial lymphoid sheath, the central artery branches quite suddenly into a number of very slender vessels called **penicillar arterioles**. These radiate from their point of origin for a distance of about 1 mm and then give rise to two or three smaller branches. Before their termination, some of these pass through a small nodule or sheath made up of two or three layers of macrophages. This is commonly called the **ellipsoid**, but some prefer the more cumbersome term periarterial macrophage sheath (Fig. 12-17). The endothelium in this segment is somewhat atypical and a basal lamina is lacking. Monocytes evidently pass through the vessel wall to become macrophages of the sheath for a time and then move on into the red pulp.

The mode of termination of these vessels has long been a subject of controversy. Some believe they continue and become confluent with the sinuses of the red pulp. This is the **closed circulation** hypothesis. Other histologists insist that they open, at their ends, into the extracellular spaces of the red pulp, permitting extravasation of erythrocytes that later find their way back into the circulation through clefts in the wall of the splenic sinuses. This is the **open circulation** hypothesis (Fig. 12-17). The open circulation is now favored for the human spleen. It seems unlikely that the spleen could be so highly efficient in clearing the blood of old and damaged erythrocytes if these did not have direct access to macrophages throughout the red pulp.

Segments of the sinuses between the cords of red pulp are lined by an atypical endothelium consisting of long fusiform cells separated by narrow intercellular clefts (Fig. 12-18). The wall of the sinus is supported by a discontinuous basal lamina, consisting of slender circumferential

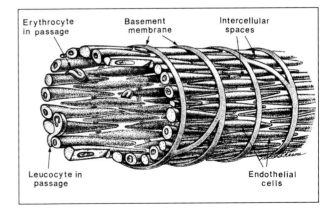

Fig. 12-18 Drawing of a splenic sinus. The endothelial cells are fusiform and are not in intimate contact, leaving intercellular spaces through which erythrocytes and leukocytes traverse the wall. The basement membrane (basal lamina) is confined to hooplike circumferential bands. (Drawing by Sylvia Collard/Keene.)

bands like the hoops on a barrel but with oblique strands connecting the successive hoops (Figs. 12-18 and 12-19 [see Plate 18]). This unusual structure permits blood cells to reenter the circulation through the clefts between the fusiform endothelial cells. From the sinuses, blood drains to short **pulp veins** that enter the trabeculae to become the **trabecular veins**. These, in turn, drain into larger veins at the hilus that converge to form the **splenic vein.**

White Pulp

Regarding the periarterial lymphoid sheaths comprising the white pulp of the spleen, their microscopic structure is comparable to that of the cortex of lymph nodes. The lymphoid nodules and their germinal centers are made up of B lymphocytes; T lymphocytes predominant elsewhere. Reticular fibers at the periphery of sheath are oriented circumferentially, and reticular cells form a boundary layer one or two layers thick. Immediately peripheral to this boundary there is an 80–100-μm transitional region called the **marginal zone**, which includes splenic sinuses, loosely aggregated lymphocytes, plasma cells, and macrophages. The marginal zone is where lymphocytes of the recirculating pool leave the blood to enter the periarterial sheaths of the white pulp. In traversing the boundary, lymphocytes come in contact with numerous dendritic reticular cells that are capable of retaining antigens on their surface for some time and presenting them to immunocompetent lymphocytes just as macrophages do elsewhere.

Red Pulp

The red pulp consists of highly tortuous splenic sinuses and the **splenic cords** between the the sinuses. The cords consist of a cellular network of reticular cells in contact with one another via long processes. The interstices of this network of reticular cells contain lymphocytes, and numerous macrophages and extravasated erythrocytes. The splenic cords vary in their configuration depending on the shape of the spaces between splenic sinuses. In some species, islands of hemopoietic tissue are normally found in the red pulp. In humans, hemopoiesis in the red pulp called **myeloid metaplasia**, occurs only in severe cases of anemia and in leukemia.

Histophysiology

The blood-filtering function of the spleen depends on the reticular structure of its red pulp and its large population of resident macrophages that monitor the quality of the blood cells passing through it. Aged, abnormal, or damaged blood cells and platelets are ingested and destroyed by the macrophages of the splenic cords. Normal cells freely return to the circulation through the intercellular clefts in the wall of the sinuses. How the macrophages recognize aging or damaged cells is not clear. The hemoglobin of the ingested erythrocytes is broken down and its iron is trasiently stored in the cytoplasm as **ferritin**; it is ultimately made available to erythroblasts of the bone marrow for synthesis of new hemoglobin. **Bilirubin** formed in the degradation of hemoglobin is transported, in the blood, to the liver and secreted in the bile.

In the presence of bacteria or their toxic products in the blood, a primary immune response is initiated in the white pulp. The secondary response is rapid and, for a time, the spleen is the body's most active organ, per unit weight, in the production of antibody, but its share of antibody production declines as the immune response spreads to the other lymphoid tissues throughout the body.

The human spleen is also an important reservoir for the storage of platelets. It is reported to contain one-third of the body's supply, and these can be returned to the circulation as needed.

QUESTIONS*

1. Which is **incorrect** about the thymus?

   A. possesses lobules
   B. has afferent lymphatics
   C. has epithelial reticular cells
   D. has Hassell's corpuscles
   E. involutes after puberty

2. The white pulp of the spleen contains

   A. lymphatic nodules
   B. central arteries
   C. diffuse lymphatic tissue
   D. reticular fibers
   E. all of the above

3. Which of the following is **incorrect** about the spleen?

   A. has a dense connective tissue capsule
   B. has trabeculae with arteries and veins
   C. has splenic cords (Billroth's cords)
   D. has sinusoids within trabeculae
   E. contains a loose net of reticular cells

4. The cell-mediated immune response is performed by

   A. B lymphocytes
   B. macrophages
   C. T lymphocytes
   D. plasma cells
   E. memory cells

5. Lymph arriving at a lymph node via an afferent lymphatic vessels goes next to a

   A. medullary sinuse
   B. subcapsular sinus
   C. cortical sinus
   D. efferent lymphatic
   E. none of the above

6. The spleen functions as

   A. a repository of monocytes
   B. a storage depot for platelets
   C. an organ for clearing blood of damaged erythrocytes
   D. a filter
   E. all of the above

7. The most common antigen-presenting cells are

   A. macrophages
   B. helper T lymphocytes
   C. reticulocytes
   D. large lymphocytes
   E. plasma cells

8. The most important immunoglobulin in immune responses is

   A. IgA
   B. IgD
   C. IgE
   D. IgG
   E. IgM

9. Which statement about T lymphocytes is **false?**

   A. They are active participants in the humoral immune response.
   B. They secrete cytokines.
   C. They have no antigen receptors on their surfaces.
   D. They stimulate differentiation of some B lymphocytes into plasma cells.
   E. They synthesize abundant amounts of antibodies.

10. The germinal center of lymph nodes

    A. has few large lymphocytes
    B. is composed primarily of T lymphocytes
    C. contains plasma cells produced in the medulla
    D. contains activated B lymphocytes
    E. is seldom involved as a site of antibody synthesis

*Answers on page 307.

13

ENDOCRINE GLANDS

KEY WORDS

Adrencorticotrophic
　Hormone
　(ACTH)
Adrenocorticotrophin
Aldosterone
Androgen
Arginine Vasotocin
Chief Cell
Cholecalciferol
Chromaffin Reaction
Chromophil
Chromophobe
Colloid
Corpora Arenacea
Corticotrope
Cortisol
Dehydroepiandroster-
　one
Diiodothyronine (T2)
Epinephrine
Epiphysis Cerebri
FSH
Glucagon
Glucocorticoid
Gonadotrope
Growth Hormone
Herring Body
Infundibulum
Insulin
Iodine
Lactogenic Hormone
Luteinizing Hormone
　(LH)
Mammotrope
Median Eminence
Melatonin
MSH
Mineralocorticoid

Monoiodothyronine
　(MT)
Neurophysin
Norepinephrine
Oxyphil Cell
Oxytocin
Parafollicular Cell
Parathyroid Hormone
　(PTH)
Paraventricular
　Nucleus
Pinealocyte
Pituicyte
Prolactin
Prolactin-Inhibiting
　Hormone
Releasing factors:
　SRH, PRH,
　GnRH, CRH,
　TRH
Somatostatin
Somatotrope
Supraoptic Nucleus
Tetraiodothyronine
　(T4)
Thyrocalcitonin
　(calcitonin)
Thyroglobulin
Thyroid Hormone
Thyroid-Stimulating
　Hormone (TSH)
Thyrotrope
Triiodothyronine (T3)
Vasopressin
Vitamin D
Zona Fasciculata
Zona Glomerulosa
Zona Reticularis

In the evolution of higher organisms, it became necessary to develop mechanisms for controlling and coordinating the functions of the various organs of the body. Two mechanisms evolved: the **nervous system** and the **endocrine system.** The nervous system exercises control by generating electrochemical signals that are transmitted over axons that synapse on the cells being regulated. The glands of the endocrine system secrete chemical agents, **hormones,** that are transported in the bloodstream to distant target cells that have specific surface **receptors** which bind the hormone. Binding triggers a cascade of intracellular reactions that change the target cell's activity.

HYPOPHYSIS

The **hypophysis (pituitary gland)** is an endocrine gland located at the base of the brain in a shallow depression of the sphenoid bone, called the **sella turcica.** It produces several hormones with wide-ranging effects on metabolism, growth, and reproduction. The gland is about 1 cm in length and width and 0.5 cm in depth and weighs 0.5 g. It has neural and vascular connections with the brain that give it a key role in the interactions of the nervous system and the endocrine system.

The hypophysis has two major subdivisions that differ in their embryological origin. The **neurohypophysis** (posterior lobe) develops as a downgrowth of the diencephalon of the brain and is composed of neural tissue. The **adenohypophysis** arises as a dorsal evagination of the embryonic pharynx and is made up of glandular tissue. From above downward, three regions of the neurohypophysis are distinguished: a slightly raised area at the base of the hypothalamus called the **median eminence;** a slender stalk extending downward from the median eminence is the **infundibulum;** and the bulbous terminal portion of this downgrowth of neural tissue is the **pars nervosa** (Fig. 13-1). The adenohypophysis consists of three subdivisions: the **pars tuberalis,** a thin layer of glandular tissue wrapped around the infundibulum; the **pars distalis** (anterior lobe), making up the greater part of the adenohypophysis; and the **pars intermedia,** a layer of epithelial cells situated between the pars nervosa and the pars distalis.

Blood Supply

Activation of the secretory cells of the adenohypophysis is dependent on **releasing factors** produced in the hypothalamus and carried to these cells in the blood. Some knowledge of the blood supply of the gland is therefore essential to an understanding of its function. Bilateral **inferior hypophyseal arteries,** arising from the internal carotid arteries, bifurcate, and their branches anastomose to form an arterial ring around the infundibular stalk of the hypothalamus. Branches descending from this ring penetrate the pars nervosa and, to a lesser extent, the pars distalis. Several **superior hypophyseal arteries,** arising from the internal carotid and anterior cerebral arteries, anastomose around the median eminence of the hypothalamus and send branches into it to form the so-called **primary plexus.** Branches of this capillary network then return to the surface, where they coalesce to form venules that course downward around the infundibular process to join an extensive network of sinusoids within the pars distalis, the **secondary plexus.** The venules connecting the primary plexus, in the median eminence, with the secondary plexus, in the pars distalis, constitute the **hypophyseoportal system.** It supplies the major part of the blood reaching the pars distalis and carries releasing factors that bind to appropriate receptors on its cells, initiating secretion of their hormones.

Pars Distalis

The pars distalis is composed of irregular cords and clusters of glandular cells in intimate relation to the thin-walled sinusoids of the secondary plexus. The sinusoids have a fenestrated endothelium. Stellate, fibroblastlike cells with long branching processes form a cellular framework throughout the gland, with the secretory cells occupying the spaces within this network.

Traditionally, histologists assigned the secretory cells to one or the other of two categories, **chromophils,** which contained secretory granules and stained deeply, and **chromophobes,** which had few or no such granules and stained very lightly. The chromophobes were interpreted

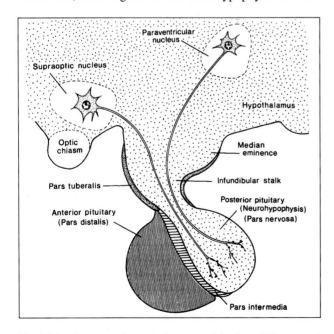

Fig. 13-1 Diagram of a sagital section of the hypothalamus and hypophysis, showing the relationship of several regions and their terminology. Two magnocellular neurones are included to show the origins of the axons that make up the bulk of the pars nervosa.

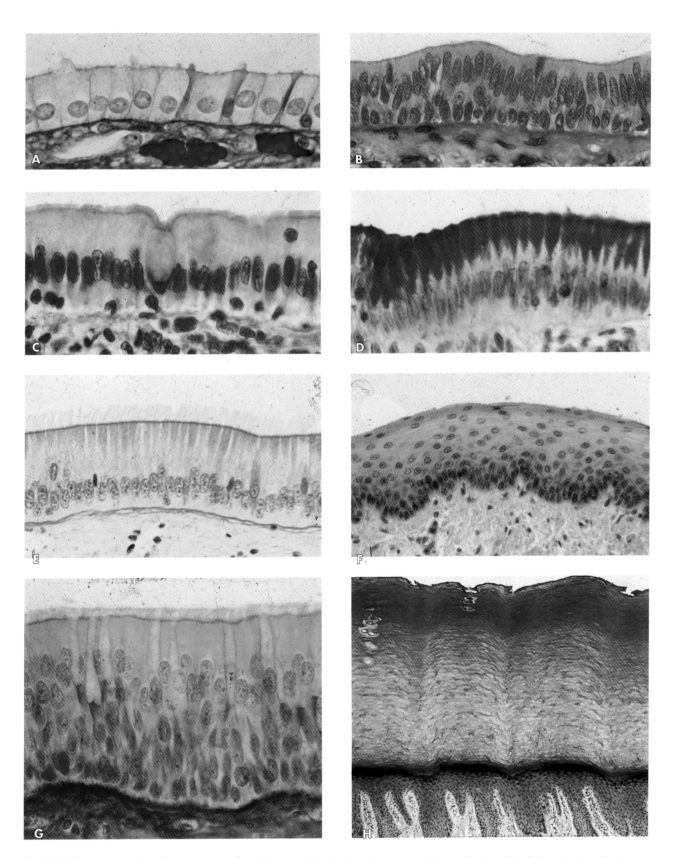

Fig. 2-7 Photomicrographs of various types of epithelium. (A) Simple low columnar epithelium of a duct of the kidney. (B) Stratified columnar epithelium of duct of um. (F) Stratified squamous epithelium of the esophagus. (G) Ciliated pseudostratified epithelium of the trachea. (H) Keratinized stratified squamous epithelium of epidermis on the sole of the foot.

Plate 1

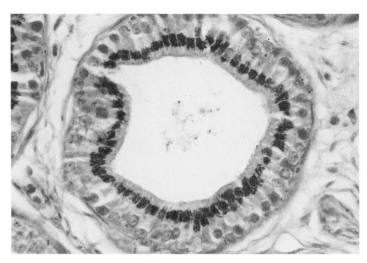

Fig. 2-8   Selective staining of the Golgi complex of a secretory epithelium. The polarity of the epithelium is apparent in the consistent supranuclear location of the Golgi complex.

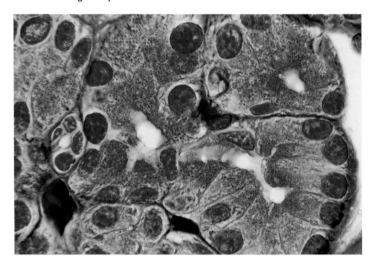

Fig. 2-20   An example of a compound acinar gland. The acini are made up of pyramidal epithelial cells around a small lumen. There is a small duct at the left.

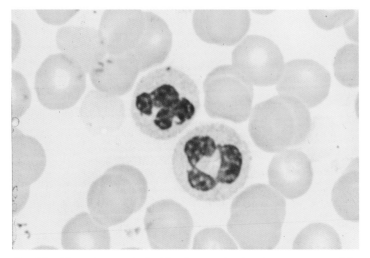

Fig. 3-1   Photomicrograph of a blood smear showing the appearance of the erythrocytes as pink disks with a slightly paler center. The two larger cells are polymorphonuclear leukocytes.

Plate 2

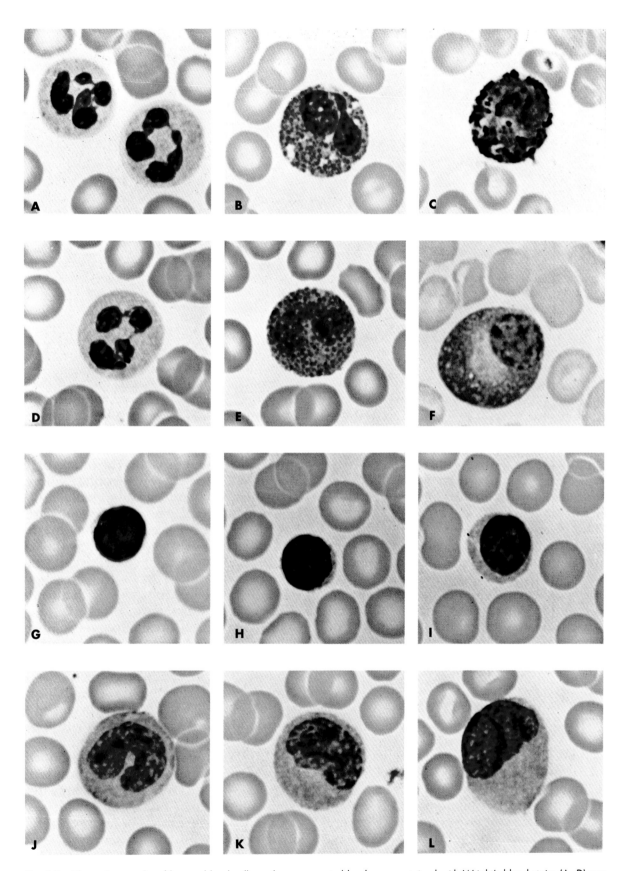

Fig. 3-7 Photomicrographs of human blood cells as they appear in blood smears stained with Wright's blood stain:.(A, D) neutrophils; (B, E) eosinophils; (G, H) small lymphocytes; (I) medium lymphocyte; (J, K, L) monocytes. The plasma cell (J) is not normally found in the blood but is common in the connective tissues. C basophil   F

Plate 3

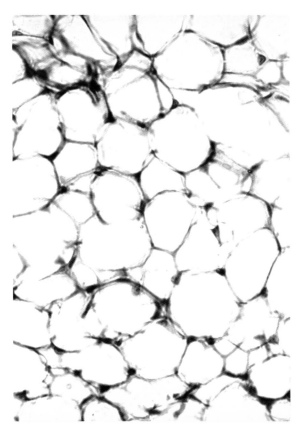

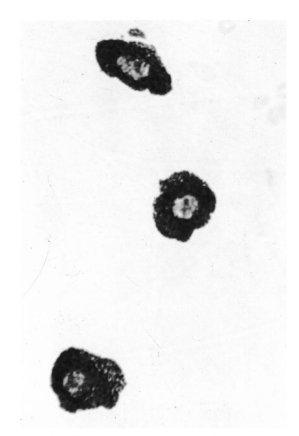

Fig. 4-9 Photomicrograph of an area of loose connective tissue in which adipose cells are the dominant cell type. (Courtesy of R.P. Jensh.)

Fig. 4-14 Three mast cells in a spread of mesentery.

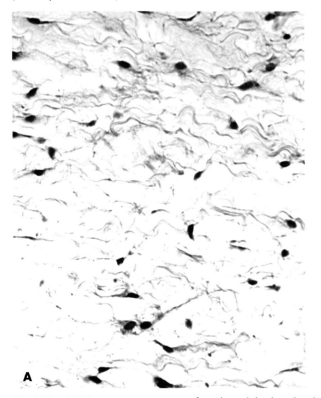

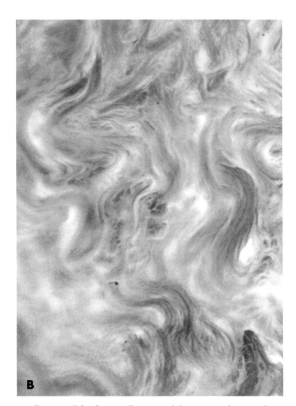

Fig. 4-17 (A) Mucous connective tissue from the umbilical cord (Wharton's jelly). Small fusiform cells are widely scattered in an abundant, amorphous, ground substance, rich in hyaluronic acid. (B) Dense irregular connective tissue from the mammary gland. Note the numerous, randomly oriented, wavy bundles of collagen. (Courtesy of R.P. Jensh.)

Plate 4

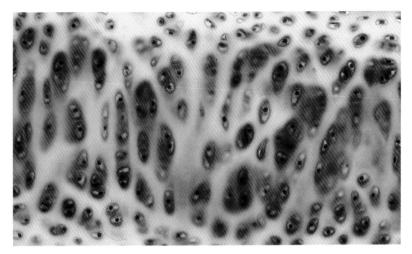

Fig. 6-3 Photomicrograph of typical hyaline cartilage. Note that the cells and their lacunae are smaller at the periphery of the cartilage, immediately beneath the perichondrium.

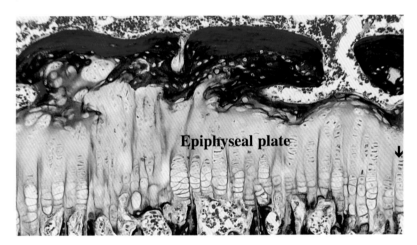

Epiphyseal plate

Fig. 6-5 Photomicrograph of the epiphyseal plate of a developing bone. The red and deep blue (above and below) are newly deposited bone. Growth in bone length depends on proliferation and degeneration of chondrocytes arranged in long columns in the plate (arrows) and their replacement by bone forming cells (osteoblasts) at the lower ends of the columns.

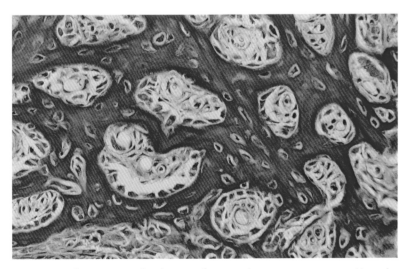

Fig. 7-10 Photomicrograph of a small area of primary spongiosa. Note the osteoblasts aligned on the surface of the anastomosing trabeculae.

Plate 5

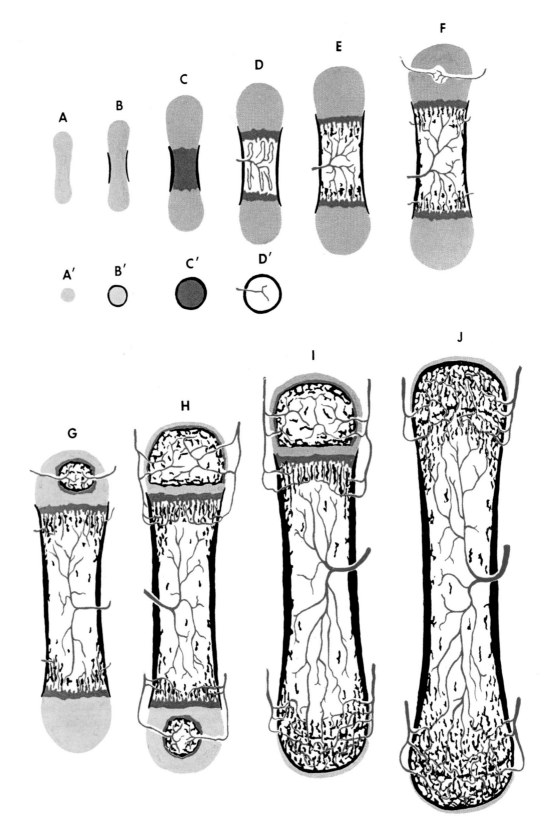

Fig. 7-13 Diagram of the development of a typical long bone as shown in longitudinal sections (A to J) and in cross sections A′, B′, C′, and D′ through the centers of A, B, C, and D. Pale blue, cartilage; purple, calcified cartilage: black, bone : red, arteries. (A) Cartilage modes (B) periosteal bone collar appears before any calcification of cartilage; (C) cartilate begins to calcify: (D) Vascular mesenchyme enters the calcified cartilage matrix and divides it into two zones of ossification (E). (F) Blood vessels and mesenchyme enter upper epiphyseal cartilage and the epiphyseal ossification center develops in it (G). A similar ossification center develops in the lower epiphyseal cartilage (H). As the bone ceases to grow in length, the lower epiphyseal plate disappears first (I) and then the upper epiphyseal plate (J). The bone marrow cavity then becomes continuous throughout the length of the bone, and the blood vessels of the diaphysis, metaphyses and epiphyses intercommunicate.

Plate 6

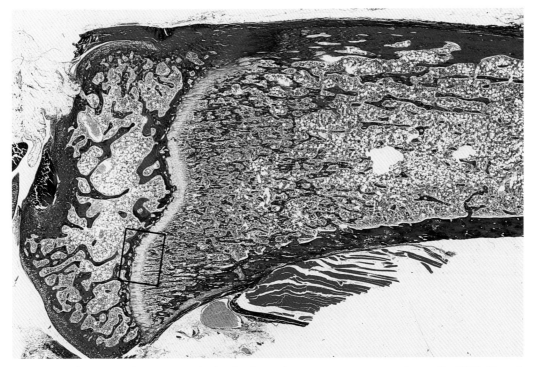

Fig. 7-14 A low-power photomicrograph of a developing bone at a state corresponding to Fig. 7-13I. The epiphysis is at the left, separated from the diaphysis by the pale-staining epiphyseal plate. The area in the box is seen at higher magnification in Fig. 7-15.

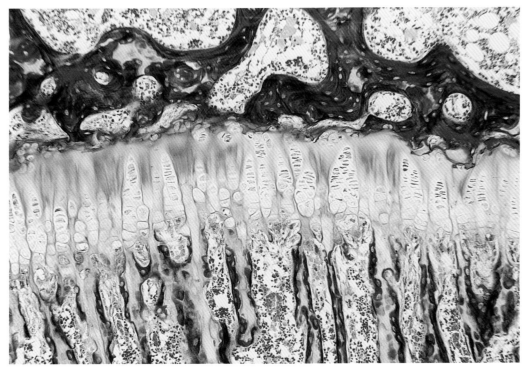

Fig. 7-15 Photomicrograph of the epiphyseal plate of a developing bone with the epiphysis above and the diaphysis below. Note the mottled appearance of the trabeculae of the diaphysis due to their centers being cartilage and their periphery newly deposited bone.

Plate 7

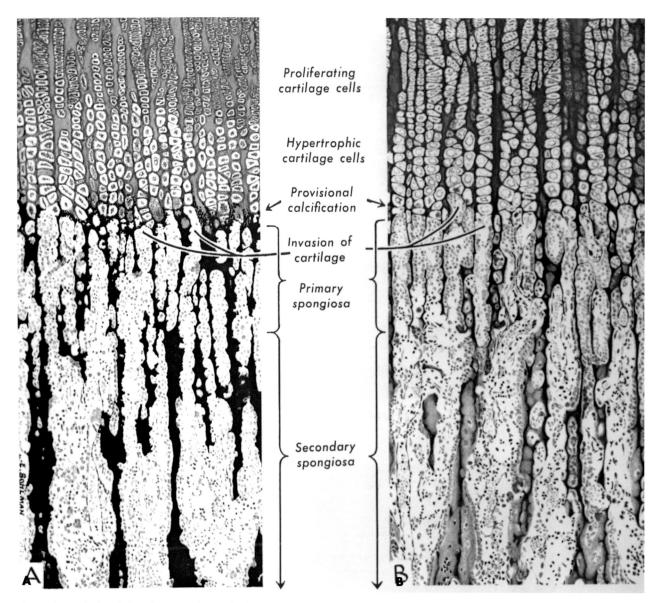

Proliferating
cartilage cells

Hypertrophic
cartilage cells

Provisional
calcification

Invasion of
cartilage

Primary
spongiosa

Secondary
spongiosa

Fig. 7-16 Endochondral ossification in longitudinal sections through the zone of epiphyseal growth of the distal end of the radius of a puppy. (A) Neutral formalin fixation; no decalcification. Von Kóssa and hematoxylin – eosin stain. All deposits of bone salt are stained black; thus, bone and calcified cartilage matrix stain alike. (B) Zenker-formol fixation; decalcified. Hematoxylin – eosin – azure II stain. Persisting cores of cartilage matrix in trabeculae of bone take a deep blue or purple stain, whereas bone stains red. It is impossible to tell where calcium deposits had been.

Plate 8

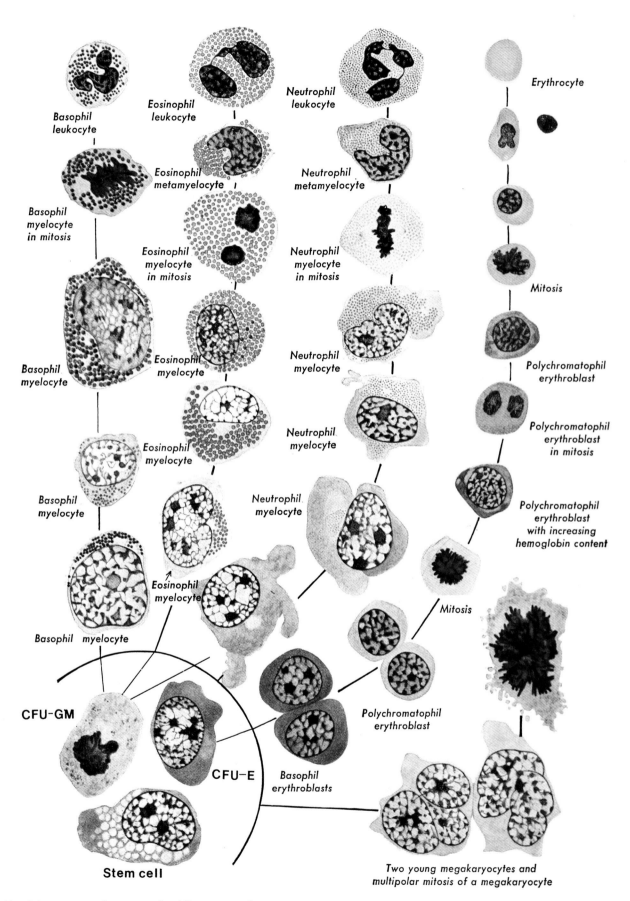

Fig. 8-3 Drawing of stages in the differentiation of eosinophils, basophils, and erythrocytes as seen with the May–Gruenwald–Giemsa stain. Monocytes and lymphocytes not shown.

Plate 9

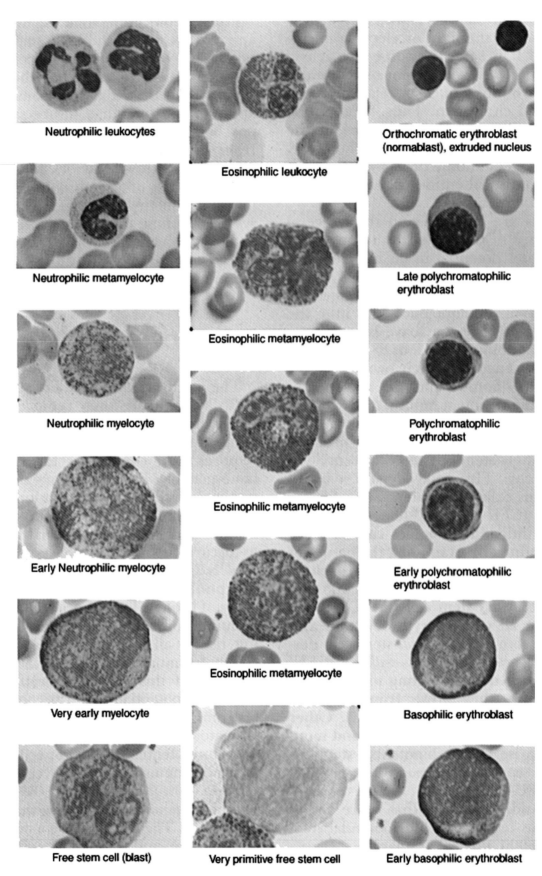

Fig. 8-4 Intermediate stages in development of neutrophils, eosinophils, and erythrocytes as seen in bone marrow smears stained with Wright's stain.

Plate 10

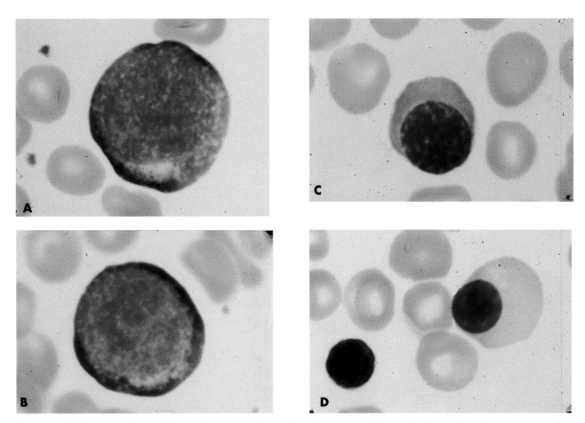

Fig. 8-5 (A) Proerythroblast; (B) basophilic erythroblast; (C) polychromatophilic erythroblast; (D) orthochromatic erythroblast, beginning to extrude its nucleus, and an extruded nucleus.

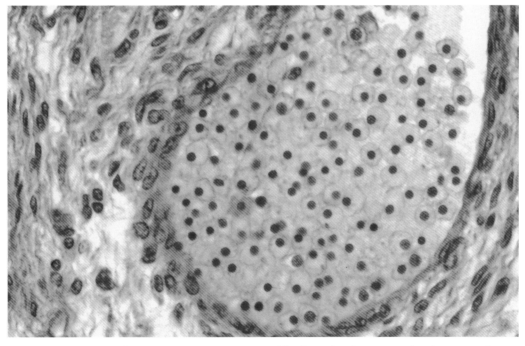

Fig. 8-7 Section from a first-trimester placenta, showing a blood vessel in the center and at the upper right containing nucleated erythrocytes of the fetus. (Courtesy of R. P. Jensh.)

Plate 11

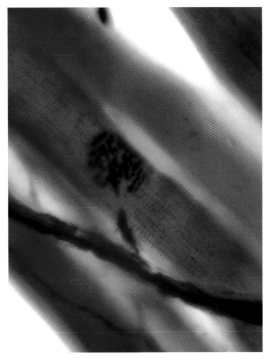

Fig. 9-15 Silver-impregnated motor nerve ending on a skeletal muscle fiber. (Courtesy of R.P. Jensh.)

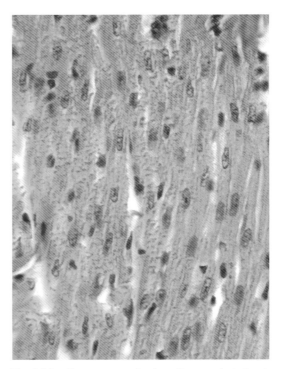

Fig. 9-18 Photomicrograph of cardiac muscle in longitudinal section. Note that, in contrast to skeletal muscle, the nuclei are in the center of the fibers. (Courtesy of R.P. Jensh.)

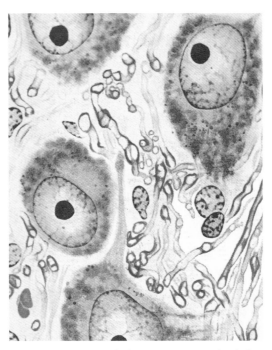

Fig. 10-2 Neurons in the human pons. Note the darker-staining clumps in the cytoplasm. These are the so-called Nissl bodies. The smaller nuclei are those of glial cells.

Plate 12

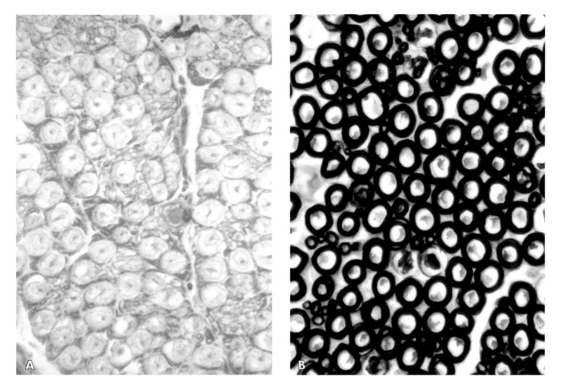

Fig. 10-7 (A) In routine preparation of histological sections, the myelin sheaths of nerves are extracted, and one sees only the axon surrounded by a round, clear area. (B) By fixing the tissue in osmium tetroxide, the myelin sheaths can be preserved and then appear as black rings around a somewhat shrunked axon. (Courtesy of R.P. Jensh.)

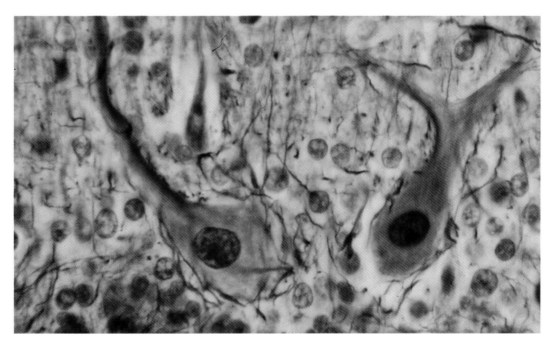

Fig. 10-15 Photomicrograph of two Purkinje cells of the cerebellum. Only the cell bodies and initial part of their dendrites are visible. The elaborate branching of their dendrites is out of this field. At the bottom of the figure, the closely crowded nuclei are those of granule cells.

Plate 13

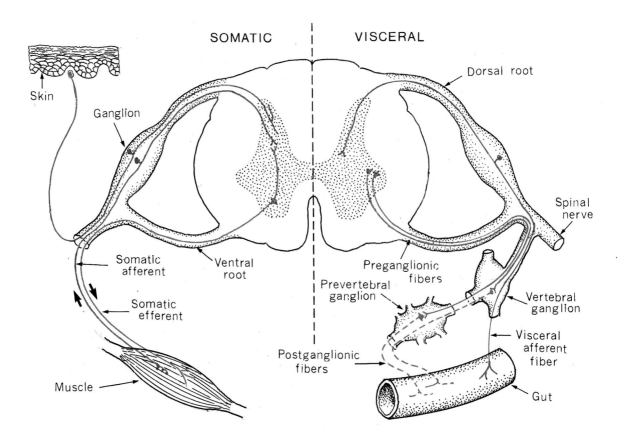

SOMATIC | VISCERAL

Skin

Ganglion

Dorsal root

Somatic
afferent

Ventral
root

Spinal
nerve

Somatic
efferent

Preganglionic
fibers

Prevertebral
ganglion

Vertebral
ganglion

Postganglionic
fibers

Visceral
afferent
fiber

Muscle

Gut

Fig. 10-16 Drawing of the spinal cord and dorsal and ventral roots of spinal nerves. The left half of the figure shows the somatic nerves and the right half shows the visceral nerves. The afferent fibers are in blue and the efferent fibers, in red. (Redrawn and modified from W. Copenhaver and R. Bunge (eds.), Bailey's Textbook of Histology, 16th ed., Williams and Wilkins, Baltimore, 1971.)

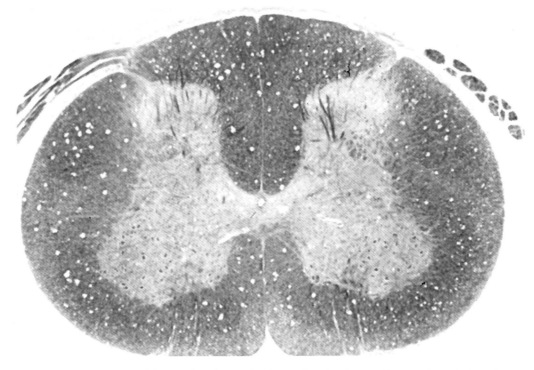

Fig. 10-17 Cross section of the spinal cord stained with Cresyl Violet, showing the central canal, the pale-staining, H-shaped, gray matter, and the dorsal and lateral columns of white matter. (Courtesy of R.P. Jensh.)

Plate 14

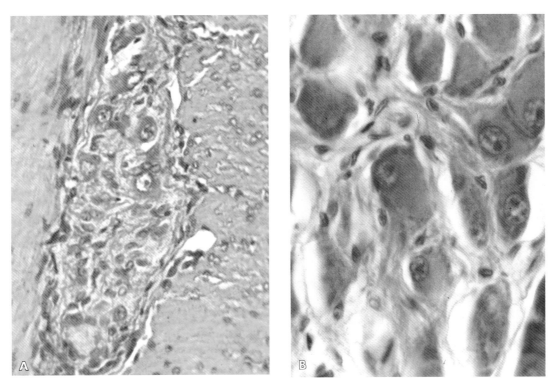

Fig. 10-19 (A) Photomicrograph of a small parasympathetic ganglion between the smooth-muscle layers of the intestinal wall. (B) Nueron cell bodies in a peripheral sympathetic ganglion. (Courtesy of R.P. Jensh.)

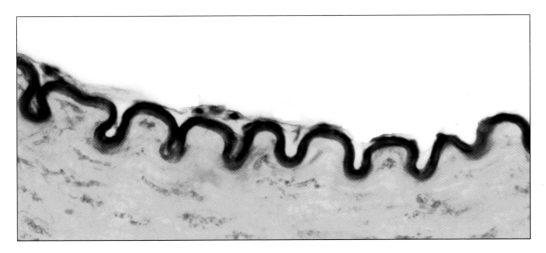

Fig. 11-5 Photomicrograph of the wall of a large artery showing a prominent elastica interna with a wavy course due to postmortem contraction of the vessel. Thinner elastic fibers can also be seen in the underlying tunica media. (Courtesy of R.P. Jensh.)

Plate 15

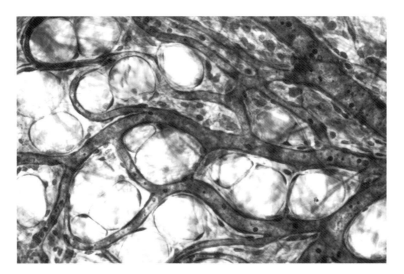

Fig. 11-10 A thick section showing a small arteriole at the upper right branching to give rise to a network of capillaries surrounding clusters of adipose cells. (Courtesy of R.P. Jensh.)

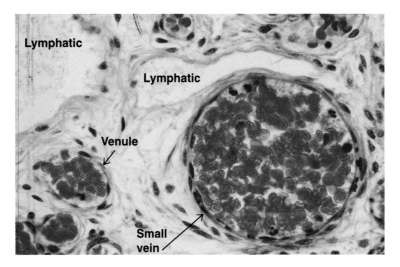

Fig. 11-16 Photomicrograph of a small vein, venules, and lymphatics in the connective tissue of an organ.

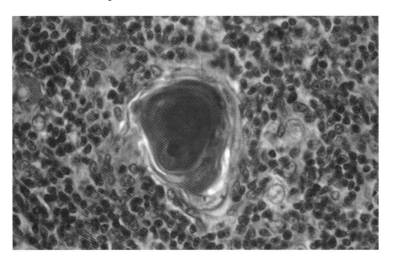

Fig. 12-10 Photomicrograph of monkey thymus. The cortex of the lobule, at the left, consists of closely packed lymphocytes. The paler-staining area at the right is part of the medulla containing three eosinophilic Hassall's corpuscles.

Plate 16

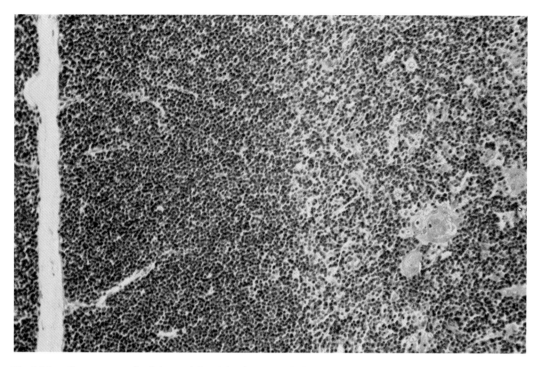

Fig. 12-9   Photomicrograph of the medulla of the thymus, including a Hassall's corpuscle in the center of the field. (Courtesy of R.P. Jensh.)

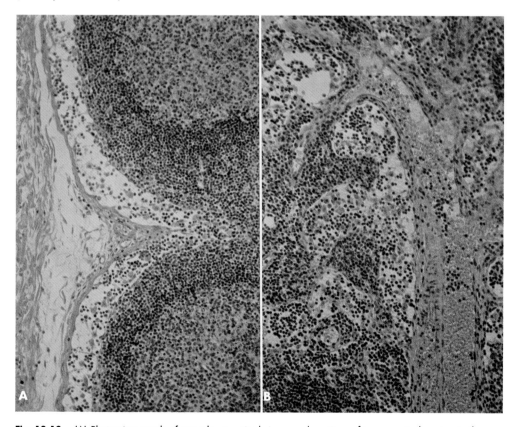

Fig. 12-13   (A) Photomicrograph of capsule, marginal sinus, and portions of two germinal centers in the cortex of a mesenteric lymph node. (B) Medullary sinuses and cords, and a trabecula containing blood vessels.

Plate 17

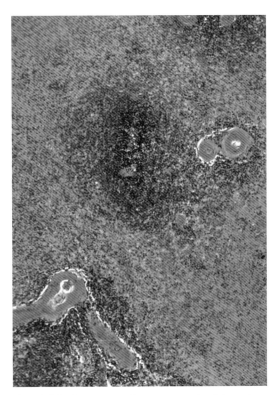

Fig. 12-15 Low-power photomicrograph of the spleen showing areas of white pulp (blue) and the red pulp (red).

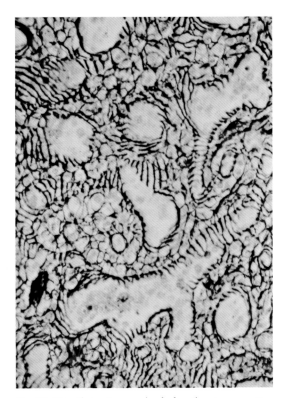

Fig. 12-19 Photomicrograph of of a silver impregnation of the spleen showing the regularly spaced hoops and reticular fibers around the endothelium of the sinusoids. (Courtesy of K. Richardson.)

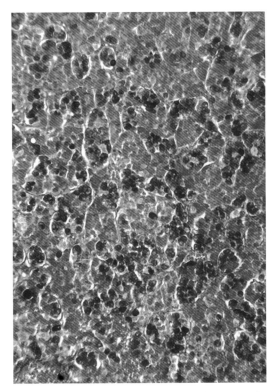

Fig. 13-2 Low-power photomicrograph of the pars distalis of the pituitary, stained by a method that permits recognition of acidophils (pink) and basophils (blue). (Courtesy of R. P. Jensh.)

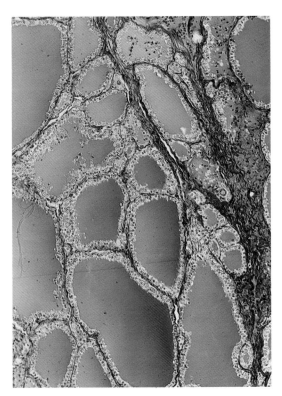

Fig. 13-7 Photomicrograph of the thyroid gland. Note the follicles of varying size, filled with colloid.

Plate 18

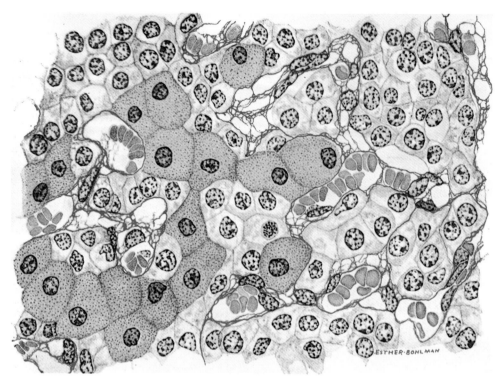

Fig. 13-12 Drawing of a small area of the parenchyma of the parathyroid gland, showing the smaller pale-staining principal cells and the larger, more deeply staining oxyphil cells.

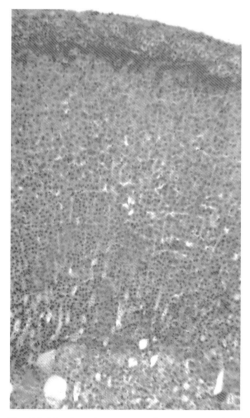

Fig. 13-13 Very-low-power photomicrograph of an adrenal gland, showing the zones of the cortex (above) and the medulla (below). (Courtesy of R. P. Jensh.)

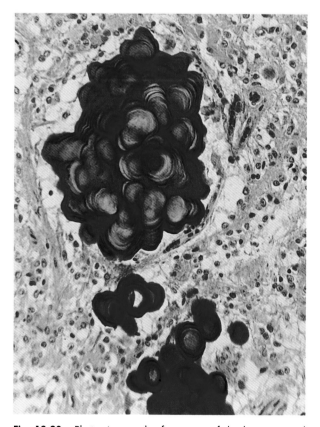

Fig. 13-20 Photomicrograph of an area of the human pineal including two corpora arenacea.

Plate 19

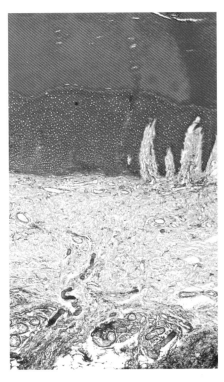

Fig. 14-1 Photomicrograph of plantar skin showing a very thick stratum corneum (bright red), a thick dermis (light blue), and a little subcutaneous adipose tissue at the bottom of the figure. (Courtesy of R. P. Jensh.)

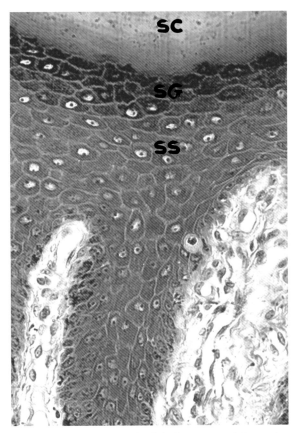

Fig. 14-3 Photomicrograph of the lower part of the epidermis of thick skin and portions of two dermal papillae. Stratum corneum (SC), stratum granulosum (SG), stratum spinosum (SS). (Courtesy of R. P. Jensh.)

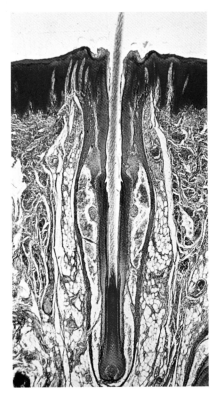

Fig. 14-12 Photomicrograph of a hair follicle. (From Anatomia Micrographica, 3rd ed., Piccin, Padova, Italy; courtesy of P. Motta.

Plate 20

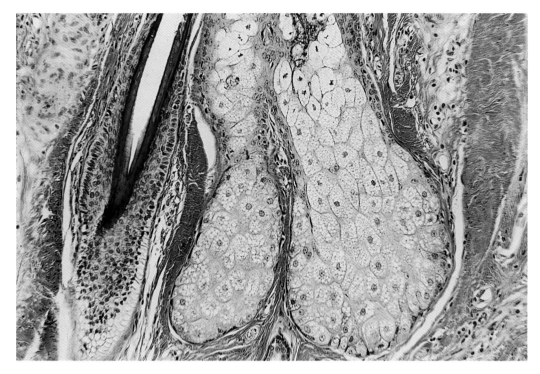

Fig. 14-16   Photomicrograph below the surface of the skin showing a hair follicle at the left and the associated seba-ceous gland.

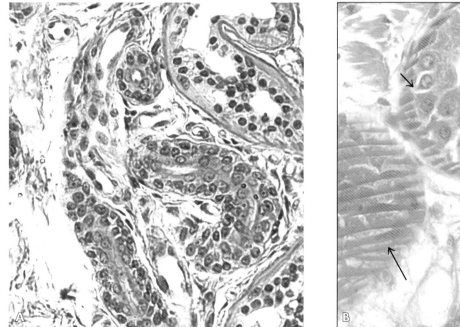

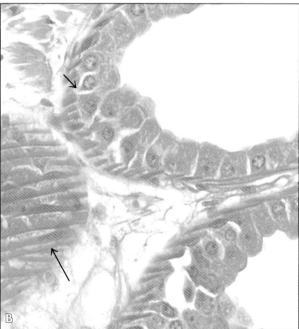

Fig. 14-17   (A) Photomicrograph of the coils of an eccrine sweat gland. (B) A slightly oblique section through tubules of an apocrine sweat gland. Note in the tangential section at the left, the parallel myoepithelial cells that are believed to play a role in expressing the secretory product into the ducts. (Courtesy of R. P. Jensh.)

Plate 21

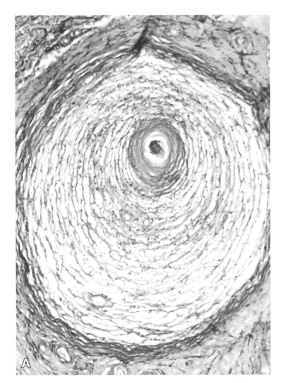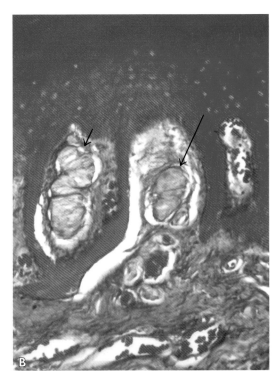

Fig. 14-20 (A) A high magnification of a Pacinian corpuscle. Note the nerve in the center and the multiple concentric layers around it. (B) A low magnification of skin in which two of the dermal papillae are occupied by Meissner's corpuscles. (Courtesy of R. P. Jensh.)

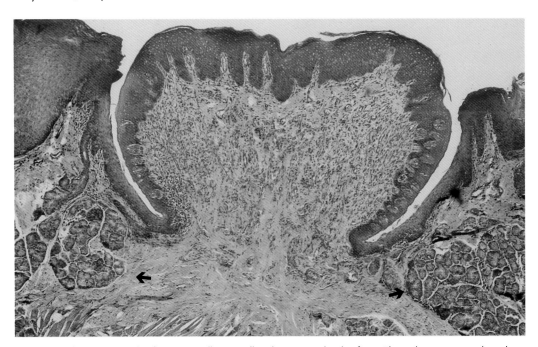

Fig. 15-3 Photomicrograph of a circumvallate papilla. The serous glands of von Ebner that open into the sulcus are indicated by arrows.

Plate 22

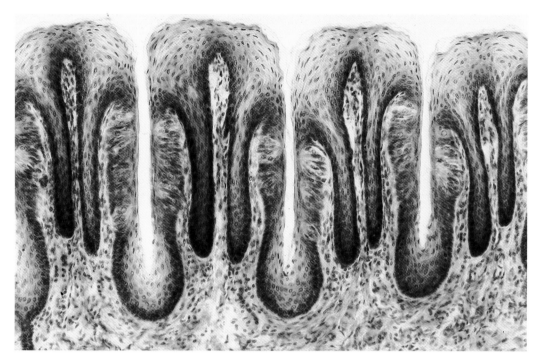

Fig. 15-4   Photomicrograph of foliate papillae of the tongue of a rabbit. Note the taste buds on the sides of the papillae.

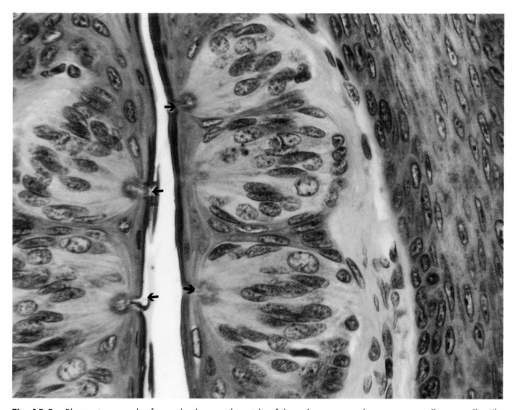

Fig. 15-5   Photomicrograph of taste buds on either side of the sulcus surrounding a circumvallate papilla. The taste pores are indicated by arrows.

Plate 23

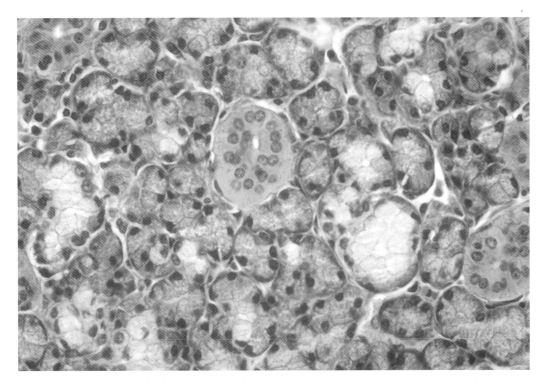

Fig. 15-16 Photomicrograph of the parotid gland. In most species, the parotid is a serous gland. In this field, the great majority of the acini are serous, but there are also two or three mucous acini. (Courtesy of R.P. Jensh.)

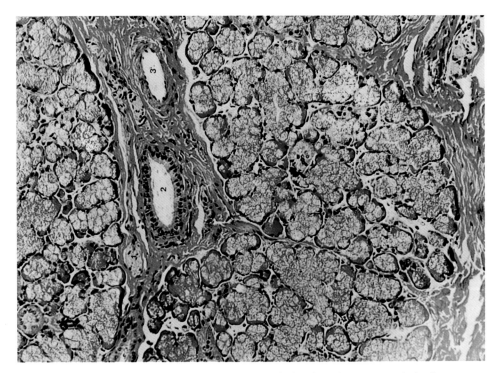

Fig. 15-17 Photomicrograph of the submandibular gland of a dog. This is a mixed gland containing both serous and mucous acini. (From Anatomia Microscopia, 3rd ed., Piccin, Padova, Italy; courtesy of P. Motta.)

Plate 24

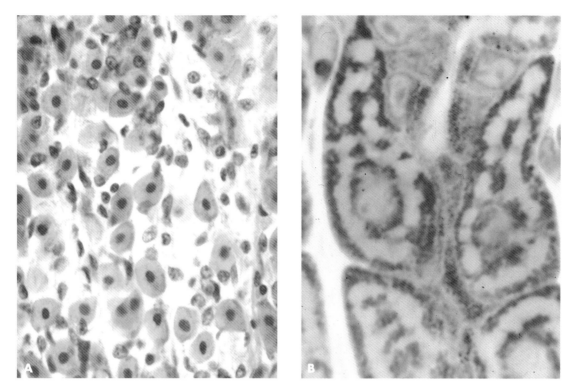

Fig. 16-7 (A) Photomicrograph of several gastric glands showing numerous intensely eosinophilic parietal cells. (Courtesy of R.P. Jensh.) (B) A high-power photomicrograph of four parietal cells showing their intracellular canaliculi.

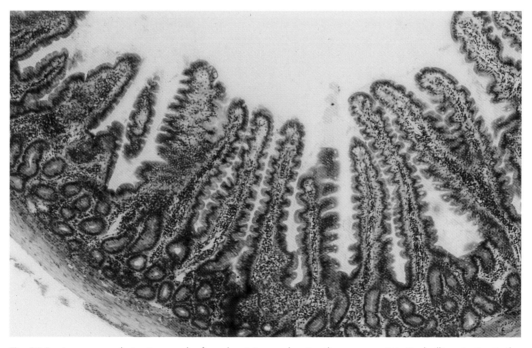

Fig. 17-1 Low-power photomicrograph of monkey jejunum showing the numerous intestinal villi projecting in the lumen.

Plate 25

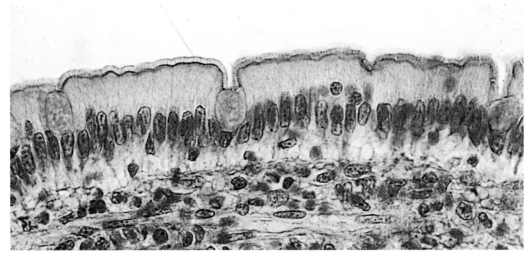

Fig. 17-3 Photomicrograph of a simple columnar epithelium of the intestine with a striated border and containing occasional mucus-secreting goblet cells.

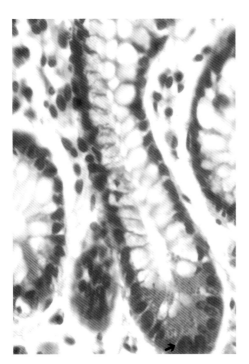

Fig. 17-8 Photomicrograph showing a cluster of Paneth cells in their usual location in the lower end of an intestinal gland. (Courtesy of R.P. Jensh.)

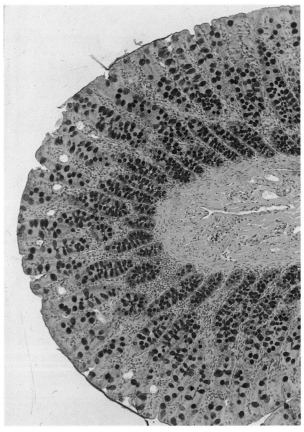

Fig. 17-13 Low-power photomicrograph of the mucosa of the colon. Observe that the number of deeply staining goblet cells increases toward the bottom of the crypts.

Plate 26

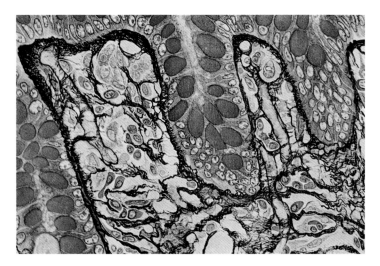

Fig. 17-14 Drawing of the upper part of the mucosa of the human colon. The section is slightly oblique and includes only a short segment of the two crypts on the right. The mucin of the goblet cells is stained blue. Note the reticular fibers (black) condensed beneath the epithelium.

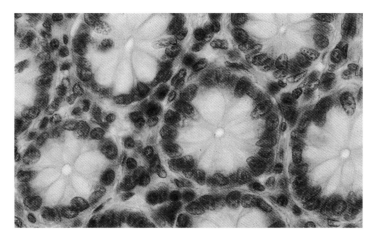

Fig. 17-15 Photomicrograph of transverse sections through the lower third of the glands of the colon. The epithelium at this level consists almost entirely of goblet cells.

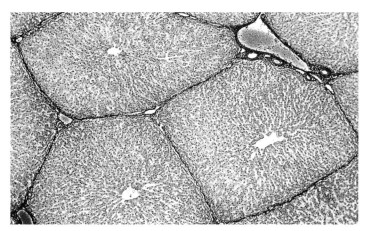

Fig. 18-1 Photomicrograph of pig liver, showing the hexagonal classical liver lobules surrounded by connective-tissue septa. Such septa are not found in the human liver. (Micrograph courtesy of P. Motta, Atlante Fotografico a colori di Anatomia Microscopia. Casa Editrice Dr Francesco Vallardi, Milan, Italy. 1972.)

Plate 27

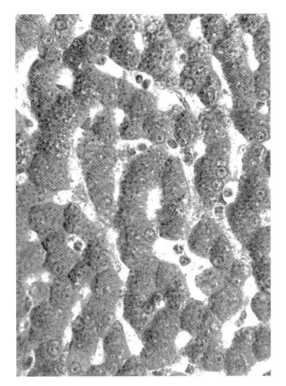

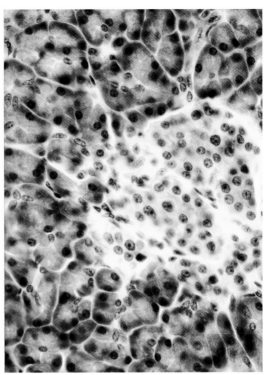

Fig. 18-11 Photomicrograph of liver stained with Best's carmine which colors glycogen deposits red. (Courtesy of R.P. Jensh.)

Fig. 19-5 Photomicrograph showing the appearance of an islet of Langerhans in a routine histological section.

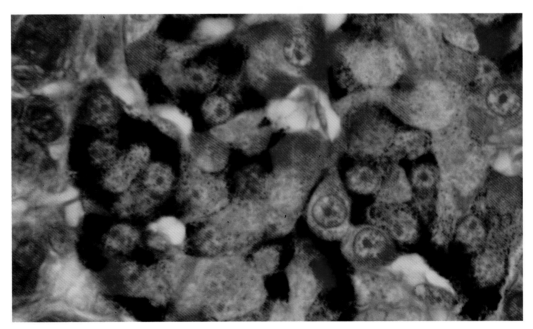

Fig. 19-6 High magnification photomicrograph of an islet of Langerhans prepared by a method that differentially stains the different endocrine cell types.

Plate 28

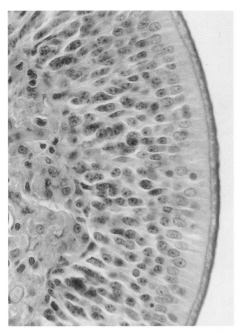

Fig. 20-1 Photomicrograph of the very tall olfactory epithelium. The darker line at the surface is a layer of mucus over the tips of the cilia.

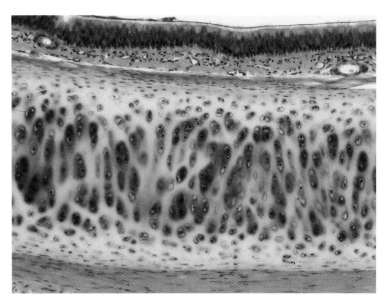

Fig. 20-4 Photomicrograph of monkey trachea. Observe the ciliated epithelium (above) underlain by lamina propria and hyaline cartilage, and at the bottom of the figure, a layer of smooth muscle.

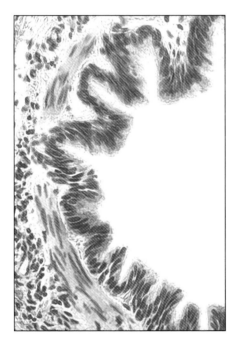

Fig. 20-5 Photomicrograph of the epithelium and smooth muscle in the wall of a bronchiole in cross section. In the living unconstricted state there is less folding of the mucosa into the lumna. (Courtesy of R.P. Jensh.)

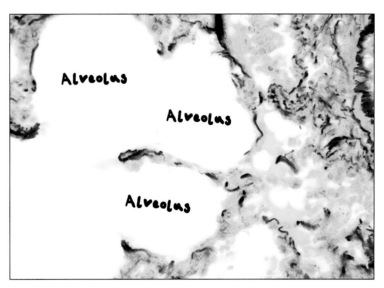

Fig. 20-11 Photomicrograph of lung prepared with a stain selective for elastin. The elastic fibers around a bronchiole at the right and in the interalveolar septa at the left are important for the elastic recoil of the lung in expiration. (Courtesy of R.P. Jensh.)

Plate 29

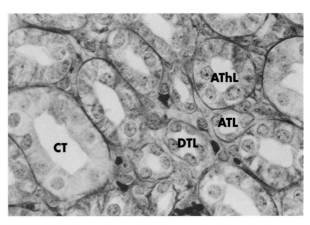

Fig. 21-13 Photomicrograph of a section through the outer medulla, showing a descending thin limb of the looper of Henle (DTL), ascending thin limbs (ATL), ascending thick limb (AThL), and a collecting tubule (CT).

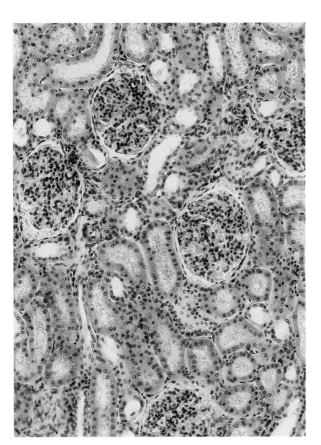

Fig. 21-3 Photomicrograph of an area of the renal cortex containing several glomeruli, and cross sections of proximal convoluted tubules.

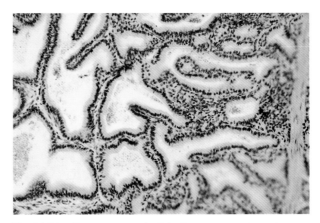

Fig. 22-17 Photomicrograph of the human seminal vesicle.

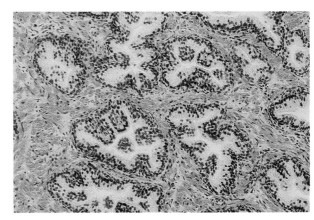

Fig. 22-18 Photomicrograph of the prostate of a young man.

Plate 30

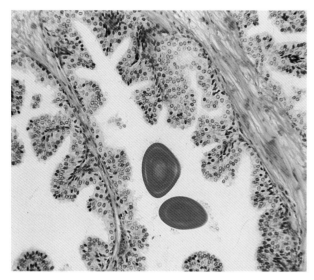

Fig. 22-19 Photomicrograph of the human prostate. Note the two corpora amylacea in the lumen.

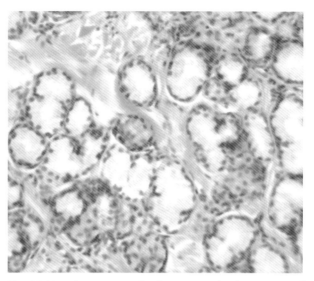

Fig. 22-20 Photomicrograph of Cowper's gland. (Courtesy of R.P. Jensh.)

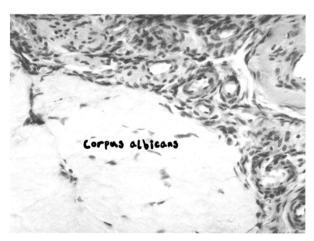

Fig. 23-9 Photomicrograph of an area in the medulla of the ovary containing, at the lower left, a corpus albicans formed in the degeneration of a corpus luteum. (Courtesy of R.P. Jensh).

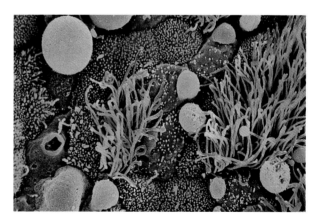

Fig. 23-12 Scanning electron micrograph of the mucosa of the endometrium. Color added. Cilia, green; microvilli, pink; globules of secretion, yellow. (Courtesy of P.M. Motta and S.A. Nottola.)

Plate 31

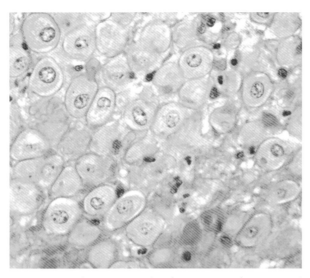

Fig. 23-20 Photomicrograph of an area of gestational endometrium, showing the large clear decidual cells that differentiate from fusiform cells of the endometrial stroma during pregnancy. (Courtesy of R.P. Jensh.)

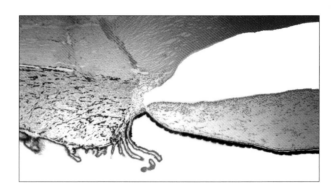

Fig. 24-5 Photomicrograph of the corneoscleral junction (above), ciliary body (lower left), and the iris extending to the right. Note Schlemm's canal (at arrow). (Courtesy of R.P. Jensh.)

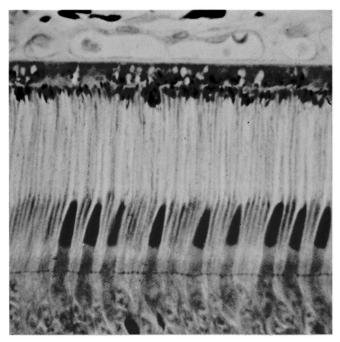

Fig. 24-10 Photomicrograph of the outermost layers of the monkey retina. The cones are easily distinguished from the rods because their inner segment is larger and more heavily stained. The arrow indicates the outer limiting membrane. (Courtesy of J. Rostgaard.)

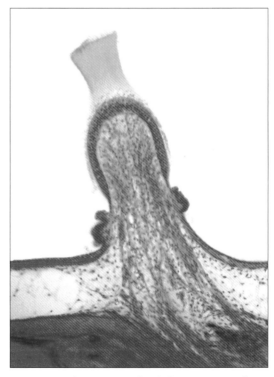

Fig. 25-6 Photomicrograph of the crista ampullaris. (Courtesy of R.P. Jensh.)

Plate 32

as undifferentiated, or resting secretory cells. The chromophils included **acidophils,** cells which stained with acidic dyes and **basophils** which stained with basic dyes. Thus, only two secretory cell types were distinguished.

The electron microscope has revealed that there is more than one cell type within each of these categories. These are distinguishable mainly on the basis of the size and shape of their secretory granules. In recent years, it has also become possible to identify the cell types by using fluorescein-labeled antibodies to their respective hormones. Of the six hormones secreted by the adenohypophysis, two are attributable to acidophils (**growth hormone** and **prolactin**) and four to basophils (**adrenocorticotropin, thyroid-stimulating hormone, follicle-stimulating hormone, luteinizing hormone**). It is now common practice to refer to the cell types of the pars distalis by terms that identify the target organ stimulated by the hormone it secretes. Thus, cells secreting thyroid-stimulating hormine (**TSH**) are called **thyrotropes;** those secreting the gonadotrophic hormones

FHS and **LH** are **gonadotropes;** cells secreting adrenocorticotrophic hormone (**ACTH**) are called **corticotropes;** those secreting growth hormone (**GH**) are **somatotropes;** and those secreting prolactin (**PL**) are **mammotropes** (Fig. 13-2 [see Plate 18]).

Somatotropes are commonly arranged in groups along the sinusoids. They contain dense spherical secretory granules 350–900 nm in diameter (Table 13-1 and Fig. 13-3). They have a large Golgi complex, but the rough endoplasmic reticulum is relatively sparse. **Mammotropes** are the dominant cell type of the pars distalis during pregnancy. They tend to occur individually in the cell cords and have a well-developed rough endoplasmic reticulum when they are actively secreting prolactin during lactation. Their ovoid secretory granules are the largest in the pars distalis, measuring up to 700 nm in diameter (Fig. 13-4). Their hormone stimulates growth of the mammary glands and secretion of milk. They are less numerous and have smaller granules (200 nm) in the nongravid female. They are also present in the male, where their function is not known. **Corticotropes** are relatively small cells occurring in groups; they sometimes form small follicles around a central mass of glycoprotein. Their granules are 200–250 nm in diameter and are usually located immediately beneath the plasma membrane (Fig. 13-3). The endoplasmic reticulum is tubular or vesicular and the Golgi complex is relatively small. They are very pale-staining and have sometimes been erroneously classified as chromophobes. Their product, adrenocorticotrophic hormone (ACTH) or corticotropin, stimulates release of the hormones of the adrenal cortex. **Thyrotropes** are elongate cells arranged in groups, usually near the center of the pars distalis. They have the smallest granules, 150–200 nm in diameter, and these are usually located at the cell periphery. They secrete thyrotropin (TSH), which stimulates the thyroid gland to release its hormone. The **gonadotropes** are large rounded cells close to the sinusoids. Their nucleus is irregular in outline, the Golgi complex is large, the granular endoplasmic reticulum is tubular or vesicular, and their secretory granules are 200–300 nm in diameter. They secrete two gonadotropic hormones: a follicle-stimulating hormone (FSH) and a luteinizing hormone (LH). In the female, FSH stimulates development of the ovarian follicles and secretion of estrogens in the female, and in the male, it promotes spermatogenesis. LH affects maturation of the ovarian follicles and their conversion to corpora lutea in the female. In the male, it stimulates the Leydig cells of the testis to secrete androgens.

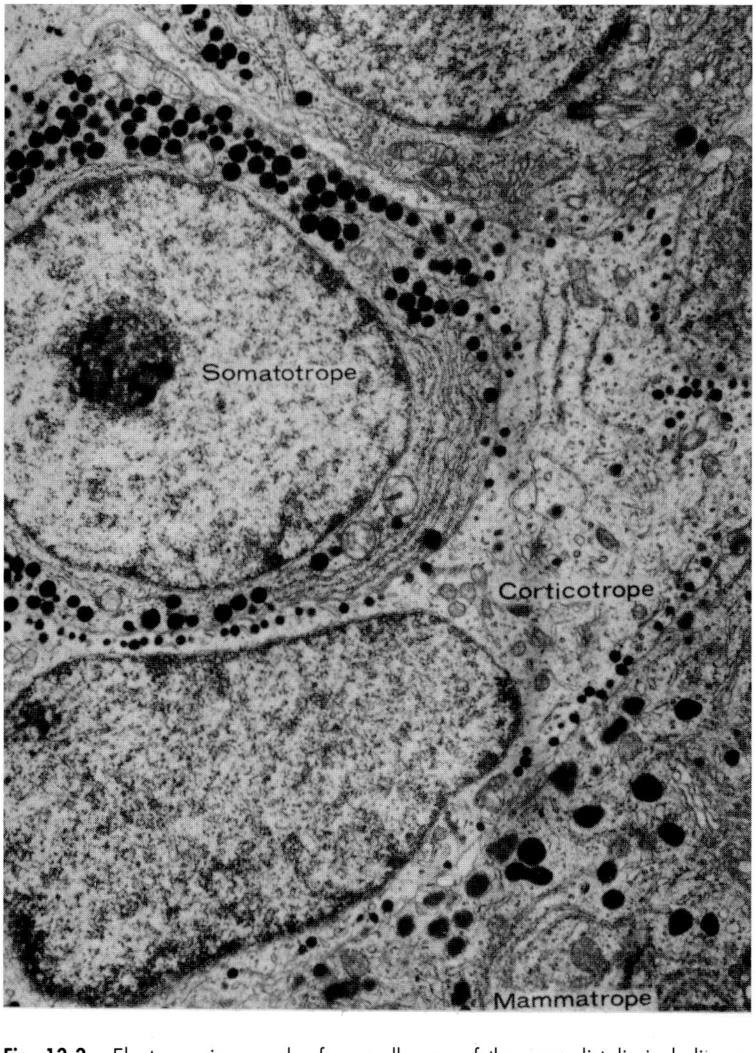

Fig. 13-3 Electron micrograph of a small area of the pars distalis including a somatotrope, a corticotrope, and a mammotrope, illustrating the difference in size of the secretory granules. (From I. Nakayama, F. A. Nickerson, and F. R. Shelton, Laboratory Investigations, 21:169, 1969.)

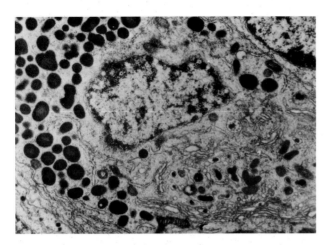

Fig. 13-4 Electron micrograph of a rat mammotrope. Note the relatively large size and irregular shape of the secretory granules. The smaller granules in the Golgi, at the lower right, coalesce to form the large dense granules seen at the upper left. (Courtesy of M. Farquhar and T. Kanaseki.)

Most of the hormones produced by the pars distalis act directly on the cells of their target organs. Somatotropin is exceptional in that its effect on growth of the body is mediated by growth factors, called **intermedins,** produced by the liver in response to somatotrophin.

A benign tumor of the pars distalis, producing excess growth hormone, in an adult, may cause **acromegaly,** *a chronic debilitating disease with overgrowth of bone and soft parts. There is enlargement of hands and feet, and a coarsening of the facial features. Surgical removal of the tumor is the treatment of choice. Excess production of growth hormone before closure of the epiphyses results in* **pituitary gigantism** *in which accelerated growth leads to abnormal stature.*

Histophysiology

In exocrine glands, the secretory cells are of the same kind throughout the gland and all are activated by the same hormone or neurotransmitter. The pars distalis of the hypophysis is unusual in the multiplicity of its cell types, each under separate control. Secretion of each of the hormones of the pars distalis is induced by a specific peptide

Cell Type	Hormone Secreted	Ultrastructure	Physiological Action	Releasing Hormone
Basophils Gonadotrope	Follicle stimulating hormone (FSH) Luteinizing hormone (LH)	Rounded cells; usually near sinusoids; 200 nm granules	Stimulates development of ovarian follicles in the female; stimulates spermatogenesis in the male	Gonadotropin-releasing hormone (GnRH)
Thyrotrope	Thyrotropin (TSH)	Angular cells; usually not near sinusoids; 140 nm granules	Stimulates thyroid hormone synthesis, storage and release	Thyrotropin-releasing hormone (TRH)
Corticotrope	Corticotropin (ACTH)	Cells pale, stellate; few large granules at cell periphery; 400–450 nm	Stimulates release of hormones of the adrenal cortex	Corticotropin-releasing hormone (CRH)
Acidophils Somatotrope	Somatotropin	Cells in groups near sinusoids; 300 nm granules	Stimulates growth of long bones, acting via liver-generated intermediates	Somatotropin-releasing hormone (SRH)
Mammotrope	Prolactin	Cells located individually in center of cords; 200 nm granules; 600 nm during lactation	Stimulates the secretion of milk	Prolactin-releasing hormone (PRH)

Table 1 Summary of Cell Types and Functions of the Pars Distalis of the Hypophysis

releasing factor produced in the hypothalamus and carried to the responding cells via the hypophyseoportal system of vessels. The releasing factors are somatotrophin-releasing hormone (SRH), prolactin-releasing hormone (PRH), gonadotrophin-releasing hormone (GnRH), corticotrophin-releasing hormone (CRH), and thyrotrophin-releasing hormone (TRH). The actions of the hypophyseal hormones will be discussed in more detail in other chapters on their target organs.

In addition to the hypothalamic releasing factors, the hypothalamus produces two inhibiting hormones: **somato-statin,** which inhibits the release of **somatotrophin,** and **prolactin-inhibiting hormone,** which suppresses the release of prolactin.

Pars Intermedia

In some mammals, the pars distalis is separated from the neurohypophysis by a cleft, lined on the juxtaneural side by a stratified epithelium of weakly basophilic cells forming the **pars intermedia.** This layer is made up of large polygonal cells, rich in mitochondria and endoplasmic reticulum, and containing numerous secretory granules. Its cells secrete **melanocyte-stimulating hormone** (MSH). This layer of epithelium is present in the human fetus, but in the adult it is no longer identifiable as a distinct layer. However, isolated groups of such cells can be found invading a short distance into the pars nervosa. These residues of the pars intermedia have no known function in man.

Pars Tuberalis

The **pars tuberalis** is a thin sleeve of epithelial cells, only 25–60 μm thick, surrounding the infundibulum of the hypophysis. This is the most highly vascular region of the gland, containing the hypophyseoportal system of venules. It consists of cords of epithelial cells occupying the spaces between the venules coursing downward to the pars distalis. The cells are cuboidal, or low columnar, and contain small dense granules, lipid droplets, and occasional colloid droplets. They are the only cells in the hypophysis that contain significant amounts of glycogen. No specific hormone is known to be secreted by the pars tuberalis, and its function remains unknown.

Neurohypophysis

The **neurohypophysis** consists of the median eminence of the hypothalamus, the infundibular process, and the pars nervosa (posterior lobe) of the hypophysis. The pars nervosa is made up of tens of thousands of unmyelinated axons of neurons whose cell bodies are in the **supraoptic nucleus** and **paraventricular nucleus** of the hypothala-

mus (Fig. 13-1). Glial cells, called **pituicytes,** form a cellular network throughout the lobe, with their long processes in communication via gap junctions. They are highly variable in size and shape and commonly contain lipid droplets and deposits of lipochrome pigment. Some of the pituicyte cell processes wrap around axons near their termination.

The hypothalamic neurons, whose axons make up the bulk of the posterior lobe, are large cells with an eccentric nucleus, abundant cytoplasm and few dendrites. The rough endoplasmic reticulum forms conspicuous parallel arrays (Nissl bodies) and the prominent Golgi complex is the site of assembly of small (120–200 nm) neurosecretory granules that are continuously transported along microtubules into the pars nervosa at a rate of 4–8 mm/h. The granules accumulate and are stored in hundreds of small dilatations along the length of each axon (Fig. 13-5). These aggregations of granules are visible with the light microscope and were traditionally called **Herring bodies.** Their constituent granules contain either **oxytocin,** or **vasopressin,** combined with a **neurophysin,** a carrier protein of a type

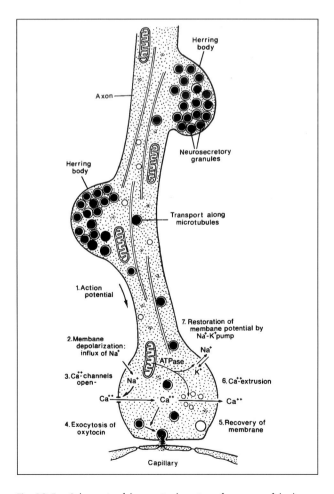

Fig. 13-5 Schematic of the terminal portion of an axon of the hypothalamohypophyseal tract in the pars nervosa. The principal events in stimulus-secretion coupling are indicated (Modified from D. W. Lincoln, in Hormonal Control of Reproduction, Cambridge University Press, Cambridge, 1984.)

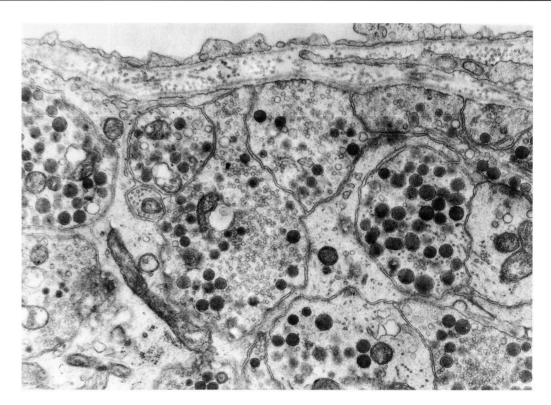

Fig. 13-6 Electron micrograph of the rat pars nervosa, showing many neurosecretory granules and small vesicles in the axoplasm of fibers of the hypothalamohypophyseal tract that are ending near a capillary (above). (Courtesy of P. Orkand and S. Palay.)

specific for each hormone. The axon terminals are closely associated with the fenestrated endothelium of sinusoids within the pars nervosa. The terminals can be recognized in electron micrographs by their content of multiple small vesicles similar to synaptic vesicles (Fig. 13-6). These vesicles, however, do not contain a neurotransmitter but are formed in the recycling of membrane added to the plasmalemma in exocytosis of the neurosecretory granules.

Histophysiology

Prior to their exocytosis, the hormones of the posterior lobe are cleaved from their neurophysin and both enter the bloodstream. The neurophysins have no known physiological function. The principal target of **oxytocin** is the pregnant uterus. Its concentration in the blood increases in the late stages of labor and stimulates contraction of the smooth muscle of the uterus. It is also involved in milk ejection from the lactating mammary gland. Stimulation of the nipple by the suckling infant sends afferent impulses to the brain that are relayed to neurons in the supraoptic and paraventricular nuclei. These respond by releasing oxytocin from their axon terminals into capillaries of the pars nervosa. Blood-borne oxytocin then stimulates contraction of myoepithelial cells around the mammary alveoli, ejecting milk into the ducts.

The principal targets of **vasopressin** are the collecting ducts of the kidney and the peripheral arterioles. Whenever the osmotic pressure of the blood rises, it acts on osmoreceptor areas in the hypothalamus that stimulate release of vasopressin from the axon terminals in the pars nervosa. The hormone binds to receptors on the cells of the distal convoluted tubules and collecting ducts of the kidney, activating a kinase that acts on a membrane protein to increase permeability of the apical plasma membrane of these cells to water. This permits increased uptake of water from the tubule lumen, thereby decreasing the volume of urine and increasing its concentration. Vasopressin is also involved in the control of blood pressure. A sudden decrease in blood volume is a potent stimulus for increased secretion of vasopressin. For example, after a severe hemorrhage, it may be secreted at 50 times the normal level. It acts on vascular smooth muscle, causing constriction of arterioles, which increases peripheral resistance in the circulatory system and thereby increases blood pressure.

The neurohypophysis may fail to respond to the normal stimuli by secreting vasopressin. This causes ***diabetes insipidus,*** *a disorder in which there is excessive thirst, excessive intake of water (polydipsia), and frequent urination (polyuria). Treatment is by injection of vasopressin or drugs with similar effects (antidiuretics).*

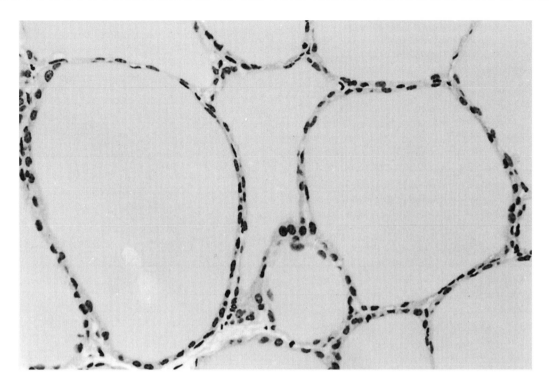

Fig. 13-8 Photomicrograph of monkey thyroid gland, showing the low cuboidal epithelium and the colloid within the follicles.

THYROID

The thyroid gland is situated in the anterior part of the neck, immediately below the larynx. It consists of two lateral lobes connected by an isthmus that crosses the trachea just below the cricoid cartilage. The secretions of the thyroid gland are important during childhood for the normal development of the central nervous and musculoskeletal systems. In the adult, its hormones play a role in thermoregulation and control of the basal metabolic rate of certain tissues.

Organization

In most endocrine glands, small amounts of hormone are stored in intracellular secretory granules. The thyroid is unique in having an organization that provides for extracellular storage of the secretory product. The gland consists of spherical **thyroid follicles** ranging in size from 0.2 to 0.9 mm in diameter. These are bounded by a simple cuboidal epithelium and filled with a gelatinous material, referred to as the **thyroid colloid** (Figs. 13-7 [see Plate 18] and 13-8).

The gland is enclosed in a moderately thick connective-tissue capsule that is continuous with the cervical fascia. Deep to this layer is looser connective tissue, from which thin septa extend into the gland separating groups of thyroid follicles. Each follicle is surrounded by a thin basal

lamina, a network of reticular fibers, and a rich plexus of capillaries (Fig. 13-9). The epithelium of the follicle is cuboidal or low columnar, depending on the state of its

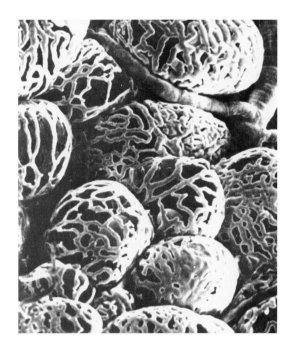

Fig. 13-9 Scanning micrograph of a portion of monkey thyroid in which the blood vessels have been injected with plastic and the tissue subsequently digested away. The dense network of capillaries around each follicle is clearly shown. (From H. Fujita and T. Murikami, *Archives of Histology Japan,* 36:181, 1974.)

activity. In electron micrographs, the cells are polarized toward the lumen and joined by typical junctional complexes. There are a few short microvilli on the free surface. The rough endoplasmic reticulum is well developed and there is a prominent supranuclear Golgi complex. Associated with the latter are many small vesicles containing newly synthesized **thyroglobulin,** the precursor of **thyroid hormone.** These vesicles move to the apex and release their content by exocytosis into the lumen of the follicle. Because of the extracellular storage of the secretory product, there is two-way traffic across the cell. In addition to the vesicles involved in adlumenal transport of thyroglobulin, there are larger vacuoles in cells of the stimulated thyroid. These are formed by endocytosis of colloid from the lumen (Fig. 13-10). Small lysosomes in the cytoplasm fuse with these vacuoles and their enzymes degrade the colloid to liberate thyroid hormone, which is released at the cell base and enters the surrounding capillaries.

> *In hyperthyroidism,* **Graves disease,** *there is thyroid enlargement (goiter) and excess production of thyroid hormones. The height of the epithelium of the follicles is increased and there are papillary infoldings of their wall. Excess hormone results in restlessness, sleeplessness, tremor, and a noticeable prominence of the eyeballs (exophthalmos). The presence of antithyroid antibodies in the blood suggests an autoimmune basis for the disease. Treatment is with radioactive iodine or subtotal thyroidectomy.*

Pale-staining **parafollicular cells** are found singly, or in small groups, at the base of the follicular epithelium. They are always separated from the lumen of the follicle by overarching portions of the neighboring thyroid follicular cells. The nucleus is round or ovoid. The cytoplasm contains tubular and cisternal profiles of the endoplasmic reticulum and a small Golgi complex. Small electron-dense secretory granules are congregated near the cell base (Fig. 13-11). These contain **thyrocalcitonin (calcitonin)**, a peptide hormone, which, in some mammalian species, is an important regulator of blood calcium. In these species, calcitonin lowers the concentration of calcium in the blood by suppressing bone resorption. In the human, it cannot be detected in the blood plasma and is of doubtful functional significance.

Histophysiology

The principal hormones of the thyroid are **thyroxine** and **triiodothyronine.** They are stored in the colloid as constituents of the very large secretory glycoprotein **thyroglobulin** (600,000 MW). After synthesis of its protein moiety in the endoplasmic reticulum, carbohydrate is

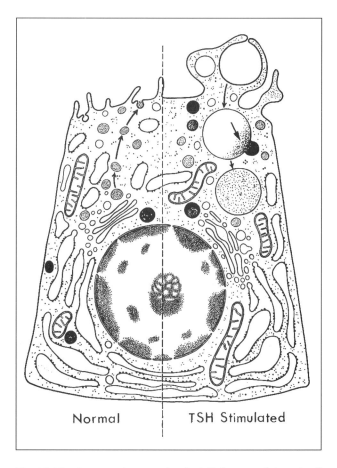

Fig. 13-10 Drawing depicting (on the left) the normal thyroid cell secreting thyroglobulin into the lumen, and (on the right) its appearance during uptake of colloid by pinocytosis after stimulation by TSH. Lysosomes fuse with the vacuoles to degrade the thyroglobulin and release thyroxine.

added in the Golgi complex and the thyroglobulin is packaged for exocytosis. The cells also synthesize a peroxidase that is located mainly in the apical plasma membrane, where it oxidizes iodide taken up at the cell base. The iodine taken up binds to tyrosine groups of the thyroglobulin to form the iodinated thyroglobulin that is stored in the colloid. In the lysosomal degradation of colloid, the products are tetraiodothyronine (T4) (thyroxine), triiodothyronine (T3), smaller amounts of diiodothyronine (DIT), and monoiodothyronine (MIT). An intracellular enzyme, iodotyrosine dehalogenase, liberates iodine from DIT and MIT for reuse by the cell in iodinization of newly synthesized thyroglobulin. Thyroxine and triiodothyronine are liberated at the cell base.

The primary control of thyroid function is mediated by the thyroid-stimulating hormone (TSH) of the hypophysis. Blood-borne TSH binds to receptors on the basolateral membranes of the follicular cells, which respond by accelerated iodine uptake, increased production of cyclic AMP, and enhanced synthesis and release of thyroid hormones.

Deficient secretion of TSH, in an adult, results in **myxedema,** *a severe form of hypothyroidism. There is weakness, drowsiness, and slowing of mental activity. There is also an accumulation of glycoprotein in the skin resulting in its thickening, with undesirable alterations in the facial features. If this condition develops in childhood, it is called* **cretinism,** *characterized by retarded bone growth, respiratory distress, and mental retardation.*

PARATHYROID

The parathyroid glands are small ovoid bodies adhering to the posterior surface of the thyroid gland. They are usually four in number and measure about 5 mm in length, 4 mm in diameter, and 2 mm in thickness. Each weighs only 20–50 mg. Accessory glands and ectopic glands located lower in the neck or in the mediastinum are not uncommon. The parathyroids are endocrine glands secreting **parathyroid hormone** (**PTH**) which acts on bone, intestines, and kidneys to maintain the necessary concentration of calcium in the blood and extracellular fluid. Calcium is an essential element in mammalian physiology. It is required for muscular contraction, glandular secretion, and blood coagulation, and for the activity of many key enzymes in intermediary metabolism.

Structure

Each gland is enclosed in a thin capsule from which thin connective-tissue trabeculae extend inward, carrying the blood vessels, nerves, and lymphatics. The parenchyma of the gland consists of branching and anastomosing cords of epithelial cells supported by a delicate framework of reticular fibers that also surround the very rich network of capillaries between the cell cords (Fig. 13-12 [see Plate 19]). Rarely, the epithelial cells may form isolated small follicles containing a colloidal material of unknown nature. The glands slowly increase in size from birth through adolescence, attaining their maximum size at age 20. The connective-tissue stroma of the gland in older individuals contains variable numbers of adipose cells, and, in the elderly, these may occupy 60% or more of the gland.

The parenchyma of the human parathyroid gland consists of two epithelial cell types: **chief cells** and **oxyphil cells** (Fig. 13-12 [see Plate 19]). The chief cells are 5–8 μm in diameter and have a centrally placed nucleus in a slightly eosinophilic cytoplasm. In electron micrographs, the cells are found to be joined by occasional desmosomes. In contrast to other glands, in which all cells exhibit the same degree of activity, parathyroid cells appear to go through their secretory cycle independently. Both active and inactive cells are found within the gland. In active cells, the cytoplasm contains elongated mitochondria, parallel cisternae of rough endoplasmic reticulum, a prominent Golgi

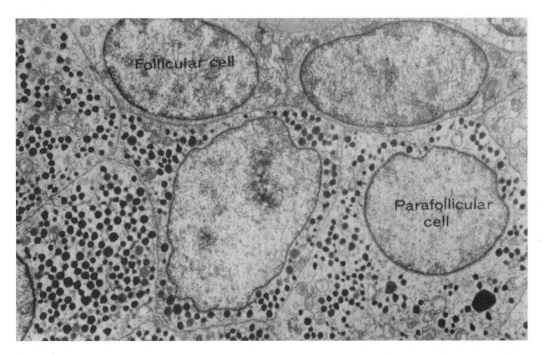

Fig. 13-11   Electron micrograph of follicular cells (above) and parafollicular cells (below). The parafollicular cells are always separated from the colloid in the lumen by follicular cells. The cells contain many small dense granules. (Courtesy of S. Wissig.)

complex and small deposits of glycogen. Conspicuous dense granules of varying shape are common and are interpreted as lipofuchsin pigment deposits. Numerous smaller granules 200–400 nm in diameter are secretory granules containing the polypeptide **parathyroid hormone.** Inactive cells contain relatively little endoplasmic reticulum, a small Golgi complex, and few secretory granules. The inactive cells outnumber the active cells.

Cells of a second type, the **oxyphil cells,** are up to 10 μm in diameter. They are clearly larger than the chief cells, and they stain more deeply with eosin (Fig. 13-12 [see Plate 19]). They are few in number and occur singly or in small clusters. In electron micrographs, the Golgi complex is small, the endoplasmic reticulum is sparse, and there are no secretory granules. They have an extraordinary number of mitochondria and these have closely spaced cristae, suggesting a high degree of metabolic activity. The small amount of space between the closely packed mitochondria is occupied by glycogen.

Histophysiology

The concentration of calcium in the body fluids is maintained in the narrow range of 8.5–10.5 mg/100 ml. Whenever the concentration falls below this level, the parathyroid glands rapidly increase their secretion of parathyroid hormone to 5–10 times the basal rate. The hormone acts on osteocytes, causing them to mobilize calcium from the bone mineral around them, a process called **osteocytic osteolysis.** This usually corrects the low blood calcium level quite rapidly. If hypocalcemia persists, precursor cells in the bones coalesce to form increased numbers of osteoclasts to erode more bone. This process, called **osteoclastic osteolysis,** is slower, taking many hours to reach effective levels of calcium release.

In addition to its action on bone, parathyroid hormone acts on the distal convoluted tubules of the kidney to increase their reabsorption of calcium from the glomerular filtrate. Calcium loss in the urine is thus reduced. Parathyroid hormone also indirectly influences the rate of calcium uptake from the lumen of the intestine. Calcium uptake from the diet is dependent on the action of **vitamin D [(1,25-(OH) cholecalciferol].** Parathyroid hormone is the principal regulator of production of this hormone by the kidney.

ADRENALS

The adrenal glands are located at the cranial pole of each kidney. They are relatively flat triangular organs, less than 1 cm thick and ranging in width from 2 cm at the apex to 5 cm at their base. On the cut surface of a transected adrenal, a thick yellow cortex is readily distinguishable from a gray medulla in the interior of the gland. The cortex and medulla are both endocrine glands, but they differ in their embryological origins and their function. The gland is enclosed by a connective-tissue capsule that sends septa into the interior of the organ.

Blood Supply

The adrenal glands have an exceptionally high rate of blood flow, and an unusual pattern of blood vessels. Each adrenal receives its blood supply from three arteries that ramify over the surface of the gland, giving rise to branches that pass through the capsule to form a dense **subcapsular plexus.** Short cortical arteries arising from this plexus ramify into a very extensive network of fenestrated sinusoidal capillaries around groups and columns of cells in the cortex. These cortical sinuses are confluent with a plexus of medullary veins (Fig. 13-13 [see Plate 19]). This plexus is drained by sizable veins in the center of the medulla that join to form the **suprarenal vein** that emerges from the hilus of the gland. In addition to the short branches of the subcortical plexus that give rise to the cortical sinusoids, there are long cortical arteries that pass unbranched through the cortex and form net-

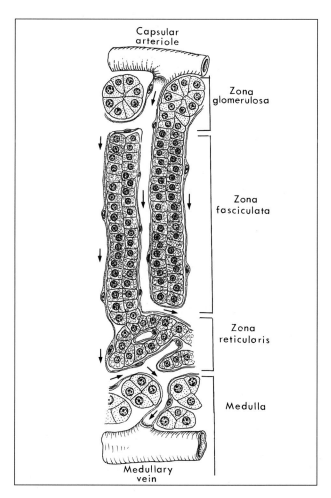

Fig. 13-14 Drawing of the various regions of the adrenal cortex and the outer medulla. The zona fasciculata is usually longer than depicted here.

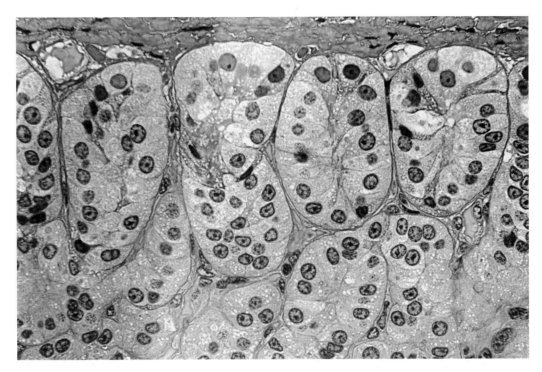

Fig. 13-15 Photomicrograph of the zona glomerulosa showing the acinar, or glomerular arrangement of the cells. These cells have fewer lipid droplets than those of the zona fasciculata, and thus appear less vacuolated after lipid extraction in specimen preparation.

works of capillaries in the medulla. Thus, the adrenal medulla has a dual blood supply, receiving blood indirectly via the cortical sinusoids and directly via the long cortical arteries.

Adrenal Cortex

Three concentric zones are distinguishable in the adrenal cortex: a thin **zona glomerulosa** immediately beneath the capsule; a broad intermediate **zona fasciculata;** and an inner **zona reticularis** adjacent to the medulla (Figs. 13-13 [see Plate 19] and 13-14). The transition from zone to zone is gradual, but their boundaries are more apparent if the blood vessels are injected with a contrast medium, for the three layers have very distinctive vascular patterns.

The zonation of the cortex is reflected in its production of different hormones in the three zones. **Aldosterone** is produced exclusively in the zona glomerulosa. **Cortisol** is secreted mainly by the zona fasciculata, and the zona reticularis is the principal site of production of **dehydroepiandrosterone.** When isolated from their natural location, cells of all three layers produce the same product. This has led to the suggestion that products of the peripheral zone carried in the blood downstream to the next zone may influence the nature of the product formed in that zone. The synthesis of a key enzyme by cells of the medulla has been shown to be dependent on their exposure to glucocorticoids reaching them in blood from the cortex. Thus, the unusual vascular pattern of the gland has physiological significance.

Zona Glomerulosa

In this zone, columnar epithelial cells form closely spaced arcades separated by thin connective-tissue septa extending inward from the capsule (Fig. 13-15). The cells have spherical, heterochromatic nuclei and an acidophilic cytoplasm containing occasional angular basophilic areas. In electron micrographs, the latter are small arrays of rough endoplasmic reticulum. There is a conspicuous network of smooth endoplasmic reticulum throughout the cytoplasm, and a few lipid droplets. A few desmosomes and occasional gap junctions are found on the cell boundaries.

Zona Fasciculata

In preparations for the light microscope, this middle zone is made up of pale-staining polyhedral cells arranged in long columns oriented radially with respect to the medulla. Capillaries, with this same orientation, run between the columns. The cells have a highly vacuolated appearance, owing to the extraction of abundant lipid droplets (Fig. 13-16). In electron micrographs, the nucleus has a prominent fibrous lamina and a large nucleolus. There are a great many lipid droplets in the cytoplasm, and mitochondria with atypical tubular or vesicular cristae. Smooth endoplasmic reticulum occupies a large part of the cytoplasm, a feature common to steroid-secreting cells.

Zona Reticularis

In this inner zone, the parallel columns of cells give way to a three-dimensional network of anastomosing

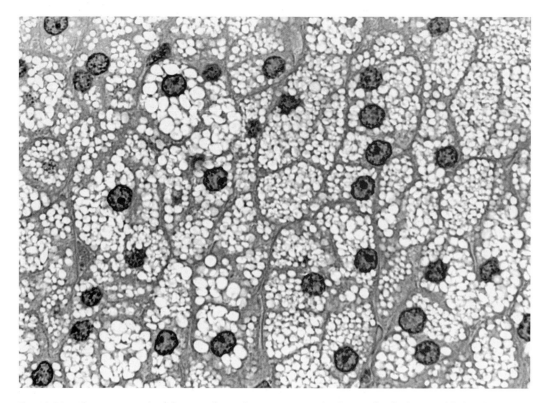

Fig. 13-16 Photomicrograph of the zona fasciculata, consisting of columns of cells that are filled with vacuoles representing extracted lipid droplets.

cords. The cells of these are somewhat smaller and stain more deeply than those of the outer zones (Fig. 13-17). In electron micrographs, lipid droplets are fewer and the smooth endoplasmic reticulum is less extensive. Large aggregations of lipochrome pigment are common. Near the medulla, there are variable numbers of "dark cells" with shrunken nuclei and dense cytoplasm. Their nuclear changes, paucity of organelles, and accumulations of pigment suggest that cell degeneration may be common in this zone.

Adrenal Medulla

The medulla is composed of large epithelioid cells in clusters, or short cords, closely related to capillaries and venules (Fig. 13-17). In electron micrographs or in tissue fixed in a solution containing potassium dichromate, many of the cells are crowded with small granules (Fig. 13-18). This staining with dichromate is called the **chromaffin reaction.** It results from oxidation and polymerization of **catecholamines** in the secretory granules. Cells exhibiting this staining are termed **chromaffin cells. Catecholamines** are compounds that serve as neurotransmitters for cells of the sympathetic nervous system. The adrenal medulla can be thought of as a modified sympathetic ganglion made up of postganglionic neurons that lack dendrites and axons. The catecholamines of the adrenal medulla are **norepinephrine**

and **epinephrine.** These are secreted in response to stimulation by preganglionic fibers from splanchnic nerves.

In the adrenal medulla, two kinds of cells giving the chromaffin reaction can be distinguished. In electron micrographs, the granules of cells that store norepinephrine have a dense core and a less dense outer zone. Cells that store epinephrine have granules with a more homogenous content of lower density. The granules also contain chromogranins and enkephalins, but these substances are of little physiological significance.

Histophysiology

The principal function of the adrenal glands is to maintain the constancy of the internal environment of the body and to make appropriate changes in its physiology in response to acute stress, injury, or prolonged deprivation of food and water. The cortex secretes three classes of steroids: **mineralocorticoids, glucocorticoids,** and **androgens.** The principal mineralocorticoid is **aldosterone,** secreted mainly by the zona glomerulosa. It controls body fluid volume by influencing the rate of reabsorption of sodium by the kidneys. Its secretion is stimulated by (1) a fall in sodium concentration in the blood; (2) by release of **adrenocorticotrophic hormone (ACTH)** of the hypophysis, or (3) by **atrial natriuretic hormone** produced by specialized cardiac muscle cells. The principal glucocorti-

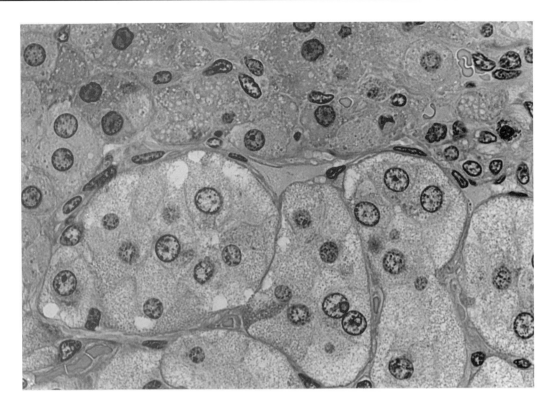

Fig. 13-17 Photomicrograph of the junction of the zona reticularis (above) with the clusters of cells of the adrenal medulla (below). With the light microscope, catecholamine granules are not visible unless a special staining method has been used.

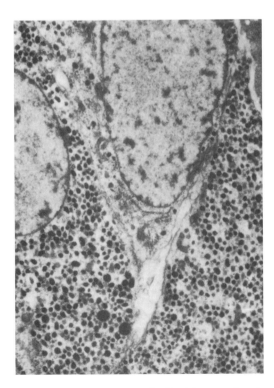

Fig. 13-18 Electron micrograph of cells of the cat adrenal medulla, showing the very numerous dense granules that are sites of storage of catecholamines. (Courtesy of R. Yates.)

coid is **cortisol,** secreted by the zona fasciculata in response to stimulation by adrenocorticotrophic hormone. It has many effects. It decreases protein synthesis, thereby increasing the circulating level of amino acids; it acts on the liver to enhance gluconeogenesis; and it mobilizes fatty acids and glycerol from adipose cells. In addition to these metabolic effects, it has anti-inflammatory effects. It stabilizes lysosomal membranes, reducing release of damaging proteolytic enzymes at sites of inflammation and it decreases capillary permeability, minimizing local swelling. These attributes make cortisol a valuable medication. Small amounts of **androgens** are secreted by the zona reticularis. The principal adrenal androgen is **dehydroepiandrosterone,** which is far less potent than testosterone and has little physiological significance.

The adrenal cortex is under hormonal control (ACTH), whereas secretory activity of the medulla is under nervous control. Centers in the hypothalamus relay impulses to the adrenal medulla via splanchnic (visceral) nerves that end among its cells. Their activation leads to secretion of **epinephrine** and **norepinephrine.** Secretion of these catecholamines in response to acute fear, or stress, results in an increase in heart rate, while the liver releases a surge of glucose into the blood as an energy source. Thus, the release of these hormones, in threatening circumstances, prepares the body for combat or flight.

*Deficiency of adrenal cortical hormones, **Addison's disease**, may be due to gradual destruction of the cortex by an autoimmune process, or by an infectious disease. There is weakness, fatigability, nausea, low blood pressure (hypotension), and pigmentation of the skin and oral mucosa. A tumor of the adrenal cortex may result in excess adrenal hormone production, **Cushing's disease**, in which there is obesity, weakness, poor wound healing, osteoporosis, and hypotension. Surgical excision of the tumor may be necessary.*

PINEAL GLAND

The pineal gland (**epiphysis cerebri**) is a small organ projecting from the roof of the diencephalon, in the midline of the brain. The gland is a conical gray body 5–8 mm in length and 3–5 mm at its greatest width (Fig. 13-

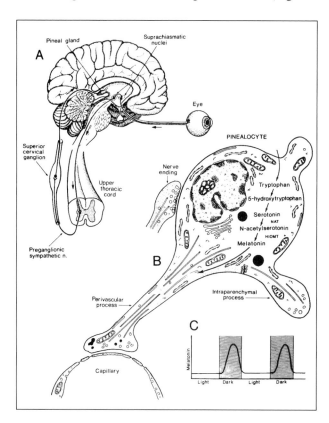

Fig. 13-19 (A) Path of information transfer from the eyes, to the pineal via retinal–hypothalamic tracts to the suprachiasmatic nucleus; relayed to the intermediolateral column of the spinal cord; then to the cervical gangion; and then by sympathetic fibers to the pineal. (B) Upon stimulation of pinealocytes, tryptophan is taken up and converted to melatonin, which is released into the blood. (C) Graph of the light–dark cycle of melatonin concentration in the blood. (Modified from R. J. Reiter in Groot's Endocrinology, W. B. Saunders, Philadelphia, 1989.)

19). The gland is invested by the pia mater, the delicate inner layer of connective tissue that covers the brain. Thin septa extend inward from this layer to surround cords, or small lobules, of cells in its interior. The parenchyma consists of pale-staining epitheloid cells, called **pinealocytes.** Their nucleus is deeply indented and may be quite irregular in outline. The cytoplasm is slightly basophilic and contains both rough and smooth endoplasmic reticulum, a small Golgi complex, and many mitochondria. It may also contain a few lipid droplets. When stained by silver-impregnation methods, the pinealocytes can be shown to have one or more long processes that terminate in bulbous expansions. The majority of these end on, or near, capillaries. Their terminations contain clusters of small vesicles that are often associated with a **synaptic ribbon,** a dense rod or lamella extending inward from the plasmalemma. Similar structures are found at synapses in sensory cells of the retina and inner ear. In the pinealocytes, they are multiple and may be found on the cell body as well as at the ends of the cell processes. Their function remains a mystery. The pinealocytes secrete the hormone **melatonin.** It is apparently released at the rate it is produced and not stored in secretory granules.

Cells of a second type, called **interstitial cells** or **astroglial cells,** are found among the pinealocytes and around capillaries. They resemble the astrocytes of the brain in having long cell processes containing an abundance of intermediate filaments. The pineal of humans contains peculiar extracellular concretions called **corpora arenacea** (so-called "brain sand") that consist of calcium phosphate and calcium carbonate in an organic matrix (Fig. 13-20 [see Plate 19]). When calcified, they are useful to the radiologist in localizing tumors of the brain that may displace the pineal from its normal midline position.

Histophysiology

The pineal is a gland that modulates gonadal function. Its biosynthetic activity exhibits a diurnal rhythmicity related to the periods of light and darkness. The plasma concentration of its hormone, **melatonin,** increases in the dark phase of the cycle. Information as to day or night is transmitted from the eyes, over retinohypothalamic tracts to nuclei in the hypothalamus, and ultimately to the pineal (Fig. 13-19). There, release of norepinephrine among the pinealocytes controls their secretory activity. Melatonin suppresses release of gonadotrophic hormones of the hypophysis. The pinealocytes also secrete **arginine vasotocin,** another peptide that has antigonadotrophic activity.

In species that are seasonal breeders, the gonads regress in the winter and only regain reproductive competence in the spring. It is the pineal that mediates this response of the reproductive system to changing day length. Increased secretion of melatonin during the longer nights of fall and winter causes regression of the testes. Longer days of sunlight, in the spring, decrease pineal secretion permitting the testes to respond to gonadotrophic hormones, with resumption of spermatogenesis. In the course of evolution, humans became continuous breeders. There is no evidence that reproductive activity of humans is subject to pineal regulation. With the invention of the electric lightbulb, day length became irrelevant.

ISLETS OF LANGERHANS

The **islets of Langerhans** secreting the hormones **insulin, glucagon, somatostatin,** and **pancreatic polypeptide** could appropriately be included in this chapter on the endocrine glands, but they do not form a separate organ. They consist of spherical aggregations of endocrine cells widely distributed within the parenchyma of an exocrine gland, the pancreas, and they will be discussed in Chapter 19.

QUESTIONS*

1. Concerning pituicytes, which one, if any, of the following statements applies?

   A. are a type of glia cell
   B. produce vasopressin
   C. are identical with Herring bodies
   D. produce prolactin
   E. none of the above

2. The most highly vascularized area of the hypophysis is the

   A. pars tuberalis
   B. pars intermedia
   C. pars nervosa
   D. pars distalis
   E. pars anterior

3. The pars intermedia secretes

   A. FSH
   B. TSH
   C. LH
   D. ACTH
   E. MSH

4. Which one, if any, of the following hormones is produced by parafollicular cells?

   A. thyroxin
   B. calcitonin
   C. parathyroid hormone
   D. angiotensin
   E. none of the above

5. Large lipid droplets are typical of which one, if any, of the following?

   A. median eminence
   B. pineal gland
   C. zona fasciculata of the adrenal cortex
   D. somatotropin cells of the pituitary
   E. none of the above

6. The adrenal medulla produces which one, if any, of the following?

   A. aldosterone
   B. melatonin
   C. norepinephrine
   D. histamine
   E. none of the above

7. Which one, if any, of the following stores the precursor of its secretion extracellularly?

   A. pars intermedia of pituitary
   B. follicular thyroid
   C. adrenal cortex
   D. adrenal medulla
   E. parathyroid oxyphil cells

8. Iodine is essential for the hormone production of which one, if any, of the following?

   A. pineal
   B. parathyroid
   C. thyroid C cells
   D. adrenal medulla
   E. thyroid

9. All of the following are involved in the regulation of calcium metabolism **except**

   A. vitamin D
   B. calcitonin
   C. parathyroid hormone
   D. melatonin
   E. cholecalciferol

10. Synthesis of which one, if any, of the following is strictly regulated by the light–dark cycle?

    A. insulin
    B. calcitonin
    C. melatonin
    D. thyroxine
    E. FSH

11. The secretion of which one, if any, of the following is controlled by hypothalamo-hypophysial feedback?

    A. calcitonin
    B. insulin
    C. thyroxine
    D. aldosterone
    E. none of the above

12. Paraganglia are closely related by their origin and functions to which one of the following?

    A. adrenal medulla
    B. adrenal cortex
    C. follicular thyroid
    D. adenohypophysis
    E. parathyroid chief cells

13. Pituicytes are found in which one, if any, of the following?

A. median eminence
B. pars distalis
C. pars nervosa
D. pars intermedia
E. none of the above

14. All of the following may be expected to occur in very high concentrations in the blood of the adrenal veins **except**

A. aldosterone
B. cortisol
C. androgens
D. melatonin
E. epinephrine

*Answers on page 307.

14

SKIN

KEY WORDS

Apocrine
Arrector Pili Muscle
Axilla
Birbeck Granule
Carotene
Corium
Cytocrine Secretion
Cytomorphosis
Dermal Papilla
Dermatoglyph
Dermis
Desmosome
Eccrine
Epidermal Melanin
    Unit
Epidermis
Eponychium
Ergosterol
Filaggrin
Hemi-desmosome
Holocrine
Hypodermis
Interleukin
Interpapillary Peg
Involucrin
Keratin

Keratinocyte
Keratohyalin
Lunula
Melanin
Melanocyte
Melanosome
Merkel Cell
Merocrine
Myoepithelial Cell
Nail Bed
Nail Root
Panniculus Adiposus
Papillary Layer
Rete Cutaneum
Rete Subpapillare
Reticular Layer
Sebaceous
Sebum
Stratum Basale
Stratum Corneum
Stratum Granulosum
Stratum Malpighii
Stratum Spinosum
Sudoriporous
Vitamin D

The **skin** is one of the body's largest organs, accounting for about 16% of body weight. It serves as a protective barrier against injury, and its impermeability to water prevents desiccation and makes life on land possible. It contains tactile sense organs that receive stimuli from the environment, and its sweat glands play an important role in the maintenance of normal body temperature.

Skin is made up of two principal layers: a surface epithelium, the **epidermis,** and a subjacent layer of connective tissue forming the **dermis,** or **corium.** Beneath the dermis, there is a layer of looser connective tissue, the **hypodermis** (Fig. 14-1 [see Plate 20]). In some regions of the body, this may consist mainly of adipose cells. It is loosely attached to the underlying deep fascia or to the periosteum of bony prominences. At the lips, nose, eyelids, and vulva, the skin is continuous, at **mucocutaneous junctions,** with the mucous membrane lining those structures.

Associated with the skin are **hair follicles** and two types of small glands: **sudoriparous glands,** which produce the watery secretion called **sweat,** and **sebaceous glands,** which have an oily secretion, the **sebum.** The epidermis varies greatly in thickness from region to region and in the number of its associated hair follicles and glands. Over much of its surface, it appears relatively smooth to the naked eye, but a pattern of shallow grooves and flexure lines is apparent at low magnification. These are deeper on thick hairless regions such as the knees, elbows, palms, and soles. On the finger pads, alternating ridges and grooves form the **dermatoglyphs,** the distinctive patterns of arches, loops, and whorls that are the basis for the individuality of the fingerprints.

EPIDERMIS

Over most of the body, the epidermis varies from 0.07 to 0.12 mm in thickness, but it may reach a thickness of 0.8 mm on the palms and 1.4 mm on the soles of the feet. At birth, it is already appreciably thicker at these sites, but continuous pressure and friction on these surfaces in postnatal life result in additional thickening.

Palms and Soles

The epidermis is a stratified squamous epithelium made up of multiple layers of cells called **keratinocytes.** These arise by continuous division of stem cells in the basal layer of the epithelium. The new cells formed there are moved slowly toward the surface by the continual generation of new cells at the base. In their transit toward the surface, they enlarge and differentiate, accumulating in their cytoplasm increasing amounts of **keratin,** a family of polypeptides ranging in molecular weight from 40,000 to 68,000. Near the surface, bundles of keratin filaments completely fill the cytoplasm, and the nucleus and cell organelles have degenerated. These flakelike, lifeless cells detach and are continually shed from the surface of the epidermis. The transit time of the keratinocytes from the basal layer to the surface is 20–30 days. The sequence of cytological changes they undergo in this period is referred to as the **cytomorphosis** of the **keratinocytes.** Their differing appearance at successive levels in the epithelium makes it possible to distinguish four zones: the **stratum basale** (stratum germinativum), the **stratum spinosum** (stratum Malpighii), the **stratum granulosum,** and the **stratum corneum** (Figs. 14-2 and 14-3 [see Plate 20]).

The **stratum basale** consists of a single layer of cells resting on a typical basal lamina. The basal cells are cuboidal, with a nucleus that is large relative to the size of the cell, and their cytoplasm is intensely basophilic. In electron micrographs, they contain the usual organelles in a matrix rich in ribosomes, and a cytoskeleton of 10-nm keratin filaments that occur singly or in small bundles. The cells are attached to neighboring cells by numerous desmosomes and to the basal lamina by regularly spaced hemidesmosomes. Mitotic figures are common in this layer.

As cells generated in the stratum basale move upward into the **stratum spinosum,** they assume a flatter, polyhedral form, with their long axis parallel to the surface of the epithelium and their nucleus elongated in the same direction. They have the usual complement of organelles in a cytoplasm that is less basophilic than that of cells in the stratum basale. A prominent feature of these cells is the presence of conspicuous bundles of keratin filaments that radiate from the perinuclear region to end in the numerous desmosomes along the highly interdigitated boundary between adjacent cells (Fig. 14-4). Cells in the upper part of the stratum spinosum and in the overlying stratum granulosum contain secretory granules 0.1–0.4 μm in diameter, referred to as **membrane-coating granules** or **lamellar granules.** These have a distinctive internal structure consisting of alternating electron-dense and electron-lucent lamellae 2–3.5 nm in thickness. Pairs of the dense lamellae are continuous at their ends, leading to the interpretation that the granules are made up of stacks of discoid flattened vesicles.

The **stratum granulosum** consists of three to five layers of cells that are considerably flatter than those of the stratum spinosum. Their most distinctive feature is the presence of irregularly shaped bodies in their cytoplasm that stain intensely with basic dyes. Unlike secretory granules, these **keratohyalin granules** do not have a limited membrane. Bundles of keratin filaments may be incorporated in their periphery or may pass through them. Their chemical nature remains unclear, but they are believed to be precursors of an interfibrillar material that is distributed throughout the cytoplasm of the fully keratinized cells of the stratum corneum. The lamellar granules, described earlier, are present in greater number in the cells of the stratum granulosum and are localized near the cell membrane. They may occupy as much as 15% of the cell volume. Their content is released by exocytosis and forms a con-

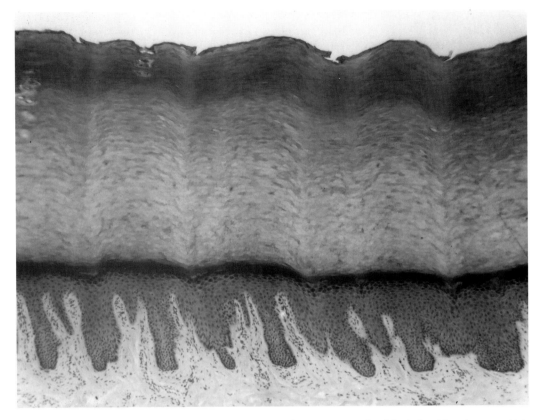

Fig. 14-2 Photomicrograph of the epidermis of the human finger, an example of thick skin. Note the great thickness of the stratum corneum and the regular spacing of dermal papillae at the base of the epithelium. The dark horizontal line below the stratum corneum is the stratum granulosum.

tinuous multilayered coating on the outside of the plasmalemma. This secretory product fills the intercellular spaces of the stratum granulosum. It is rich in lipids and serves as a waterproof sealant, making it a major component of the epidermal permeability barrier.

> *Pemphigus is an autoimmune skin disease seen most often in the elderly. There is a loss of cohesion between cell layers of the epidermis resulting in the formation of fluid-filled blisters that rupture easily, leaving denuded areas. The blood contains autoantibodies directed against keratinocyte surface antigens. At the periphery of the lesions, deposits of IgG and its complement can be demonstrated on the kertinocytes. The lesions may be spread over much of the body, and if infected, the disease can become life threatening. Treatment is with glucocorticoids.*

In the thick skin of the palms and soles, the **stratum lucidum** consists of four to six rows of very thin, pale-staining, eosinophilic cells, located between the stratum granulosum and the overlying stratum corneum. This stratum is not identifiable in the thinner skin over the rest of the body. Nuclear degeneration, which begins in the outer part of the stratum granulosum, is completed in cells of the stratum lucidum. The cytoplasm consists of closely aggregated keratin filaments embedded in an electron-dense

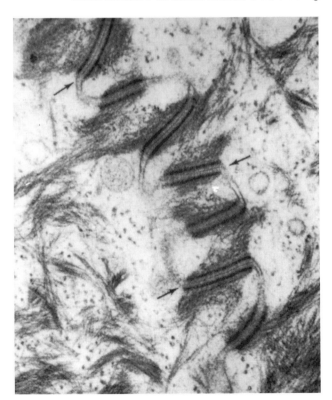

Fig. 14-4 Electron micrograph of the boundary between two cells of the stratum spinosum. Prominent desmosomes occur between short interdigitating processes of the two cells. Bundles of keratin filaments terminate in the dense plaques of the desmosomes.

matrix. The filaments are generally oriented parallel to the surface of the skin.

The **stratum corneum** of thick skin consists of many layers of very flat, devitalized cells containing no nucleus or cytoplasmic organelles. The plasmalemma appears thickened and the entire cell is filled with keratin filaments embedded in an amorphous matrix. The lowermost cells of stratum are still closely adherent, but their desmosomes have been greatly altered. In the outer layers, desmosomes are no longer identifiable and the heavily keratinized dead cells loosen from one another and desquamate. For this reason, this superficial portion of the stratum corneum is sometimes called the stratum disjunctum, but its cells are identical to those deeper in the stratum and its designation as a separate layer serves no useful purpose.

The epidermis is a remarkable epithelium. During their differentiation, its cells synthesize a variety of structural proteins. The most abundant of these are the **keratins.** Biochemists have identified at least 20 molecular species of keratin that are designated by the letter K and a number. At least four of these occur in the epidermis. The cytoskeleton of the basal cells consists of a loose network of keratins K5 and K14. Upon reaching the stratum spinosum, the cells synthesize two new keratins, K1 and K10, that form coarser bundles. The cells of this stratum also produce **involucrin** and other envelope proteins that are deposited on the inner side of the plasmalemma. They also synthesize the **membrane-coating granules** that will later release complex lipids and lipoproteins into the intercellular spaces, contributing to the permeability barrier of the epidermis. As the cells move into the stratum granulosum, they cease to produce keratins and, instead, synthesize **filaggrin,** a basic protein involved in the assembly and binding of keratin filaments into coarser bundles.

Thin Skin

The thin epidermis over most of the body is similar to that of the palms and soles in its basic organization, but the various strata are less obvious. There is a much thinner stratum corneum (Fig. 14-5). A thin stratum spinosum is always present. A stratum granulosum is usually identifiable, but it is only two or three cells thick. A distinct stratum lucidum is usually lacking. The contour of the dermo-epidermal junction is less complex than that of thick skin (see below).

Melanocytes

Skin color depends on varying amounts of three components. The tissue has an inherent yellowish color attributable, in part, to its content of **carotene,** a precursor of vitamin A. In addition, a pink tint is imparted to the skin by the oxygenated **hemoglobin** of blood in the dermal capillary bed. Shades of brown to black are due to varying amounts of the pigment **melanin** produced by **melanocytes,** specialized cells present in varying number in the basal layer of the epidermis and, occasionally, in the underlying dermis. These cells arise from the neural crest of the embryo and their shape is reminiscent of that of cells in the central nervous system. Radiating from their rounded cell body are numerous branching processes, called dendrites, that extend between the surrounding keratinocytes. Melanin occurs in their cytoplasm in ellipsoidal granules, 1 µm in length, and 0.4 µm in width, called **melanosomes.** When newly formed, these have a characteristic fine structure consisting of longitudinally oriented parallel filaments with a 10-nm periodicity. In mature melanosomes, this sub-

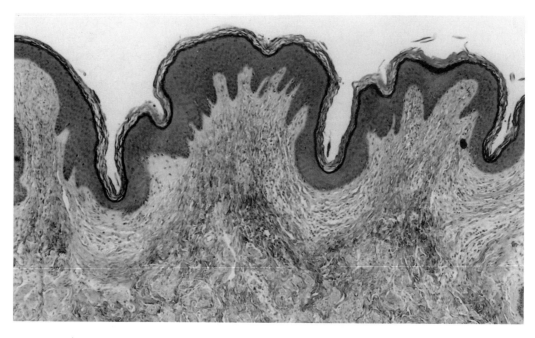

Fig. 14-5 Photomicrograph of thin skin of the abdomen. Observe how thin the stratum corneum is compared to that of thick skin in Fig. 14-2.

structure is obliterated by the accumulation of dense melanin pigment on the filaments. Vesicles containing multiple melanosomes are pinched off from the tips of the melanocyte dendrites and these fuse with the plasmalemma of neighboring keratinocytes, transferring melanosomes to their cytoplasm (Fig. 14-6). This unique process is called **cytocrine secretion.** A melanocyte and its satellite epidermal cells collectively constitute an **epidermal melanin unit.** Because of their continual transfer of pigment, the melanocytes may contain fewer melanosomes than the neighboring keratinocytes.

The number of melanocytes varies in different regions of the body. They may be as few as $1000/mm^2$ on the arms and thighs and as many as $4000/mm^2$ on the face and neck. The racial differences in color are not attributable simply to differing numbers of melanocytes but to the amount of melanin they produce and transfer. In Caucasians, the melanosomes are largely confined to the keratinocytes of the stratum basale. In Negroids, they are somewhat larger, more numerous, and are found in keratinocytes throughout the epidermis.

> *Chronic exposure of light-skinned individuals to solar radiation increases the possibility of developing the skin cancers* ***squamous carcinoma*** *and* ***malignant melanoma.*** *Pigmentation is protective, and blacks are at very much lower risk of developing one of these malignancies. Ultraviolet rays also appear to interfere with antigen presentation by the Langerhans cells, impairing the skin's immunological defenses.*

Langerhans Cells

A solitary cell type widely distributed in the epidermis is the **Langerhans cell.** These are stellate cells with a dark-staining nucleus of very irregular shape, surrounded by a pale-staining cytoplasm. In electron micrographs, the cytoplasm is of low density and contains few mitochondria and little endoplasmic reticulum (Fig. 14-7). They contain small membrane-bounded granules of unusual shape, called **Birbeck granules.** These are discoid in form, but in section appear as rodlike profiles 15–50 nm in length and about 4 nm in thickness. Langerhans cells can be distinguished from keratinocytes by their nuclear shape, their lack of bundles of keratin filaments, and the absence of desmosomes on their surface. They are usually located in the upper layers of the stratum spinosum. They may number as high as $800/mm^2$ and make up 3–8% of the cell population of the epithelium. They arise from precursors in the bone marrow, which are transported in the blood to the dermis and migrate into the epidermis.

The Langerhans cells participate in the body's immune responses. They have surface receptors and immunological markers similar to those of T lymphocytes and macro-

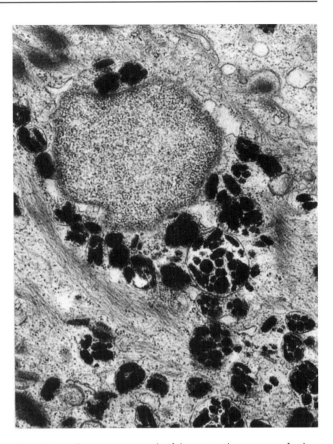

Fig. 14-6 Electron micrograph of the perinuclear region of a keratinocyte from the stratum spinosum of human skin, showing the clusters of melanosomes. Some clusters are enclosed in a membrane.

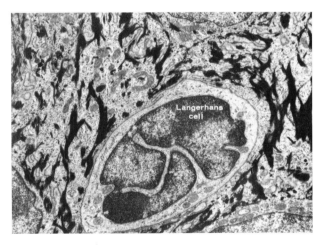

Fig. 14-7 Electron micrograph of a Langerhans cell surrounded by keratinocytes containing dense bundles of keratin filaments. A polymorphous nucleus and multiple cell processes are characteristic of this cell type. None of the processes are included in this plane of section. (Courtesy of G. Szabo.)

phages. They bind the *Fc* fragment of IgG, IgA, and the C3 component of complement. At sites of allergic contact dermatitis, they are believed to take up antigen and present it to lymphocytes in a form to which they can respond. Langerhans cells occur in other stratified squamous epithelia, including those of the oral cavity, esophagus, and vagina.

Merkel Cells

Small numbers of **Merkel cells** are found in the basal layer of the epidermis over the entire body (Fig. 14-8). They are more abundant in areas such as the fingertips, which have an important role in sensory reception. The naked terminals of myelinated afferent nerves end in apposition to these cells, forming **Merkel cell–neurite complexes.** The long axis of the Merkel cells is usually parallel to the basal lamina and their cell processes extend between the overlying keratinocytes, to which they may be attached by desmosomes. The nucleus is deeply invaginated and the cytoplasm contains many dense-cored granules 80–130 nm in diameter and intermediate filaments of keratins K8, K18, and K19 which differ from those of the surrounding keratinocytes. It is postulated that the Merkel cell–neurite

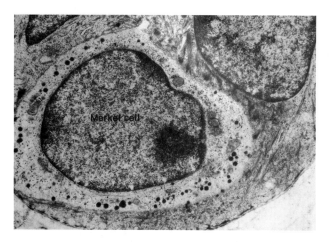

Fig. 14-8 Electron micrograph at the base of human epidermis including a Merkel cell. Note its pale cytoplasm and small dense secretory granules. (Courtesy of G. Szabo.)

complexes have a mechanoreceptor function, but this has yet to be firmly established. Merkel cells also occur in the epithelium of the oral mucosa.

MUCOCUTANEOUS JUNCTIONS

Mucocutaneous junctions are the transitions from skin to the mucous membrane lining the mouth and anus. Like skin, they have a stratified squamous epithelium, but it has a very thin stratum corneum and lacks hairs, sebaceous glands, and sweat glands. The surface is moistened by secretions of mucous glands situated deeper in these orifices. Because of the thinness of the stratum corneum, the color of the blood in the underlying capillary bed shows through the epithelium, giving mucocutaneous junctions a red tint, as seen in the lips.

DERMIS

The **dermis** is the tough layer of connective tissue immediately beneath the epidermis. It makes up the greater part of the thickness of the skin, ranging from 0.6 mm in the thin skin of the eyelids, to 3 mm or more on the palms and soles (Fig. 14-1 [see Plate 20]). It is generally thinner in women than in men. The interface between the dermis and epidermis is very irregular in contour and varies greatly from region to region. It is best studied in scanning micrographs of dermis from which the epithelium has been separated by immersion in a calcium-chelating agent (Fig. 14-9). In such preparations, the upper surface of the dermis exhibits a pattern of **primary ridges** separated by deep **primary grooves** formerly occupied by

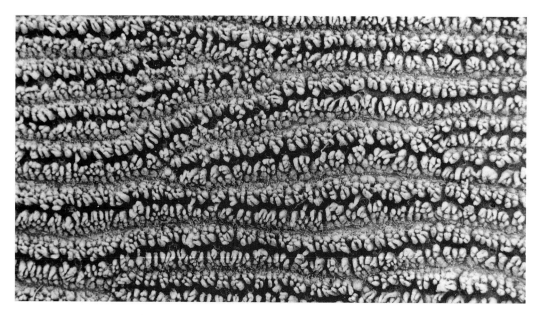

Fig. 14-9 Low-power scanning micrograph of human plantar dermis, viewed from above, after removal of the epidermis. The dark grooves are between the primary ridges of the dermis. On each ridge are two rows of dermal papillae separated by a shallow groove. (Courtesy of D. K. MacCallum, Anatomy Record, 211:142, 1985.)

ridgelike thickenings of the epidermis that were inappropriately called interpapillary "pegs" before their true form was revealed by scanning microscopy. In the midline of each primary ridge, there is a shallow **secondary groove,** which divides it into two **secondary ridges.** Rows of conical **dermal papillae,** 0.1–0.2 mm in height, project upward from these secondary ridges, occupying conforming concavities in the underside of the epidermis (Figs. 14-10A and 14-10B). The papillae, which number about 80/mm² occur in groups of three to five that share a common base. Regularly spaced, dark circular areas in the floor of the primary grooves represent openings of channels that were occupied by the ducts of sweat glands pulled out of the dermis in the removal of the epidermis (Figs. 14-10A and 14-10B). In thin skin, lacking a dermatoglyphic pattern on its outer surface, the configuration of the dermo-epidermal junction is much simpler than that described above for thick skin. The dermal papillae are shorter, broader, and fewer, and they are not arranged in rows corresponding to ridges on the skin surface, as they are in the thick skin of the palms.

Two layers are identified in the dermis: a superficial **papillary layer,** adjacent to the epidermis, consists of fibroblasts widely dispersed among thin bundles of type III collagen fibers and a loose network of elastic fibers. This layer contains many capillaries. The deeper and thicker **reticular layer** is made up of closely packed coarser bundles of type I collagen fibers. The interstices between fiber bundles are occupied by an amorphous matrix rich in dermatan sulfate and other glycosaminoglycans. Cell types other than fibroblasts include macrophages, lymphocytes, mast cells, and occasional clusters of adipose cells.

SUBCUTANEOUS TISSUE

The **subcutaneous tissue** (or **hypodermis**), deep to the reticular layer of the dermis, is a loose connective tissue in which the bundles of collagen fibers course mainly parallel to the skin surface. In some regions, this layer permits movement of the skin over the underlying structures. In others, fibers crossing into the dermis are more abundant and the skin is relatively immobile. Adipose cells tend to accumulate in this layer on the abdomen and buttocks which may reach a thickness of 3 cm or more. Where this has occurred, this subcutaneous layer of fat is called the **panniculus adiposus.**

SKIN APPENDAGES

Hairs

Hairs (Fig. 14-11) develop from cells lining deep invaginations of the epidermis, called **hair follicles.** Their base extends down into the dermis and sometimes a short

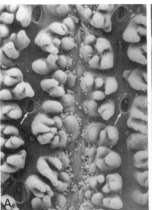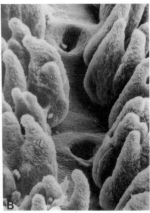

Fig. 14-10 (A) Scanning micrograph of one of the primary ridges shown in Fig. 14-9, at higher magnification. The openings in the grooves on either side were occupied by ducts of sweat glands (arrows). (B) An oblique view along one of the grooves at higher magnification. In this view, the shape of the dermal papillae is more apparent. (Courtesy D. K. MacCallum, Anatomical Record 211:142, 1985.)

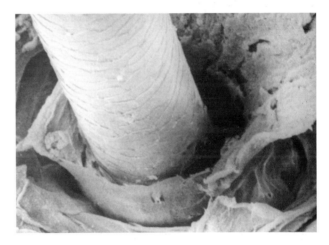

Fig. 14-11 Scanning electron micrograph of a hair emerging from the human scalp. Note the exfoliating cells of the stratum corneum around its base. (Courtesy of T. Fujita.)

distance into the subcutaneous tissue (Fig. 14-12 [see Plate 20]). Although humans appear to be largely hairless, the number of their hairs does not differ appreciably from the number on other primates. However, over much of the body, they are very small and colorless and go unnoticed. Hairs are absent only on the palms and soles, lateral aspect of the feet, the glans penis, clitoris, and the labia minora. There are about 800 hairs/mm² on the face, but on the rest of the body, they number only about 60/mm². On the eyelid, hairs do not project beyond their follicle, but on the head, they may grow to well over 1 m in length.

An active hair follicle has a terminal expansion called the **hair bulb,** which has, on its under side, a deep recess occupied by a **papilla** of dermal connective tissue (Fig. 14-13). Nutrients diffusing from capillaries of the papilla are essential for normal hair growth, and cells of the papilla have inductive properties that influence the activity of the follicle. The epithelial cells of the follicle adjacent to the

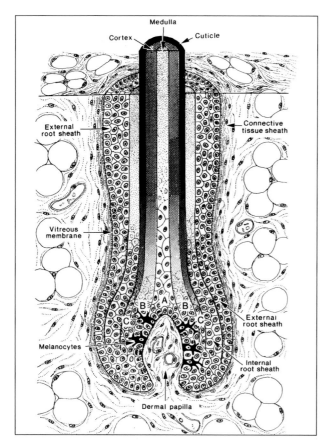

Fig. 14-13 A simplified drawing of a hair follicle. The expanded lower end of the follicle contains a dermal papilla. Growth of the hair depends on proliferation of cells overlying the papilla. Cells over its tip (A) form the medulla, Those on its sides (B) give rise to the cortex, and cells lateral to these (C) form the hair cuticle. The most peripheral cells of the bulb form the internal and external root sheaths. The color of the hair depends on the activity of melanocytes in the epithelium over the papilla. (Redrawn from L. C. Junquiera, J. Carniero, R. O. Kelley, Norwalk, Conn., Basic Histology, Appleton and Lange Medical Publications, 1972.)

papilla are comparable to those of the stratum basale of the epidermis. Among them are a few large melanocytes whose long dendrites contribute melanosomes to the cells that will form the cortex of the hair. The graying of the hair in old age is attributed to a gradual loss in the capacity of these cells to synthesize melanin.

A mass of epithelial cells in the hair bulb over and around the papilla constitute its **cell matrix.** Proliferation of those immediately overlying the apex of the papilla produces large vacuolated cells that form the **medulla** of the hair. Further lateral, proliferation and differentiation of cells give rise to heavily keratinized cells that make up its **cortex.** Lateral to these is a layer of cells that form the hair **cuticle.** The cells arising in this layer are initially cuboidal, but, higher in the shaft, they become highly keratinized, change their orientation, and are transformed into flat, imbricated, shinglelike cells that have their free edges directed downward. Further toward the periphery of the bulb are the cells that form an **internal root sheath** which

completely surrounds the proximal part of the hair shaft. The outermost layer of cells in the bulb form the **external root sheath,** which is initially only one cell thick but becomes several cells thick higher on the hair shaft. This layer is continuous with the basal layer of the epidermis. The hair follicle is surrounded by a condensation of the fibrous components of the dermis. Interposed between these and the epithelium of the external root sheath is an acellular **vitreous layer** (glassy layer) which appears to be an exceptionally thick basal lamina of the follicular epithelium.

Hair growth is cyclical and three phases of the cycle are recognized: the **growth phase, regression phase,** and **resting phase** (Fig. 14-14B). On the human scalp, the growth phase may last for 2–6 years, the regressing phase for 2–3 weeks, and the resting phase for 3–4 months. After the resting phase, the old hair is shed and a new hair shaft is formed. The bulb of the hair follicle undergoes considerable atrophy during the regressing and resting phases (Fig. 14-14B) and is restored at the beginning of the next growth phase.

Bound to the connective-tissue sheath of the hair follicle are one or more bundles of smooth-muscle fibers forming the **arrector pili muscle** (Fig. 14-14A). These extend diagonally upward from the follicle to the papillary layer of the dermis. In animals with a dense coat of hair, their contraction serves to erect the hairs, increasing the efficiency of the fur as a thermal barrier. In the human, their contraction, in response to cold, results in slight depressions of the skin over their sites of attachment, and an elevation of the site of emergence of the hair. This results in a roughening of the surface commonly described as "goose-flesh."

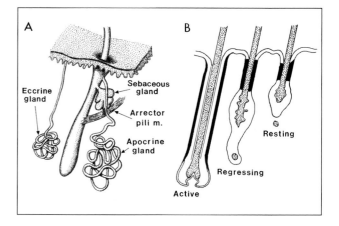

Fig. 14-14 (A) Hair follicle and its associated structures. The ducts of the sebaceous and apocrine glands open into the infundibulum of the follicle. Eccrine sweat glands are not associated with the hair follicles, but open onto the skin surface separately. (B) Hair follicles go through a growth cycle, passing successively through a growth phase, followed by regression and a resting phase, before again becoming active. (Redrawn from W. Montagna and P. F. Parakkel, Structure and Function of the Skin, Academic Press, New York, 1974.)

Nails

Nails are plates of closely compacted hard keratin, formed by proliferation and keratinization of epithelial cells in a **nail matrix** that is comparable to the hair matrix but simpler in its organization. The **nail root** and its matrix are located under a fold of skin, called the **proximal nail fold** (Fig. 14-15). The stratum corneum of the epidermis on this fold may extend for 0.5–1 mm onto the upper surface of the nail, forming a thin covering called the **eponychium.** Where the **lateral nail folds** turn inward into the **lateral nail grooves** their epidermis loses its stratum corneum and continues under the nail plate as the **nail bed.** There, the epidermis consists of a stratum basale and stratum spinosum, with the nail replacing the stratum corneum. It is continuous proximally with the **nail matrix** that extends some distance under the proximal nail fold. Growth of the nail from the nail matrix slides the nail over the epidermis of the nail bed, which makes no contribution to its formation. The anterior portion of the nail matrix can be seen through the nail as an opaque white crescent, called the **lunula.** As in the hair matrix, the cells of the nail matrix synthesize large amounts of keratin. As these cells are incorporated into the nail root, they are transformed into extremely flat, anuclear structures consisting of keratin embedded in a hard interfibrillar matrix. Nails grow at a rate of about 0.5 mm per week. Fingernails grow about four times as fast as toenails.

Sebaceous Glands

Sebaceous glands are appendages of the hair follicles and are found throughout the dermis, except where hairs are lacking on the palms, soles, and sides of the feet. One or two are associated with each follicle (Fig. 14-14A). They number 400–800/cm² on the face, forehead, and scalp, but over the rest of the body their number is very much lower. The glands are 0.2–2 mm in diameter and are located above the insertion of the arrector pili muscle, with their duct

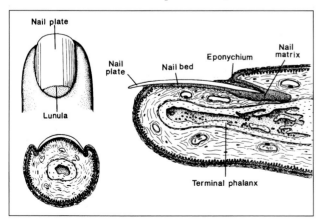

Fig. 14-15 Drawing of fingernail, nail bed, nail matrix, and associated structures.

opening into the follicular canal around the hair shaft. Their secretion, called **sebum,** is a mixture of triglycerides, cholesterol, and waxes. It is thought to maintain the soft texture of thin skin and the flexibility of the hairs.

Sebaceous glands have several small lobules consisting of sizable elongated acini that are continuous with a short duct (Fig. 14-16 [see Plate 21]). The acini have no lumen. Their basal cells are relatively small with round nuclei and a cytoplasm containing both rough and smooth endoplasmic reticulum, abundant glycogen, and numerous small lipid droplets. Production of sebum involves loss of whole cells and their content and is an example of **holocrine secretion.** Cells nearest to the duct die and break down, with their lipid and cell residues constituting the sebum. The cells more centrally situated in the acini are in various stages of degeneration with pycnotic nuclei and coalescing lipid droplets. The ducts of the gland are lined by stratified squamous epithelium that is continuous with that lining the infundibulum of a hair follicle.

*There is an increase in the amount of sebum released from the sebaceous glands after puberty and many teenagers suffer from **acne vulgaris.** The lesions are largely confined to the face but may also be found on the chest. They are small elevations of the skin (papules or pimples) that may contain pus. There are also small white lesions (comedones) that are collections of sebum and dead cells retained in a hair follicle or in the duct of a sebaceous gland. The disease is self-limiting, but antibiotics may be helpful in preventing superimposed bacterial infection.*

Eccrine Sweat Glands

Eccrine sweat glands are widely distributed throughout the integument. They are coiled tubular glands, with their secretory portion deep in the dermis or in the hypodermis. Their slender duct ascends through these layers to open at a **sweat pore** on the surface of the skin. The secretory portion of the gland is lined by cuboidal, or low-columnar, epithelium containing two cell types, designated **light cells** (clear cells) and **dark cells** on the basis of their appearance in stained histological sections. Between the epithelium and its basal lamina are **myoepithelial cells** that contract to promote discharge of the secretion (Fig. 14-17B [see Plate 21]).

The light cells are pyramidal in form with their base in contact with the basal lamina between myoepithelial cells (Fig. 14-18). As in other cells involved in transepithelial fluid transport, the plasmalemma at the cell base is elaborately infolded. The egress of their secretion is via intercellular canaliculi that open into the duct. Their cytoplasm is rich in glycogen but contains no secretory granules. The dark cells have the form of inverted pyramids with a broad

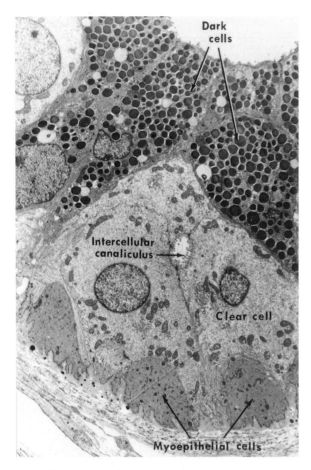

Fig. 14-18 Low-power micrograph of a portion of the wall of an eccrine sweat gland. Mucus-secreting dark cells line the lumen and pale serous cells are more deeply situated in the epithelium. These release their secretion via intercellular canaliculi. Note the myoepithelial cells at the base of the epithelium. (Courtesy of R. E. Ellis.)

adlumenal end tapering down to a slender ablumenal end that does not reach the basal lamina. They have a small, dark-staining nucleus, a prominent Golgi complex, long mitochondria, and a few cisternae of rough endoplasmic reticulum. The apical cytoplasm contains many moderately dense secretory granules. Their chemical composition is not known, but their staining suggests that their content is glycoprotein in nature. The long duct of the gland is lined by an epithelium consisting of two layers of cuboidal cells. The cells adjacent to the basal lamina have a comparatively large heterochromatic nucleus and abundant mitochondria. Those bordering on the lumen have an irregularly shaped nucleus and relatively little cytoplasm, containing few organelles. There is a conspicuous terminal web beneath their apical plasmalemma.

Because of the wide spacing of the eccrine sweat glands, there is a tendency to underestimate their total mass and their physiological importance. They number between 3 and 4 million, and their aggregate weight is roughly equivalent to that of a kidney. Humans engaged in

vigorous physical activity in a warm environment may perspire as much as 10 liters a day. This volume of secretion exceeds that of some of the largest exocrine glands.

Apocrine Sweat Glands

A second kind of sweat gland is found in the axilla, on the mons pubis, and in the circumanal region. These **apocrine sweat glands,** located deep in the dermis, are larger than the eccrine sweat glands. Their mode of secretion is actually merocrine. Their original designation as "apocrine" was based on an artifact of specimen preparation, but, unfortunately, the name has persisted. As in sebaceous glands, their duct opens into the canal of a hair follicle. The tubular secretory portion is lined by cells that are usually cuboidal, but they may be squamous if the gland is distended with secretion. Their apical cytoplasm contains rather large secretory granules. The chemical nature of the secretion has been little studied. It is a slightly viscous fluid that is odorless when secreted, but after modification by the resident bacteria of the skin, it acquires an odor that is considered socially offensive. The secretory activity of apocrine sweat glands does not begin until puberty. In women, there is an enlargement of the cells and of the lumen of axillary apocrine sweat glands during the premenstrual phase of the cycle, followed by regression during menses. The apocrine sweat glands are innervated by adrenergic nerves, whereas the eccrine glands are innervated by cholinergic nerves.

BLOOD VESSELS AND LYMPHATICS

The skin receives its blood from large vessels in the subcutaneous tissue. Ascending branches of these ramify to form a plexus, the **rete cutaneum,** at the boundary between the dermis and hypodermis. Ascending branches from this rete form a second plexus, the **rete subpapillare** in the papillary layer of the dermis. Its branches form a capillary network in each papilla and around the sebaceous glands and the sheath of the hair follicle. The capillaries of the dermis drain into a venous **rete subpapillare** and then to a venous rete associated with the rete cutaneum. There are numerous **arteriovenous anastomoses** in the system that are of physiological importance in controlling blood flow to the superficial layers of the skin where heat is lost to the environment.

A blind-ending lymphatic capillary from each dermal papilla joins a lymphatic plexus below the dermo-epidermal junction. From there, branches descend to a deeper lymphatic plexus associated with the rete cutaneum. Larger lymphatics, possessing valves, arise from this plexus and follow the course of the veins through the subcutaneous tissue.

NERVES

Free Endings

Abundant efferent nerves activate the glands of the skin and control blood flow by changing the caliber of its small arteries. There are also many afferent sensory nerves with a variety of endings (Fig. 14-19). Unspecialized **free endings** penetrate the epidermis and terminate in the stratum granulosum. These free endings are thought to be pain receptors or thermoreceptors. The axons of other myelinated nerves end in disklike expansions, called **Merkel endings** in contact with Merkel cells at the base of the epithelium. Their function is still unknown.

Encapsulated Endings

There are also sensory nerves with more complex encapsulated endings. The **Pacinian corpuscles** in the dermis and hypodermis are ovoid structures up to a millimeter in length. The axon of a myelinated nerve continues into the core of the corpuscle, where it is surrounded by 20–60 concentric lamellae consisting of very thin flat cells separated by narrow spaces filled with a gellike material. The corpuscle resembles an onion in cross section (Fig. 14-20A [see Plate 22]). **Meissner's corpuscles** are pear-shaped structures made up of flattened cells oriented transversely, resulting in a ladderlike cross-striation of the corpuscle. The axon of a myelinated nerve loses its sheath, enters one pole of the corpuscle, and pursues a spiral or zigzag course among the flat cells in its interior. Meissner's corpuscles occupy occasional dermal papillae. Such endings are probably mechanoreceptors sensing slight deformations of the skin. **Kraus's end-bulbs** are small spheroidal bodies in the papillary layer of the dermis. They bear a superficial resemblance to Pacinian corpuscles but are much smaller and lack concentric lamellae. Their sensory modality is unclear.

HISTOPHYSIOLOGY

The skin has many functions. Although in the human, it lacks the thick fur, feathers, scales, or spines found on some other creatures, it still has a significant protective function. The heavy keratinization of the stratum corneum provides some degree of protection against mechanical damage. The lipid-rich intercellular material in this stratum prevents loss of fluid and electrolytes and bars entry of toxins from the environment.

The rich innervation of the skin, with endings sensitive to touch, pain, heat, and cold, protects by initiating evasive action. Skin protects against the harmful effects of excessive

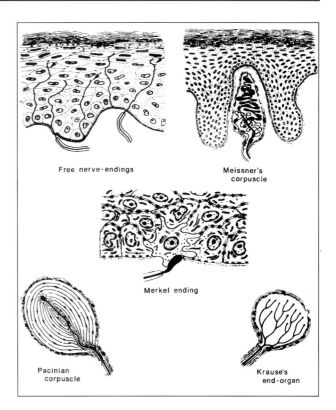

Fig. 14-19 Drawings of some of the free nerve endings and encapsulated endings found in the skin.

solar irradiation by increasing the number of melanosomes that absorb or scatter light of this wavelength.

Skin is an effective mechanical barrier against entry of pathogenic bacteria, and its Langerhans cells and lymphocytes are important components of the immune system. Langerhans cells present antigen to intradermal lymphocytes that respond with the production of antibodies. Although the number of lymphocytes observed in the epidermis seems small, their total number in this large organ is probably as great as their number in the blood. The basal keratinocytes also participate in immune responses. When reacting to an immunological challenge, they produce interleukin-1 that induces lymphocyte proliferation, and a thrombopoietin-like molecule that promotes their activation.

Skin is a major agent of temperature regulation. When the ambient temperature is higher than normal body temperature, evaporation is the only method of heat dissipation subject to physiological control. It depends on enhanced secretory activity of some 3 million sweat glands. An elevated ambient temperature also results in vasodilation and opening of arteriovenous anastomoses to conduct deep body heat to the surface. In a hot environment, cutaneous blood flow may increase to 2–3 liter/m/min. When exposed to extreme cold, vasoconstriction and closure of arteriovenous anastomoses may reduce flow to 50 ml/m/min.

QUESTIONS*

1. The function(s) of the integument is (are) to

   A. sense the external environment
   B. aid in metabolic homeostasis
   C. retard diffusion of liquids and gases
   D. act as a solar radiation barrier
   E. all of the above

2. The arteriovenous shunts found in the hypodermis function primarily for

   A. thermoregulation
   B. selective nutrition to epithelial elements
   C. shunting blood to viscera after eating
   D. stimulation of hair growth

3. The reticular and papillary layers of the skin contain the following **except**

   A. blood vessels
   B. keratohyalin
   C. nerves
   D. glands
   E. arrector pili muscles

4. The term "cytomorphosis" relates to the following items **except**

   A. keratinization
   B. disappearance of the nucleus
   C. formation of melanosomes
   D. cellular movement toward the surface of the skin
   E. disappearance of organelles

5. Cytomorphosis may be characterized as

   A. dynamic morphological exchange between cells
   B. replacement of cytoplasm by melanosomes
   C. an integral part of the process of keratinization
   D. progressive thickening of the membrane of adjacent cells in the stratum spinosum
   E. all of the above

6. The melanocyte system is primarily associated with

   A. rete papillare
   B. stratum germinativum
   C. disulfide bonding with cystine
   D. holocrine secretion
   E. stratum corneum

7. The epidermis contains the following layers **except**

   A. stratum lucidum
   B. stratum Malpighii
   C. stratum corneum
   D. stratum reticularis
   E. stratum germinativum

8. The epidermis contains all of the following **except**

   A. free nerve ends
   B. keratohyalin granules
   C. desmosomes
   D. melanin
   E. blood vessels

9. Langerhans cells are found primarily in the

   A. stratum germinativum
   B. stratum spinosum
   C. stratum granulosum
   D. stratum lucidum
   E. stratum corneum

10. Myoepithelial cells are most commonly associated with

   A. eccrine (sweat) glands
   B. hair follicles
   C. arteriovenous shunts
   D. Langerhans cells
   E. melanocytes

11. Cytocrine secretion refers to

   A. the process by which DOPA is produced
   B. the production of type IV collagen
   C. the process by which melanin is transferred to keratinocytes
   D. the production of fatty substances in apocrine glands
   E. the production of eleidin by keratinocytes

12. Skin coloration is due to

   A. natural tissue color
   B. oxyhemoglobin
   C. eumelanin
   D. carotene
   E. all of the above

*Answers on page 307.

15

ORAL CAVITY

CHAPTER OUTLINE

Tongue
    Lingual Papillae
    Taste Buds
Lymphoid Tissue
Teeth
    Dentin
    Enamel
    Cementum
    Periodontal Ligament
    Gingiva
    Tooth Development
Salivary Glands
    Major Salivary Glands
    Minor Salivary Glands
    Histophysiology

KEY WORDS

Ameloblast	Molar
Canine	Mucus
Cementocyte	Myoepithelial
Cementum	Odontoblast
Circumvallate Papilla	Palatine Tonsil
Crown	Parotid Gland
Deciduous Teeth	Periodontal Ligament
Demilune	Periodontal
Dental Lamina	Membrane
Dentin	Predentin
Enamel	Pharyngeal Tonsil
Enamel Organ	Root
Excretory Duct	Root Canal
Facial Nerve	Saliva
Filiform Papilla	Serous
Fungiform Papilla	Striated Duct
Gingiva	Sublingual Gland
Glossopharyngeal	Submandibular Gland
Nerve	Taste Bud
Intercalated Duct	Taste Pore
Kallikrein	Tome's Process
Lingual Papilla	Tonsillar Crypt
Lingual Tonsil	Tooth Bud
	von Ebner Glands

The digestive tract includes the oral cavity, esophagus, stomach, duodenum, small intestine, colon, rectum, and anus. Each segment is specialized for its particular role in the processing, or absorption of nutrients to meet the energy needs of the body. In the oral cavity, the food is mechanically fragmented by the teeth, chemically modified, and lubricated by the secretions of the salivary glands for its passage through the esophagus to the stomach.

The oral cavity is bounded above by the hard and soft palate, laterally by the cheeks, and below by the tongue and floor of the mouth. It is lined by stratified squamous epithelium throughout, but the epithelium varies in its thickness and degree of keratinization from region to region. On the floor of the mouth and underside of the tongue, it is thin and mobile. Where it is reflected onto the alveolar processes to form the **gingiva** (gums), it is thick and firmly fixed to the periosteum of the underlying bone. On the dorsum of the tongue, the inner aspect of the cheeks, and the palate, it is moderately thick and heavily keratinized to withstand the abrasion to which these regions are subjected during mastication of food. There are many small glands in the submucosa of the palate, cheeks, and floor of the mouth.

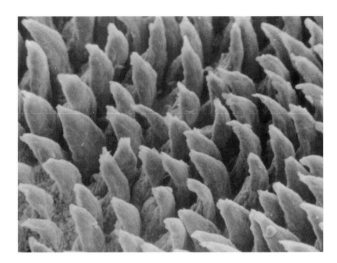

Fig. 15-1 Scanning electron micrograph of the filiform papillae on the tongue of a rabbit. Their form is similar in the human. (Courtesy of F. Fujita.)

TONGUE

The bulk of the tongue consists of intersecting vertical and horizontal bundles of striated muscle that provide it with the mobility required for speech, chewing, and swallowing. Its dorsal surface is covered with a multitude of small specializations of the epithelium called the **lingual papillae.** These are of four types: **filiform, fungiform, circumvallate,** and **foliate.**

Lingual Papillae

Filiform papillae are slender conical projections of the epithelium, 2–3 mm in length, with their tips pointing toward the back of the tongue (Fig. 15-1). They are the most numerous of the lingual papillae, covering most of the upper surface of the tongue. The heavily keratinized cells at their tips are continuously exfoliated. **Fungiform papillae,** 0.5–1.0 mm in diameter, have a relatively narrow base and a hemispherical upper portion. They are widely scattered among the filiform papillae. They have a connective-tissue core and **taste buds** in the epithelium on their sides. **Circumvallate papillae** number only 6–14 and are confined to the posterior portion of the tongue. They are 1–2 mm in diameter and are thus considerably larger than the fungiform papillae. Each is surrounded by a circular furrow or sulcus (Figs. 15-2 and 15-3 [see Plate 22]). The squamous epithelium on the free surface is smooth and unspecialized. That on the sides contains taste buds, estimated to number over 100 on each papilla. In the underly-

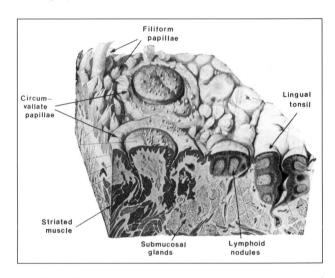

Fig. 15-2 Drawing of the dorsal surface of the posterior portion of the tongue, showing the large circumvallate papillae and the lingual tonsils. (Modified from Braus H., Anatomie des Menchen Springer-Verlag, Berlin 1924.)

ing submucosa, there are small **serous glands of von Ebner.** Their ducts open into the sulcus around the papilla, and their secretion keeps the sulcus rinsed. **Foliate papillae** are well developed in many mammals but are rudimentary in the human. They are located on the sides of the tongue and consist of several parallel ridges separated by intervening clefts (Fig. 15-4 [see Plate 23]). The ducts of small serous glands in the underlying connective tissue open into the clefts between ridges. Taste buds are numerous on the sides of the ridges.

Taste Buds

The taste buds are small neurosensory bodies in the epithelium of the fungiform and circumvallate papillae.

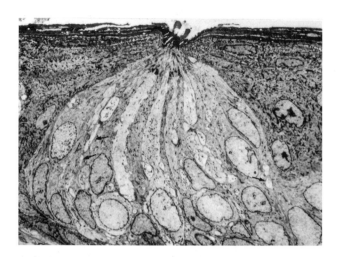

Fig. 15-6 Electron micrograph of a rabbit taste bud. The nerves penetrating the bud are indicated by arrows. The cell types differ slightly in density. There is some disagreement as to which are sensory. (Courtesy of S.M. Royer.)

There are about 3000 on the human tongue. They appear as pale ovoid bodies, 50–80 µm in height and 30–50 µm in width (Figs. 15-5 [see Plate 23] and 15-6). They consist of 50–75 cells, with tapering apices that converge on a small depression in the surface of the epithelium called the **taste pore.** Three types of cells are distinguishable by differences in their staining properties. Slender, **dark cells** (type I cells) at the periphery of the bud have microvilli that project into the taste pore. Their cytoplasm is rich in fine filaments and contains small secretory granules of unknown chemical nature. The **light cells** (type II cells) are less numerous and have a cytoplasm containing some smooth endoplasmic reticulum and relatively few filaments. Central to these are still-paler cells (type III cells). In electron micrographs, their cytoplasm contains longitudinally oriented microtubules and some smooth endoplasmic reticulum. In the basal cytoplasm there are small vesicles, resembling synaptic vesicles. These cells have a single club-shaped apical process that projects into the taste pore. This unusual apical structure and the presence of small vesicles near nerve axons penetrating the epithelium have fostered the belief that this cell type is the principal taste receptor, but this is a subject of dispute. Near the basal lamina, there are small dark cells interpreted as stem cells capable of differentiating into any of the other cell types. There are four basic tastes: sweet, bitter, sour, and salty. Physiologists have postulated four kinds of taste buds corresponding to these flavors, but histologists find no differences among them.

Nerve axons form a plexus around each taste bud, sending branches inward between the cells. Gustatory sensation in the anterior portion of the tongue is transmitted over the chorda tympani branch of the **facial nerve** (cranial nerve VII). In the posterior portion of the tongue, the taste buds are innervated by the lingual branch of the **glossopharyngeal nerve** (cranial nerve IX).

LYMPHOID TISSUE

The oral cavity is continuous posteriorly with the **pharynx,** the chamber through which air passes from the nasal cavity to the larynx and food passes from the oral cavity to the esophagus. On either side of the transition from oral cavity to pharynx, there are large subepithelial accumulations of lymphoid tissue forming the **palatine tonsils.** The overlying stratified squamous epithelium is deeply invaginated to form 15 or more **tonsillar crypts.** A thin connective-tissue capsule surrounds the tonsil and thin partitions extend from it into the lymphoid tissue. Mast cells and plasma cells abound in this connective tissue, and infiltrating polymorphonuclear leukocytes may become very numerous when the tonsils are inflamed (tonsillitis). Immediately beneath the epithelium lining the crypts, there are many closely spaced lymphoid nodules, resembling those in lymph nodes. The space between them is occupied by diffuse lymphoid tissue. The lumen of the crypts contains many lymphocytes, exfoliated epithelial cells, bacteria, and cellular debris. In chronic inflammation of the tonsils, semisolid masses of this material may accumulate in the crypts.

Tonsillitis is a streptococcal infection of the lymphoid tissue of the palatine tonsils. They become red and swollen. Degenerating neutrophils and lymphocytes accumulate in the crypts as "pus," which may appear as yellow spots on the surface of the tonsil. The infection usually responds to antibiotics, but recurrent attacks may make tonsillectomy advisable.

In the posterosuperior wall of the pharynx, there is a single **pharyngeal tonsil.** It is normally covered by ciliated pseudostratified epithelium, but patches of stratified squamous epithelium are not uncommon. The epithelium is often plicated into surface folds that are infiltrated with lymphocytes. The underlying lymphoid tissue is 2–3 mm in thickness and indistinguishable from that of the palatine tonsils.

On the posterior third of the tongue are small areas of epithelium free of papillae. These smooth areas overlay **lingual tonsils** consisting of lymphoid nodules and diffuse lymphoid tissue around a single crypt (Fig. 15-2). All of the tonsils of the oral cavity reach their greatest development in childhood and begin their involution at age 15 or younger.

TEETH

The adult human has 32 permanent teeth, of which 16 are in the alveolar arch of the maxilla and 16 in the alveolar arch of the mandible. These are preceded by a set of 20 **deciduous teeth** which are shed at various times between the 6th and 16th year and are gradually replaced by the 4 incisors, 2 canines, 4 premolars, and 6 molars that make up

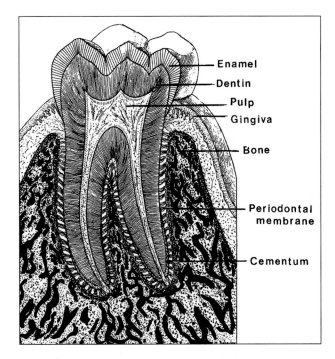

Enamel
Dentin
Pulp
Gingiva
Bone
Periodontal membrane
Cementum

Fig. 15-7 Drawing of a section of a human lower first molar tooth. (Courtesy of I. Schour.)

the adult dentition. Each of these types of teeth has a distinctive shape, adapted to its specific function. Thus, the chisellike **incisors** are specialized for cutting or shearing; the pointed **canines,** for puncturing and holding; and the **molars,** for crushing and grinding. The portion of each tooth that projects above the gum is called the **crown.** The lower portion, the **root** (or roots), occupy a socket of conforming shape in the underlying bone (Fig. 15-7). The bulk of the tooth consists of **dentin,** which is covered over the crown by a thick layer of **enamel.** In the root, enamel is lacking and the dentin is enveloped by a thin layer of **cementum,** which is enclosed in a **periodontal membrane** that binds the root to the surrounding alveolar bone (Fig. 15-7). A tooth has a small central **pulp cavity** that continues down into each root as the **root canal.** The pulp cavity is occupied by loose connective tissue, supplied with capillaries and nerve fibers that enter through an apical foramen at the tip of each root. Teeth are studied in histological sections of decalcified material, or in thin ground sections, in which the calcium salts are retained.

Dentin

Dentin is an avascular mineralized tissue harder than bone, but similar in composition. Eighty percent of its mass is made up of crystals of **hydroxyapatite,** and 20% is organic matter, consisting of type I collagen and glycosaminoglycans. During tooth development, **predentin** is secreted around long apical processes of cells called **odontoblasts.** Subsequent deposition of hydroxyapatite crystals in the predentin around these processes forms the **dentinal tubules.** An **odontoblast process** initially occupies each dentinal

tubule, but these may be withdrawn in old age. In histological sections, dentin has a radially striated appearance, due to the presence of innumerable, parallel dentinal tubules that radiate from the pulp cavity toward the enamel (Fig. 15-7).

The tall columnar cell bodies of the odontoblasts line the pulp cavity but are less closely adherent than in a typical epithelium. The nucleus is in the lower half of the cell. There is a large supranuclear Golgi complex, abundant rough endoplasmic reticulum, and numerous mitochondria (Fig. 15-8A). The apical portion of the cell tapers down to the slender odontoblast process (Fig. 15-9), which contains mitochondria and many secretory vesicles that fuse with the plasmalemma to discharge their content of procollagen. Converted to tropocollagen extracellularly, it polymerizes into the small randomly oriented collagen fibers of the predentin. The frontier between the uncalcified predentin and the outer zone of mineralized dentin is abrupt (Fig. 15-10). In the mature dentin the collagen fibers, are obscured by the hydroxyapatite crystals. They are randomly oriented except in the wall of the dentinal tubules, where they are oriented parallel to the long axis of the odontoblast process. Dentin continues to be formed slowly throughout life and the pulp cavity is narrowed with advancing age.

Enamel

Enamel is the hardest substance in the body. Ninety-nine percent of its mass is made up of large hydroxyapatite crystals. Viewed with the light microscope, enamel consists of thin **enamel rods (enamel prisms)** that radiate from the dentin with a slight inclination toward the occlusal surface (the surface that contacts the opposing tooth). Around each rod is a very thin layer of organic matrix called the **prismatic rod sheath.** Each rod extends through the entire thickness of the enamel. The small angular spaces between parallel enamel rods are **interrod enamel,** which is similar in composition but has its hydroxyapatite crystals oriented differently from those of enamel rods (Fig. 15-11).

Enamel is produced by a layer of columnar cells called **ameloblasts.** These must be studied before eruption of the tooth, for this layer of cells is no longer present in mature teeth. In sections of developing teeth, the ameloblasts form an epithelium of very tall columnar cells over the outer surface of the dentin. The apex of each cell tapers down to a long conical process, called **Tome's process.** The ameloblasts have a basal nucleus and their cytoplasm contains a large supranuclear Golgi complex surrounded by cisternae of rough endoplasmic reticulum (Fig. 15-8B). Associated with the Golgi complex, and in the apical cytoplasm, there are numerous small, dense, secretory granules that contain **amelogenin** and **enamelin,** proteins of the organic matrix of enamel. The Tome's process of each ameloblast secretes the matrix of an enamel rod, and lateral branches of the process near its base secrete the matrix of the interrod enamel. In subsequent calcification, the

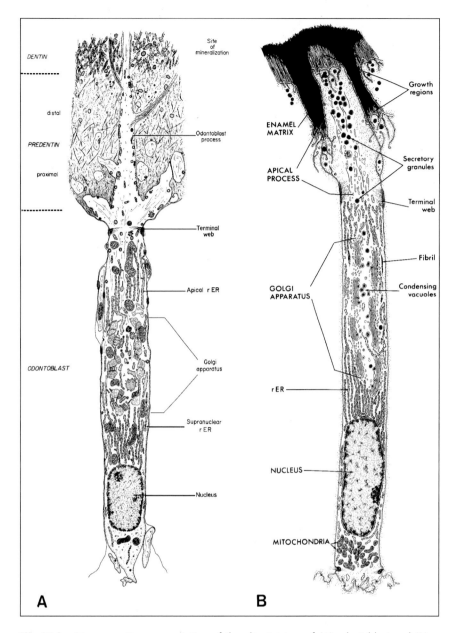

Fig. 15-8 Diagrammatic representation of the ultrastructure of (A) odontoblast and (B) a secretory ameloblast from a developing rat incisor. Both are very tall columnar cells. (From M. Weinstock and C.P. Leblond, Journal of Cell Biology 51:26, 1971.)

hydroxyapatite crystals formed in the interrod matrix are more random in their orientation than those of the rod enamel (Fig. 15-11). When formation of the enamel is complete, the ameloblasts degenerate.

Cementum

Enamel is confined to the crown of the tooth, and the dentin of the root is covered by a thin layer of **cementum** that meets the enamel in a sharp line, the **cemento-enamel junction,** which marks the boundary between the crown and the root. The cementum is similar to bone in its composition. Its cells, called **cementocytes,** occupy lacunae that communicate via minute radiating canaliculi.

However, there are no haversian systems in cementum. On its outer surface, there is a discontinuous layer of **cementoblasts** that are comparable to the osteoblasts on the surface of bone. Production of cementum maintains close contact between the root and the tooth socket.

Periodontal Ligament

The roots of a tooth are enveloped by a dense layer of collagen, forming the **periodontal membrane** or **periodontal ligament** interposed between the cementum and the surrounding alveolar bone. In it, collagen fibers run obliquely from the cementum into the alveolar bone, so that pressure on the tooth applies tension to the fibers

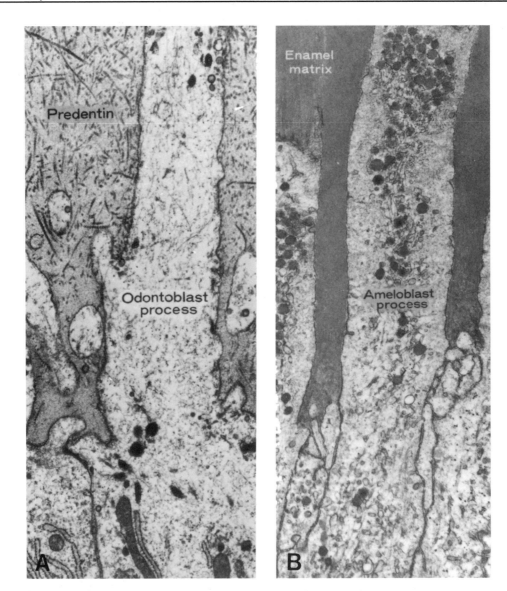

Fig. 15-9 (A) Electron micrograph of the apical process of an odontoblast and the surrounding fibrous and amorphous components of the predentin. (B) Apical process (Tome's process) of an ameloblast from a developing rat incisor. (From M. Weinstock and C.P. Leblond, Journal of Cell Biology 60:92, 1974; from Journal of Cell Biology 51:26, 1971.)

inserting into bone. The periodontal ligament firmly anchors the tooth to its socket while providing a limited degree of mobility.

*The oral cavity has a large and varied bacterial flora. Streptococcus mutans and other bacteria may accumulate on a tooth in an adherent layer (bacterial plaque). The underlying enamel and dentin are demineralized, resulting in **dental caries**. If not arrested, this may lead to a painful infection of the pulp. Other bacteria proliferating in the gingival cleft may destroy the periodontal ligament and cause resorption of surrounding alveolar bone and loosening of the teeth.*

Gingiva

The **gingiva** is the thicker portion of the oral mucous membrane that is firmly bound to the periosteum of the alveolar ridges of the maxilla and mandible. Around the base of the crown of each tooth, the gingiva is separated from the enamel by a shallow furrow called the **gingival crevice.** In the depths of the crevice, the epithelium is bound to the enamel by an intervening layer of material resembling that of a basal lamina. The superficial squamous cells of the gingival epithelium are bound to this layer by hemi-desmosomes. This seal between the epithelium and the enamel usually prevents entry of bacteria into the periodontal tissues.

Tooth Development

Tooth formation begins in the 6th week of gestation, when mesenchymal cells of neural crest origin aggregate at 10 sites beneath the epithelium covering the dental arches. These induce proliferation of the overlying epithelium to form **tooth buds.** At each of these sites, an invagination of the epithelium expands to form a cap-shaped structure connected to the surface by a stalk called the **dental lamina** (Fig. 15-12A). The epithelium on the underside of this cap thickens and invaginates further into the cap, forming the **inner enamel epithelium.** With further deepening of the concavity of the tooth bud, it takes on a bell shape (Fig. 15-12B). The outer layer of the cap (**outer dental epithelium**) remains relatively thin. The space between these layers contains a loose network of stellate cells derived from the epithelium. The cap, as a whole, is called the **enamel organ,** for it will later form the enamel on the crown of a tooth. The rim of the bell, where the outer enamel epithelium is continuous with the inner enamel epithelium, is called the **cervical loop.** This region will later form the region of the tooth, between the crown and the root. The concavity of the bell, which is designed to form the pulp cavity, is occupied by mesoderm.

Late in the bell stage, the columnar cells of the inner enamel epithelium begin to differentiate into ameloblasts. In the **dental papilla,** beneath the bell, this change induces mesenchymal cells to differentiate into odontoblasts. These gather on the underside of the basal lamina

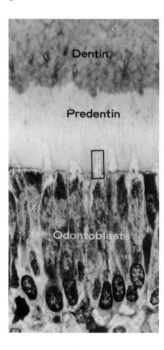

Fig. 15-10 Photomicrograph from a growing rat incisor, showing the relationships of the odontoblasts (bottom) to the predentin and dentin (above). An area such as that in the rectangle is shown in Fig. 15-9A. (From M. Weinstock and C.P. Leblond, Journal of Cell Biology 60:92, 1974.)

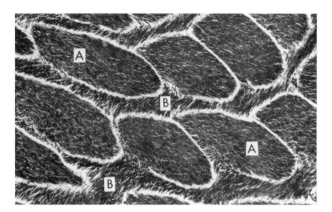

Fig. 15-11 Electron micrograph of a slightly oblique section of undecalcified bovine enamel, showing (A) the enamel rods or prisms and (B) the interprismatic enamel. Note the regular orientation of the hydroxyapatite crystals in the rods, and the differing orientation of the crystals in the interprismatic enamel. (Courtesy of E.J. Daniel and J.J. Glimcher.)

of the inner enamel epithelium and begin to secrete dentin (Fig. 15-12C). This, in turn, induces the ameloblasts to change their original polarity and begin to secrete enamel matrix at the end toward the basal lamina (Fig. 15-13). Thereafter, this end is called the **functional apex** of the ameloblast. Progressive thickening and calcification of both enamel and dentin completes formation of the crown of the tooth, and the overlying layer of ameloblasts then degenerate.

Formation of the root of the tooth depends on proliferation of cells in the cervical loop that results in elongation of the juxtaposed inner and outer dental epithelia in this region to form **Hertwig's epithelial root sheath.** As the sheath lengthens, the length of the dental papilla in its interior is increased and cells in its interior differentiate into odontoblasts. These secrete a layer of root dentin that is continuous above with the dentin of the crown. No ameloblasts are formed; hence, no enamel layer is formed on the root. When the root has attained its definitive length, the root sheath breaks down and the dentin is exposed to the surrounding connective tissue. Some of its fibroblasts then differentiate into cementoblasts that deposit a layer of cementum on the outside of the root dentin.

SALIVARY GLANDS

Glands are described as **simple** or **compound.** Simple glands are composed entirely of secretory cells or have a secretory segment at the end of an unbranched duct. Compound glands consist of multiple acini at the ends of a highly branched duct system (Fig. 15-14). An **acinus** is a grouping of secretory cells arranged around a narrow lumen. Two categories of salivary glands secrete into the oral cavity: the **minor salivary glands,** which are widely

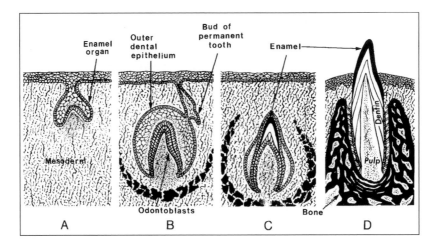

Fig. 15-12 Diagram of the stages of development of a human deciduous tooth. (A) cap stage; (B) bell stage; (C) beginning calcification of enamel (black) and dentin (white); (D) the erupted tooth.

distributed in the oral submucosa, and the **major salivary glands,** which are much larger and not confined to the submucosa.

Major Salivary Glands

The largest of these are two **parotid glands** each weighing about 25 g. They are located subcutaneously on either side of the face anterior to the ears. Their long duct opens into the oral cavity opposite the second upper molar tooth, on either side. Two **submandibular glands,** about 3 cm in diameter are located beneath the mandible on either side of the mid-line. Their ducts open onto the floor of the mouth near the frenulum of the tongue. The **sublingual glands** lie beneath the floor of the mouth near the symphysis of the mandible and their ducts open onto ridges of the mucosa near the frenulum.

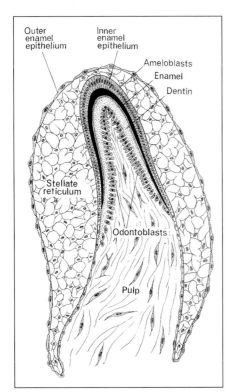

Fig. 15-13 Drawing of the primordium of a lower central incisor of a 6.5-month fetus.

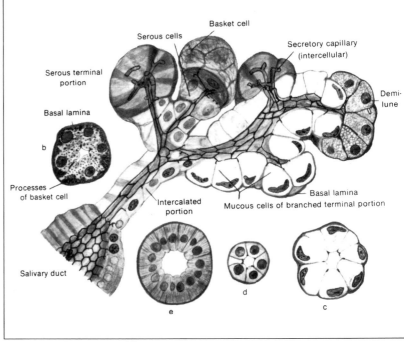

Fig. 15-14 Drawing of a terminal branch of a compound salivary gland and its ducts. (b) Cross section of a serous acinus; (c) cross section of a mucous acinus; (d) cross section of an intercalated duct, (e) cross section of a striated duct. (From Braus, H. Anatomie des Menschen, Springer Verlag, Berlin, 1924.)

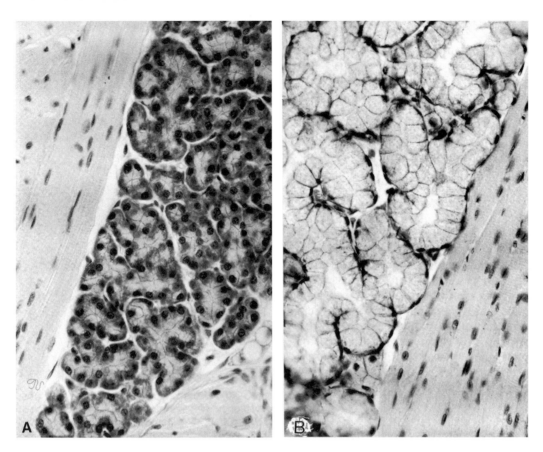

Fig. 15-15 Lingual glands, examples of minor salivary glands. (A) A serous gland and (B) a mucous gland. Note the basal displacement of the nuclei. Both glands are between bundles of striated muscle of the tongue.

*The common childhood disease called **mumps** is a viral infection of the parotid gland. The gland becomes swollen and tender for a week or more and then subsides. The virus may spread to the submandibular and sublingual glands. The disease is usually self-limiting; but, rarely, in males, blood-borne spread of the virus to the testes (**orchitis**) is a painful and serious complication.*

The major salivary glands are all compound glands consisting of large numbers of acini at the ends of a duct system with many orders of branching. The acini are described as **serous** and **mucous.** Serous is the term applied to those in which the cells have electron-dense apical secretory granules and produce a watery secretion rich in enzymes (Fig. 15-15A). Mucous is the descriptive term applied to cells with abundant homogenous electron-lucent secretory droplets, that tend to deform the cell nucleus and displace it to the basal plasmalemma (Fig. 15-15B). Their secretion, **mucin** (mucus), is a viscous mixture of glycoproteins.

The **parotid gland** consists entirely of acini made up of pyramidal cells surrounding a narrow lumen (Fig. 15-16 [see Plate 24]). The cells have abundant rough endoplasmic reticulum. Interposed between the secretory cells and the

basal lamina are inconspicuous highly branched **myoepithelial cells** (basket cells). The neighboring processes of these cells are adherent at desmosomes. Their cytoplasm is rich in actin and contaction of these cells helps to expel the secretory product from the lumen of the acinus.

The **submandibular glands** contain both serous and mucous acini (Fig. 15-17 [see Plate 24]). In addition, many of the elongated mucous acini have, capping their end, a crescentic layer of serous cells that is called a **serous demilune** (Fig. 15-18). The secretion of these serous cells reaches the lumen of the acinus via intercellular canaliculi between the underlying mucous cells.

The **sublingual glands,** in the floor of the mouth, are made up predominantly of mucous acini with serous demilunes, but serous acini are also present in limited numbers.

Salivary ducts

The acini of the major salivary glands are at the ends of slender branching **intercalated ducts** that are lined by simple cuboidal epithelium. The intercalated ducts are branches of larger **striated ducts,** lined by low columnar epithelium (Fig. 15-14). In electron micrographs, these cells have deep invaginations of the plasmalemma at the

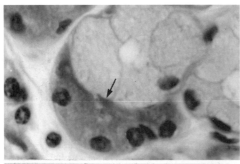

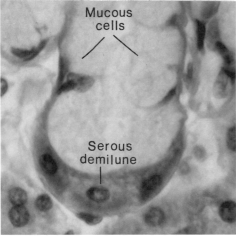

Fig. 15-18 Photomicrographs of mixed acini from human submandibular gland, showing mucous cells and serous demilunes.

cell base. The striations observed with the light microscope are due to the vertical alignment of long mitochondria in the cytoplasm between these invaginations. This specialization greatly increases the area of membrane associated with mitochondria that provide the energy for efficient active transport of water and ions to modify the secretory product during its passage through the ducts. The striated ducts draining the separate lobules of the gland converge upon interlobular **excretory ducts,** lined by stratified cuboidal epithelium. These, in turn, are branches of the long **main duct,** which is lined by columnar epithelium. This is transformed to stratified squamous epithelium as the duct approaches its opening into the oral cavity.

Minor Salivary glands

Among the minor salivary glands are small glands between the bundles of striated muscle in the tongue. Some of these are serous and others are mucous glands (Fig. 15-15). Numerous smaller glands, found in the submucosa of the cheeks and floor of the mouth, are made up of highly branched tubules. In some glands, these are lined by serous cells, in others by mucous cells. The mucous glands greatly outnumber the serous. Both open onto the surface of the oral epithelium via short ducts lined by unspecialized cuboidal epithelium. These glands are believed to secrete continuously contributing to the saliva that moistens and lubricates the oral mucosa.

Histophysiology

Between meals, the major salivary glands secrete continuously at a slow rate of 0.5–1 ml/min. Upon ingestion of food, the flow is greatly increased due to activation of the glands by sympathetic and parasympathetic nerves. The serous cells of the glands secrete a variety of enzymes, including amylase, lysozyme, peroxidase, desoxyribnuclease, and ribonuclease. The sympathetic neurotransmitter also causes serous cells and intercalated duct cells to release **kallikrein,** which causes a vasodilatation within the glands that contributes to their production of an increased volume of saliva.

QUESTIONS*

1. Which statement is **incorrect** about the periodontal membrane?

   A. It contains collagenous fibers.
   B. It is located between the cement and alveolar socket.
   C. It helps hold the tooth in its socket.
   D. All of the above
   E. None of the above

2. Which matched pair is **incorrect?**

   A. dental lamina/enamel organ
   B. odontoblasts/enamel
   C. ameloblasts/ectoderm
   D. dentin/tubules
   E. cementum/no haversian canals

3. Which statement is **incorrect** concerning the submandibular gland?

   A. It contains intercalated ducts.
   B. It contains striated ducts.
   C. It contains demilunes.
   D. It contains myoepithelial cells.
   E. None of the above

4. Dentine is produced by

   A. cementoblasts
   B. fibrocytes
   C. periodontal membrane
   D. ameloblasts
   E. odontoblasts

5. Which of the glands listed below is almost entirely composed of serous elements?

   A. sublingual
   B. liver
   C. parotid
   D. submandibular
   E. Brunner's gland

6. Which immunoglobulin is most abundant in saliva?

   A. IgE
   B. IgM
   C. IgG
   D. IgA
   E. None of the above

7. Von Ebner's glands are associated with

   A. gastric mucosa
   B. circumvallate papillae
   C. esophagus
   D. anus
   E. None of the above

8. The dental lamina comes from

   A. mesodermal derivative
   B. endodermal derivative
   C. epidermal derivative
   D. mesenchymal derivative
   E. None of the above

9. Serous cells which form a cap over a mucous secretory unit are properly known as a

   A. serous capping unit
   B. serous demilune
   C. serous secreting unit
   D. serous acinus
   E. serous gland

10. Which statement is **false** concerning oral lymphatic tissue?

    A. The single palatine tonsil is located on the posterior roof of the mouth.
    B. Epithelium overlying the pharyngeal tonsil may be of more than one type.
    C. Crypts can be observed in the palatine tonsil but not in the pharyngeal tonsil.
    D. Mast cells and plasma cells are easily seen when tonsils are inflamed.
    E. Tonsils reach their greatest development in childhood.

*Answers on page 307.

16

ESOPHAGUS AND STOMACH

CHAPTER OUTLINE

KEY WORDS

A Cell
Argentaffin Cell
Auerbach's Plexus
Cardia
Cardiac Gland
Chief Cell
Chyme
Corpus
D Cell
EC Cell
Enteroendocrine Cell
Esophageal Gland
Foveolae
Fundus
G Cell
Gastric Intrinsic
   Factor
Gastric Pit

Gastrin
Glucagon
Langerhans Cell
Meissner's Plexus
Mucous Neck Cell
Oxyntic Cell
Oxyntic Gland
Paracrine
Parietal Cell
Pepsinogen
Peristalsis
Pyloric Antrum
Pyloric Canal
Pyloris
Rugae
Serotonin
Somatostatin
Zymogenic Cell

After mechanical fragmentation of the ingested food and initiation of its digestion by salivary enzymes, it passes through the esophagus to the stomach for further processing. Beyond the oral cavity, the wall of the alimentary tract has four layers: **mucosa, submucosa, muscularis,** and the **serosa** (Fig. 16-1).

The **mucosa** consists of (1) an epithelium of a type appropriate to the function of that segment, (2) a thin lamina propria beneath the epithelium, consisting of a highly vascular connective tissue containing macrophages, plasma cells, and lymphocytes concerned with immunological defense against the intralumenal bacterial flora, and (3) a **muscularis mucosae,** a layer of smooth-muscle cells that is able to change the surface contour of the mucosa.

The **submucosa** is a denser connective-tissue layer that contains most of the blood vessels supplying the mucosa and a network of sympathetic nerves, **Meissner's plexus,** that controls the intrinsic motility of the tract. This layer also contains scattered lymphoid nodules involved in immunological defenses of the mucosa. In some segments of the tract, there are also mucus-secreting submucosal glands that deliver their product into the gut lumen.

The **serosa,** the outermost layer of the alimentary tract, is **mesothelium,** the squamous epithelium that lines the body cavities and covers all the organs within them. There is a very thin layer of loose connective tissue between the mesothelium and the muscularis. In some segments of the tract, adipose cells accumulate in this layer, making it much thicker.

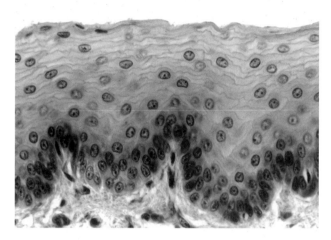

Fig. 16-2 Photomicrograph of the stratified squamous epithelium of the esophagus.

ESOPHAGUS

The esophagus is the tubular organ that conveys the ingested food from the pharynx to the stomach. It plays no role in food digestion. The greater part of its length (25 cm) is within the thorax, but it passes through the diaphragm, and its short terminal segment (2–4 cm), within the abdomen, is continuous with the stomach. The esophageal mucosa is 300–400 μm thick and covered by stratified squamous epithelium (Fig. 16-2). Its stratum corneum is only three or four cells in thickness and is not heavily keratinized. Occasional **Langerhans cells** can be found among the cells of its stratum germinativum. These migratory antigen-presenting cells are involved in immunological responses to bacterial antigens reaching them from the lumen. At the junction of the esophagus with the stomach, there is an abrupt transition from stratified squamous epithelium to the simple columnar epithelium of the gastric mucosa.

In the upper portion of the esophagus, the muscularis mucosae is represented by only scattered fascicles of smooth-muscle cells, predominantly longitudinal in their orientation. Lower down, near the stomach, these come together to form a thin continuous layer. The esophageal submucosa contains numerous blood vessels, interlacing collagen fibers and elastic fibers. The latter are important in maintaining the surface configuration of the mucosa. In the undistended esophagus, longitudinally oriented folds of the mucosa and submucosa give the lumen a highly irregular outline. As a bolus of food passes down the esophagus, these folds are transiently obliterated and then rapidly restored by the recoil of the elastic fibers of the submucosa.

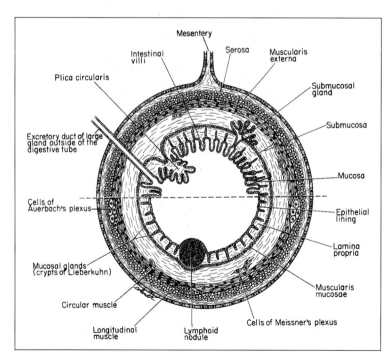

Fig. 16-1 Schematic representation of the organization of the gastrointestinal tract. The concentric layers, serosa, muscularis, and mucosa, are common to all regions of the tract. In the upper half of the figure, the mucosa is shown with glands and villi, as in the small intestine. In the lower half, it is shown with glands and no villi, as in the colon.

The muscularis of the esophagus consists of outer longitudinal and inner circular layers. Swallowing is a voluntary act, and this is reflected in the type of muscle fibers in the muscularis. In the upper third of the esophagus, the muscularis is made up of striated muscle. In the middle third, it is a mixture of smooth and striated fibers, and in the lower third, both outer and inner layers consist entirely of smooth muscle, as in more distal parts of the alimentary tract.

Two categories of mucus-secreting glands are found in the wall of the esophagus. The **mucosal esophageal glands** (esophageal cardiac glands) are confined to the lamina propria. They are present in small numbers in the upper esophagus and near its junction with the stomach. The longer **submucosal esophageal glands** extend into the submucosa and are more widespread. Both types are branched tubular glands containing mucous cells only. The apical cytoplasm of the cells is distended with pale-staining secretory granules that deform and displace the nucleus to the base of the cell (Fig. 16-3). The principal function of these glands is to provide a lubricating layer of mucus to facilitate transport of food to the stomach.

*In some individuals, the muscularis of the lower esophagus fails to maintain the state of partial contraction that normally prevents reflux of gastric contents into the esophagus. **Gastroesophageal reflux** is a rather common disorder attended by recurrent "heartburn." The esophageal mucosa lacks an adequate protective blanket of mucus. The highly acid gastric juices irritate it, causing painful esophagitis.*

STOMACH

Gross anatomists assign separate terms to five regions of the stomach (Fig. 16-4A). A narrow zone around the junction of the esophagus is the **cardia.** A dome-shaped region above this is the **fundus,** and a large central segment is the **corpus.** This is continuous below with a conical region, called the **pyloric antrum,** which narrows to the **pyloric canal** and this terminates in the **pyloris,** which contains the **pyloric sphincter** that relaxes to allow the contents of the stomach to pass into the duodenum (Fig. 16-4). Histologists are able to distinguish only three regions on the basis of differences in microscopic structure of the mucosa: the **cardia,** a narrow zone 2–3 cm wide around the esophageal orifice; a **fundic region,** which is coextensive with the fundus and corpus of the gross anatomist; and the **pyloric region,** which includes the pyloric antrum, pyloric canal, and pyloris.

When the empty stomach is opened, its inner surface presents branching longitudinal folds of the mucosa and underlying submucosa called **rugae** or **plicae mucosae**

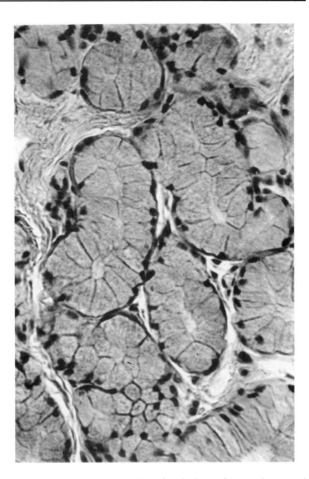

Fig. 16-3 Photomicrograph of tubules of a submucosal esophageal gland. Note that the nuclei are displaced to the base by the accumulated mucus secretion.

(Fig. 16-4B). During a meal, the pyloric sphincter is closed, and as the organ becomes distended with food, the rugae are obliterated. Closure of the pyloric sphincter and generation of waves of contraction by the muscularis of the fundic region of the organ reduce the ingested food to a viscous semifluid mass, referred to as the **chyme.** In this process, food is mixed with hydrochloric acid and **pepsin,** a protease secreted by the mucosa to initiate the digestion of proteins.

Gastric Mucosa

The epithelium of the gastric mucosa is invaginated to form myriad closely spaced **gastric pits,** or **foveolae.** From the bottom of each of these, several slender **gastric glands** extend downward, occupying the greater part of the thickness of the mucosa (Fig. 16-5). The number of foveolae in the human stomach is estimated to be about 3.5 million, and the number of glands 15 million. The spaces between the glands are occupied by the loose connective tissue constituting the **lamina propria.** The surface epithelium and that lining the gastric pits consists of tall, columnar, mucus-secreting cells. These produce a thick blanket

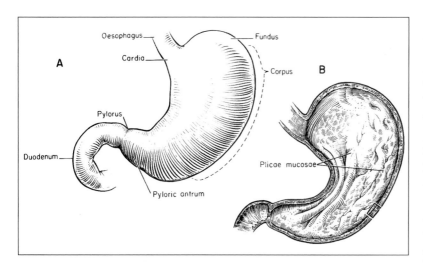

narrow band 10–40 mm wide around the esophageal orifice, the cardia, the foveolae are relatively shallow, occupying only about one-fourth the thickness of the mucosa. Their associated **cardiac glands** are branched and coiled. They contain a few undifferentiated cells in their necks, but the greater part of the gland is made up of mucus-secreting cells indistinguishable from those lining the foveolae. There are also a few **enteroendocrine cells** that secrete **gastrin,** a hormone that influences gastric motility and stimulates the secretory activity of the glands. These are abundant in glands of the corpus but are uncommon in the cardiac glands.

Fig. 16-4 (A) Drawing of the gross anatomical regions of the stomach. (B) A hemisected stomach showing the plicae mucosae.

of mucus that lubricates the mucosa and protects it from damage by the strongly acidic (pH 2) and hydrolytic components of the chyme.

Cardiac Glands

The depth of the foveolae, the shapes of their glands, and the relative proportions of the several glandular cell types differ somewhat in the three regions of the stomach. In a

Gastric Glands

In the mucosa of the fundic region, the foveolae are relatively short and the glands arising from them are long and straight. These so-called **gastric glands** (oxyntic glands) make a major contribution to the gastric juice. Their epithelium contains five cell types: **stem cells, mucous neck cells, parietal cells** (oxyntic cells), **chief cells** (zymogenic cells), and **enteroendocrine cells** (Fig. 16-6).

The **stem cells** are small basophilic cells confined to the neck of the gland. They are often found in mitosis. Their

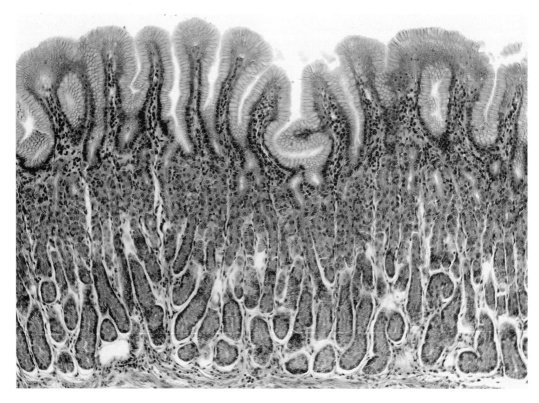

Fig. 16-5 Photomicrograph of the gastric mucosa of a macaque showing the long tubular gastric glands, opening into the gastric pits, or foveolae.

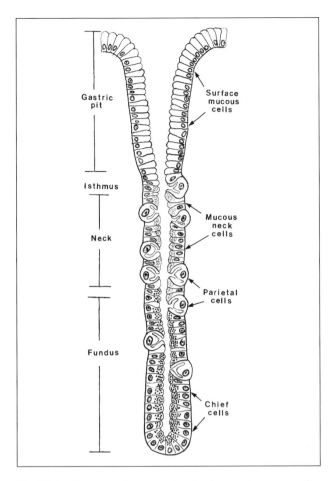

Fig. 16-6 Diagram of an oxyntic gland from the corpus of a mamalian stomach, showing the isthmus, base, and neck.

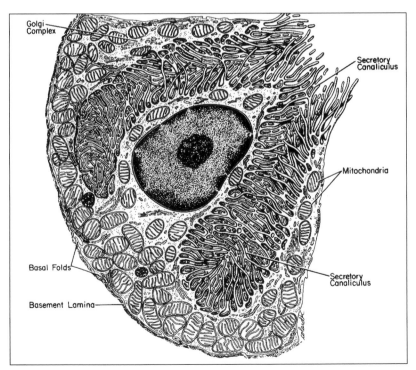

Fig. 16-8 Drawing of the ultrastructure of an active parietal cell. It is a large cell with an exceptional number of mitochondria and a prominent intracellular canaliculus lined with microvilli. (Courtesy of S. Ito.)

proliferation is responsible for the continuous renewal of the gastric mucosa. Some of their progeny, moving upward, differentiate to replace the mucous cells of the gastric pits. Others migrate deeper into the glands, where they differentiate into any of the cell types found there.

The numerous **mucous neck cells** in the neck region of the glands are irregular in shape, with a basal nucleus and apical secretory granules that have histochemical characteristics distinct from those of the mucus-secreting cells of the surface epithelium. The glycoproteins they produce are more acidic. The physiological significance of production of two kinds of mucus by the gastric mucosa is not understood.

The **parietal cells** (oxyntic cells) are large, rounded cells that are more numerous in the upper half of the gland but are interspersed among the other cell types along its entire length (Figs. 16-6 and 16-7 [see Plate 25]). They have a centrally placed nucleus and an intensely eosinophilic cytoplasm. In electron micrographs, their most distinctive feature is the presence of a deep invagination of the apical membrane forming a **secretory canaliculus,** which partially encircles the nucleus and extends nearly to the cell base (Fig. 16-7B [see Plate 25]). Like the apical plasmalemma, the membrane lining the canaliculus bears numerous microvilli that project into its lumen. There are no secretory granules and the Golgi complex is relatively small. Some 40% of the cytoplasmic volume is occupied by large mitochondria possessing numerous cristae. The cytoplasm around the canaliculus contains numerous membrane-limited tubules and vesicles comprising the **tubulovesicular system** of the parietal cell (Fig. 16-9). These are not elements of the smooth endoplasmic reticulum but are interiorized portions of the plasmalemma. When the cell is stimulated, they fuse with the membrane of the canaliculus increasing its surface area and thereby enhancing the efficiency of the cell in secreting the **hydrochloric acid** (HCl) of the gastric juice. A large part of the protein in the membrane added to the surface is a specific H+K+-ATPase, which serves as a proton pump moving H+ ions from the cell to the lumen and K+ ions from the lumen into the cell. For each H+ ion secreted, a bicarbonate ion (HCO_3-) is released into the gastric venous circulation. H+ ions are at a concentration 3 million times their concentration in the blood plasma. Between meals, the size of the secretory canaliculus is reduced, as membrane is withdrawn from its surface to regenerate the tubulovesicular system of the cytoplasm. Acid secretion is stimulated by **gastrin** secreted by enteroendocrine cells and by **histamine** released by mast cells in the lamina propria. In addition to hydrochloric acid, parietal

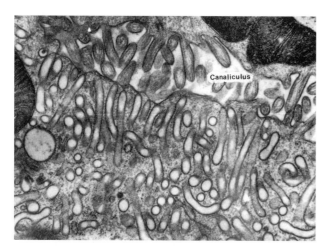

Fig. 16-9 Electron micrograph of a portion of a parietal cell including a segment of the secretory canaliculus. (Courtesy of N. Sugai and A. Ichikawa.)

cells secrete **gastric intrinsic factor,** a glycoprotein necessary for intestinal absorption of vitamin B_{12}, which is required for erythrocyte production in the bone marrow.

> *The gastric mucus of a third or more of the population is inhabited by bacteria of the genus **Helicobacter pylori**. These produce toxins that cause **chronic gastritis**. A bacterial enzyme, urease, breaks down urea to CO2 and ammonia, which neutralizes gastric HCl. Muscosal glands may counteract this effect by formation of nearly twice the normal number of parietal cells. Some of these patients subsequently develop **gastric** or **duodenal ulcer** and are more likely to have gastric cancer in later years.*

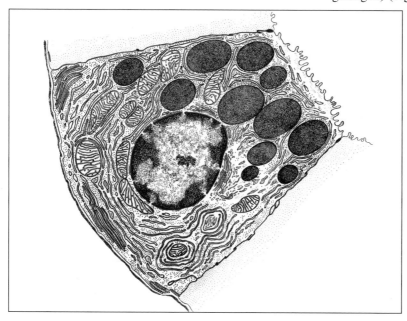

Fig. 16-10 Drawing of a gastric chief cell (zymogenic cell) as seen with the electron microscope. (From S. Ito and R. J. Winchester, Jour-nal of Cell Biology 16:541, 1963.)

The **chief cells** (zymogenic cells) are the predominant cell type of the lower third of gastric glands in the fundic region. They have a strongly basophilic cytoplasm and conspicuous secretory granules. In electron micrographs, they have the abundant granular endoplasmic reticulum and prominent Golgi complex characteristic of protein-secreting cells (Figs. 16-10 and 16-11). The secretory granules contain **pepsinogen,** the precursor of the proteolytic enzyme **pepsin.** When released into the acid environment in the gastric lumen, pepsinogen is converted to the active enzyme. These cells also secrete small amounts of a **lipase** to initiate the degradation of lipids to fatty acids.

Enteroendocrine cells, previously mentioned, are widely scattered among the exocrine cells of the gastric glands and throughout the intestinal tract. They are small, ovoid, or pyramidal cells. They were initially recognized in histological sections by their ability to reduce silver salts and were formerly called **argentaffin cells.** Some have secretory granules that are located at the cell apex. Such cells evidently release their product into the gland lumen to stimulate other cells of the gland (a **paracrine** action). Others have their granules at the cell base, and their product presumably diffuses into the blood vessels of the lamina propria to be transported to more distant target cells (an **endocrine** action). The different types of these cells are not easily identifiable in histological sections, but by taking advantage of improved extraction techniques and immunocytological methods, it has been possible to distinguish 15 types of enteroendocrine cells in the alimentary tract. Their products include a wide variety of amines, polypeptides, and more complex hormones. The number and kind of enteroendocrine cells vary in different segments of the stomach. The so-called **A cells** (secreting glucagon) (Fig. 16-12), are confined to the upper third of the stomach, **EC cells** (secreting serotonin) occur throughout the mucosa, and **G cells** (secreting gastrin) are most abundant in the antrum. **D cells** (secreting somatostatin) are widely distributed, but absent from the midportion of the stomach. They play a role in regulating the activity of the A cells and G cells.

Pyloric Glands

The foveolae in the pyloric region are unusually deep, occupying half to two-thirds the thickness of the mucosa. The relatively short **pyloric glands** originating from them are branched, highly tortuous, and have a larger lumen than the glands of the fundic region. Mucus-secreting cells predominate. In addition to mucin, these glands secrete appreciable amounts of the bacteriolytic enzyme, **lysozyme.** Parietal cells are relatively few in these glands, but enteroendocrine cells are common.

Lamina Propria

The interspaces between the glands of the gastric mucosa are occupied by the **lamina propria.** It is a typical loose connective tissue containing fibroblasts, scattered eosinophils, macrophages, plasma cells, and mast cells. In addition, there are slender vertical strands of smooth-muscle cells that extend upward from the muscularis mucosae into the lamina propria. It is speculated that intermittent contraction of these muscle cells may slightly compress the mucosa, promoting discharge of secretion from its glands.

Submucosa

The **submucosa** is a denser layer of connective tissue deep to the thin muscularis mucosae. It contains bundles of collagen fibers, a network of lymphatics, a plexus of veins, and numerous arterioles from which capillaries course vertically to form a network around the glands of the mucosa. This network is drained into the venous plexus in the submucosa.

Muscularis

The muscularis of the stomach has three layers of smooth muscle instead of the usual two. Cells of the outermost layer are oriented longitudinally, those of the middle layer are circular, and those in the inner layer are oblique. The outer layer is incomplete, being present along the greater and lesser curvature of the stomach but thin or absent on its dorsal and ventral surfaces. It thins out and ends before reaching the pyloris. The middle layer of circular fibers is complete. It is greatly thickened around the pyloric canal to form the **pyloric sphincter.**

Histophysiology

The principal functions of the stomach are the mixing of the ingested food with the gastric secretions. With the pylorus closed, mixing is accomplished by waves of contraction of the muscularis sweeping over the stomach every 20 s. When the gastric phase of digestion is complete, the pyloric sphincter opens and stronger contractions of the muscularis eject the chyme into the duodenum.

The enteroendocrine cells play an important role in controlling the secretory activity of the gastric mucosa. In the fasting stomach, the pH of its contents is relatively low and secretion of somatostatin by the D cells exerts a paracrine inhibitory effect upon release of the peptide hormone gastrin from the G cells. Filling of the stomach with food raises the pH, and the D cells are inactivated, permitting the G cells to release gastrin which, in turn, increases gastric motility and stimulates acid secretion by the parietal cells. The resulting lowering of the pH creates the conditions necessary for activation of the enzyme pepsin, secreted by the chief cells. This enzyme is then able to digest nearly all of the proteins of the chyme. Upon emptying of the stomach, the pH returns to its fasting level and gastrin secretion by the G cells is again inhibited.

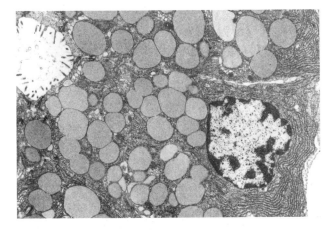

Fig. 16-11 Electron micrograph of three chief cells (zymogenic cells) around the lumen of an oxyntic gland. The cell bases are occupied by cisternae of the rough endoplasmic reticulum, and the cell apices are crowded with pale-staining secretory granules. (Courtesy of S. Ito.)

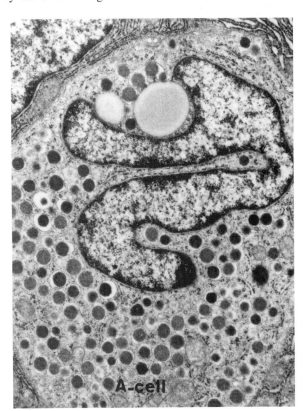

Fig. 16-12 Electron micrograph of an enteroendocrine A cell secreting glucagon.

QUESTIONS*

1. A smooth surfaced system of tubules and vesicles is associated with which of the following cell types?

   A. chief cell of the stomach
   B. Paneth cell
   C. acinar cell of the parotid
   D. acinar cell of the pancreas
   E. oxyntic cell

2. Which of the following statements is **incorrect?**

   A. The gastric pits are shallow in the corpus stomach compared with the pylorus.
   B. Gastrin is produced in the body (corpus) of the stomach.
   C. Gastrin is a polypeptide hormone.
   D. The terminal four amino acids account for the activity of gastrin.
   E. Gastrin is produced by an APUD type cell.

3. Which of the following does **not** belong in the mucosa of the corpus stomach?

   A. smooth muscle
   B. mucigenous-bordered epithelium
   C. oxyntic cells
   D. goblet cells
   E. chief cells

4. A well-developed rough surfaced endoplasmic reticulum is **not** associated with

   A. body chief cell of the stomach
   B. Paneth cell
   C. acinar cell of the parotid
   D. acinar cell of the pancreas
   E. oxyntic cell

5. Which of the following statements is **incorrect?**

   A. The gastric pits (foveolae) are deep in the corpus stomach compared with the pylorus.
   B. Gastrin is produced in the antrum of the stomach.
   C. Gastrin is a polypeptide hormone.
   D. The terminal four amino acids account for the activity of gastrin.
   E. None of the above

6. Regeneration of epithelial cell types in the stomach comes from differentiation of

   A. surface mucigenous-bordered cells
   B. isthmus mucous cells
   C. mucous neck cells
   D. body chief (peptic) cells
   E. oxyntic cells

7. A gastric pit is surrounded by which of the following cell types?

   A. body chief cells
   B. oxyntic cells
   C. APUD cells
   D. mucigenous-bordered cells
   E. None of the above

8. A surgical specimen of the esophagus whose muscularis externa contains smooth muscle only

   A. was obtained from the pharyngoesophageal region
   B. was obtained from the central region of the esophagus
   C. was obtained from the distal end of the esophagus
   D. could have been obtained from any region of the esophagus
   E. has been incorrectly labeled, as the muscularis externa of the esophagus consists entirely of striated muscle

9. Pepsinogen production is associated with which of the following cell types?

   A. Paneth cell
   B. body chief cell
   C. oxyntic cell
   D. pyloric gland cell
   E. None of the above

10. Which statement about the esophagus is **false?**

    A. The esophagus contains two categories of mucous-secreting glands.
    B. The esophagus contains both smooth and striated muscle types.
    C. Mucus produced in the esophagus can be either neutral or acidic.
    D. The esophagus contains a muscularis externa arranged in three layers.
    E. The principal function of esophageal glands is lubrication.

*Answers on page 307.

17

INTESTINES

CHAPTER OUTLINE

KEY WORDS

Anal Sphincter
Appendices
  Epiploicae
Auerbach's Plexus
Brunner's Glands
Caecum
Cholecystokinin
Chylomicron
Cisterna Chyli
Colon
Columns of Morgagni
Cryptin
Crypts
Crypts of Lieberkuhn
D Cell
Duodenum
Enteroendocrine Cell
Enteroglycogen
G Cell
Glycocalyx
Haustrae
I Cell
Ileocecal Sphincter

Ileum
Immune Exclusion
Jejunum
L Cell
Lacteal
M Cell
Meissner's Plexus
Microvilli
MO Cell
Motilin
Paneth Cell
Peritoneum
Peyer's Patch
Plicae Circulares
S Cell
Secretin
Somatostatin
Striated Border
Taeniae Coli
Thoracic Duct
Valve of Kirkring
Villi

SMALL INTESTINE

Digestion of food begins in the mouth and stomach, but there is little absorption of metabolites in those organs. Digestion is continued in the small intestine by enzymes secreted by its mucosa, supplimented by enzymes reaching it from the pancreas. However, the major function of the small intestine is the absorption of the products of digestion (monosaccharides, amino acids, fatty acids, and monoglycerides).

The small intestine is a convoluted tube about 5 m in length, divided, for descriptive purposes, into three segments distinguishable by minor differences in the microscopic structure of their mucosa. The initial segment, the **duodenum,** about 12 cm in length, is firmly fixed to the posterior abdominal wall. It has a C-shaped course around the head of the pancreas. At its distal end, it is continuous with the **jejunum,** which is not fixed but is suspended from the dorsal wall on a mesentery. The jejunum, comprising about two-fifths of the total length of the small intestine, is followed by the **ileum,** which makes up the distal three-fifths. The transition among the three segments is gradual. Throughout its length, the wall of the intestine is made up of the four layers described previously: the mucosa, submucosa, the muscularis, and the serosa.

Mucosa

Efficient absorption of nutrients is promoted by several devices that increase the total area of the mucosal surface. The first of these is the great length of the organ (5–7 m). The next level of surface amplification, the **plicae circulares** (valves of Kirkring) are transversely oriented folds of the mucosa and submucosa that project into the lumen. They are 8–10 mm in height, 3–4 mm in thickness, and readily visible to the naked eye. Unlike the rugae of the stomach, the plicae are permanent structures that are not obliterated by distension of the intestine. They are most conspicuous in the first portion of the jejunum but diminish in number and height more distally and are seldom found in the ileum. They slow the passage of the intestinal contents and probably increase the surface area of the mucosa about threefold. The next level of surface amplification is the presence of myriad **intestinal villi,** 0.1–0.5 mm in length, and numbering 10–40/mm^2 of mucosa (Fig. 17-1 [see Plate 25]). They are narrow, foliate structures parallel to the long axis of the intestine. They are longest in the duodenum and proximal jejunum and become shorter and more cylindrical in form in the distal jejunum and ileum. They achieve an additional eightfold increase in surface area. The core of each villus consists of loose connective tissue containing a subepithelial network of fenestrated

capillaries and a central **lacteal.** This is a blind-ending lymphatic vessel that drains into a plexus of lymphatics in the underlying lamina propria (Fig. 17-2). The lacteals in the villi, and the larger lymphatics in the wall of the gut, provide an important pathway for transport of absorbed lipids from the intestinal mucosa to the blood vascular system.

The epithelium covering the intestinal villi (Fig. 17-3 [see Plate 26]) has a striated border consisting of up to 3000 **microvilli** per cell, resulting in an additional 30-fold increase in surface area. The total surface area of the intestinal mucosa is estimated to be about 200 m^2. Between the bases of the intestinal villi, the epithelium is invaginated to form short **intestinal glands,** also called **crypts of Lieberkuhn** (Fig. 17-1 [see Plate 25]).

The epithelium covering the intestinal villi contains four principal cell types: **absorptive cells, goblet cells, enteroendocrine cells,** and **Paneth cells.** All of the cells of the intestinal epithelium are short-lived and are constantly renewed. They arise from pluripotential **stem cells** situated in the necks of the intestinal glands (crypts). These undergo frequent divisions, and their progeny slowly move upward along the sides of the villi as they differentiate into absorptive cells and goblet cells, to replace spent cells that are constantly being exfoliated at the tips of the villi. Other cells arising from the stem cells move downward into the crypts, differentiating into enteroendocrine cells and Paneth cells. Paneth cells reside in the base of the crypts for about 20 days and then undergo apoptosis (programmed cell death). The rapid turnover of the intestinal epithelium can be demonstrated by injecting a rat with tritiated thymidine, which labels the dividing cells in the necks of the intestinal glands. In histological sections, labeled cells can be found on the sides of the villi 1 day later, and by the fifth day after the injection, labeled cells are being exfoliated at the villus tips. The rate of cell turnover in the human intestine is probably only slightly slower.

Absorptive cells of the villi are tall columnar cells with a prominent brush-border consisting of microvilli with a core of actin filaments. The microvilli have been observed to shorten from time to time, and this activity may promote movement of absorbed nutrients into the cytoplasm. Exceedingly thin, branching filaments of molecular dimensions project from the tips of the villi and intermingle to form a continuous surface coat, called the **glycocalyx** (Fig. 17-4). The filaments are extensions of integral proteins of the plasmalemma and consist of a core polypeptide with oligosacharide side chains. There is evidence that intralumenal enzymes that hydrolyze disaccharides and dipeptides are adsorbed onto the filaments of the glycocalyx. The monosaccharides and amino acids resulting from their activity then diffuse or are actively transported into the cell, and then into the subepithelial capillaries.

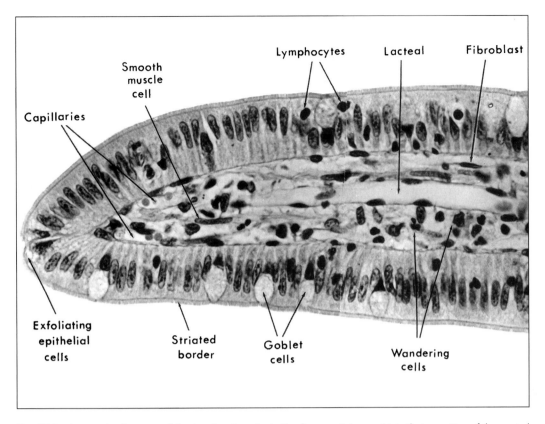

Fig. 17-2   Longitudinal section of the tip of an intestinal villus from cat jejunum. Note that a portion of the central lacteal is included in the section.

*Hydrolysis of disaccharides takes place on or in the brush-border of the intestinal mucosa. In **disaccharidase deficiency syndrome**, one of the hydrolytic enzymes involved is lacking. The commonest of these inherited disorders is **lactase deficiency** manifested by intolerance to milk with symptoms of cramping, bloating, and diarrhea. It is managed by avoidance of milk in the diet.*

Below the prominent terminal web of the absorptive cells, the cytoplasm contains abundant smooth endoplasmic reticulum, an organelle that plays an important role in the absorption of lipids. Intralumenal digestion of fats depends on their emulsification by bile and their degradation to fatty acids and monoglycerides by lipase secreted into the duodenum by the pancreas. The smooth endoplasmic reticulum of the absorptive cells contains the enzymes necessary for synthesis of triglycerides from the fatty acids and monoglycerides that diffuse across the plasmalemma from the intestinal lumen. In histological sections of intestine from fasting animals, the absorptive cells are free of lipid inclusions, but during the absorption of fat, droplets of triglyceride appear in the reticulum and are transported in vesicles to the Golgi complex, where they are combined with a lipoprotein to form lipid droplets called **chylomicrons** (Fig. 17-5). These are transported in vesicles to the

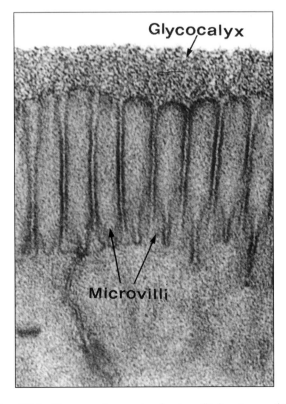

Fig. 17-4   Electron micrograph of microvilli bearing a thick glycocalyx, consisting of oligosaccharide chains of glycoproteins of the membrane of the intestinal cell. (Courtesy of S. Ito.)

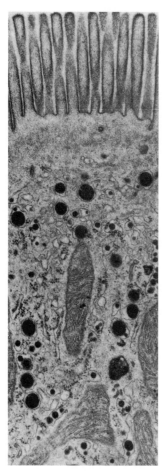

Fig. 17-5 Electron micrograph of an intestinal cell during lipid absorption. Note the numerous lipid droplets in the apical cytoplasm.

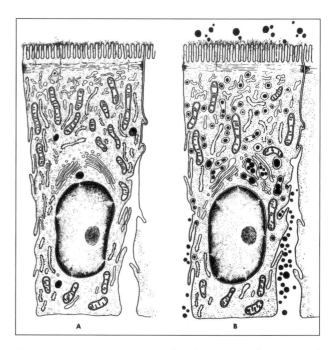

Fig. 17-6 Drawings presenting the ultrastructure of an intestinal absorptive cell (A) in the fasting state and (B) after a lipid-rich meal. (Redrawn from R. Cardell, S. Badenhausen, and K.R. Porter, Journal of Cell Biology 34:123, 1967.)

lateral cell membrane and are released into the intercellular spaces of the epithelium (Figs. 17-6 and 17-7). Moving into the core of the villus, they enter the lacteal and then slowly flow through the larger lymphatics to the cisterna chyli and then via the thoracic duct to the bloodstream.

Goblet cells, scattered among the absorptive cells, secrete mucus. Accumulation of pale droplets of mucus expand the apical portion of the cell and displace the nucleus into a narrower cell base, resulting in the shape that gives the cell its name. Below the mucin droplets, there is a Golgi complex and rough endoplasmic reticulum. Goblet cells are relatively few in the duodenum but become more numerous in the jejunum. The mucus that they secrete serves to lubricate the surface of the intestinal mucosa, protecting it from abrasion and preventing adherence and invasion by the numerous bacteria in the lumen.

Enteroendocrine cells of several types are found scattered individually between epithelial cells on the villi and in the glands. They have previously been described in Chapter 16. They are small cells at the base of the epithelium containing dense argyrophilic granules, usually on the side near the basal lamina. The different types secrete

different peptide hormones that modulate various activities of the intestinal tract. Their number and type vary along the length of the intestine. **G cells** (secreting gastrin) are numerous in the duodenum, fewer in the jejunum, and absent in the ileum. **S cells** (secreting secretin), **I cells** (cholecystokinin), **D cells** (somatostatin) and **MO cells** (secreting motilin) are found in the duodenum and jejunum but are rare in the ileum. **L cells** (secreting enteroglucagon) occur throughout the small and large intestines.

Paneth cells occur in clusters at the base of the intestinal glands (Figs. 17-7 and 17-8 [see Plate 26]). They have a moderately basophilic cytoplasm and large eosinophilic secretory granules. In electron micrographs, the cytoplasm is rich in rough endoplasmic reticulum and contains many lysosomes. Paneth cells are believed to have an important role in controlling the bacterial flora of the gut. They contain elevated levels of **lysozyme,** an enzyme capable of digesting bacterial cell walls. Whether this enzyme is confined to the lysosomes or also present in their secretory granules is unclear. They also secrete other antimicrobial peptides, called **cryptdins.**

Lamina Propria

The **lamina propria** of the intestine consists of areolar tissue surrounding the intestinal glands and forming the core of the intestinal villi. In addition to fibroblasts, it contains many lymphocytes, macrophages, and plasma cells. Immediately beneath the epithelium, there is a layer of stellate cells that are rich in actin and myosin and are

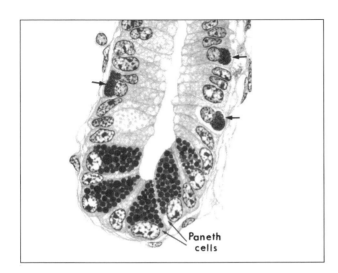

Fig. 17-7 Drawing illustrating the Paneth cells at the base of an intestinal gland. Note three enteroendocrine cells higher in the gland.

believed to be contractile. A very slender strand of smooth-muscle cells extends vertically from the muscularis mucosae into the core of each villus.

The intestinal mucosa is exposed to a lumen containing toxic substances and an immense and varied flora of potentially invasive bacteria. The constant threat of their penetration of the epithelial barrier has been countered by the development of special immunological defenses. In addition to the population of lymphocytes, plasma cells, and macrophages normally present in the lamina propria, there are occasional **solitary lymph nodules.** In the ileum, groups of these coalesce into **aggregated lymphoid nodules (Peyer's patches)** that are much larger and extend into the submucosa (Fig. 17-9). Immediately overlying these are specialized **M cells** that are not found elsewhere in the epithelium. They are broad cells with few microvilli, and their base is invaginated to form deep recesses occupied by lymphocytes and macrophages of the underlying lymphoid tissue (Fig. 17-10). Bacteria are often observed adhering to the lumenal surface of the M cells. Antigens are constantly taken up from the lumen and transported across the cell to macrophages that present the antigens to lymphocytes capable of generating a specific antibody. Having interacted with antigen, the lymphocytes migrate to regional lymph nodes, and from there to the circulation via the thoracic duct. From the circulation, they home back into the lamina propria of the intestine where they differentiate into **plasma cells** that secrete **IgA-type antibodies** specific for the antigens previously presented to their lymphocyte precursors by macrophages and dendritic cells beneath the M cells. This so-called **secretory immune system** depending on the IgA class of antibodies differs from the general immunological defenses of the body which produce the IgG class of antibodies. The IgA antibodies formed by plasma cells of the lamina propria bind to receptors on the base of the epithelial cells and are transported across the cells to be released into the lumen, where they are adsorbed onto the glycocalyx. There, they are ideally situated to neutralize virus and toxins and to inhibit bacterial adherence to the epithelium. This mechanism is called **immune exclusion.**

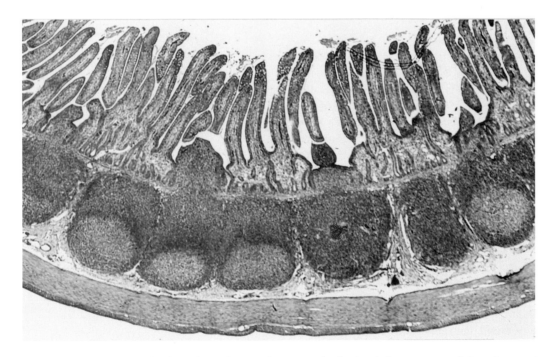

Fig. 17-9 Photomicrograph of cat ileum showing the intestinal villi, the shallow crypts, and the submucosal lymphoid nodules (Peyer's patches).

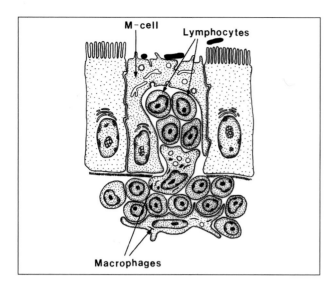

Fig. 17-10 Diagram of an M cell showing lymphocytes and macrophages occupying a deep recess in its base. Bacteria adhere selectively to the M cell, which transports bacterial antigen to lymphocytes in the basal pocket. (Redrawn from M.R. Neutra and J.P. Kraehenbuhl, *Trends in Cell Biology* 2:134, 1992.)

Muscularis Mucosae

The **muscularis mucosae** is similar to that previously described for the stomach (Chap. 16). Its contraction may contribute to movements of villi that can be observed in the jejunal mucosa in the living state. This layer is thin or absent where aggregated lymphoid nodules underlie the mucosa of the ileum.

Submucosa

The **submucosa** in the greater part of the length of the intestine consists of connective tissue that contains more collagen and elastic fibers than that of the lamina propria. In addition to fibroblasts, it may contain small clusters of adipose cells. In the duodenum, it is largely replaced by the **submucosal glands of Brunner** (Fig. 17-11). The ducts of these tubuloacinar glands traverse the muscularis mucosae and open into the gut lumen. The coiled tubules of the glands are lined by cuboidal cells with a prominent Golgi complex, rough endoplasmic reticulum, and pale-staining apical secretory granules. The secretion of the Brunner's glands is a clear alkaline mucin (pH 8.2–9.3) with a high content of bicarbonate. Its principal function is to protect the duodenal mucosa against the potentially damaging effects of the strongly acidic chyme discharged into the duodenum from the stomach. It raises the pH of the intestinal content into the optimal range for the pancreatic enzymes released into this segment of the tract. Brunner's glands form a nearly continuous layer in the submucosa of the initial portion of the duodenum, but they diminish in number and end at its junction with the jejunum.

Within the connective tissue of the submucosa, there is a network of ganglia and interconnecting nerve bundles forming the **submucous plexus (Meissner's plexus).** Its efferent fibers innervate the muscularis mucosae and smooth-muscle fibers in the core of the intestinal villi.

Muscularis Externa

The **muscularis** of the small intestine consists of outer longitudinal and inner circular layers of smooth muscle. Some thin strands of muscle may pass from one layer to the other. The muscularis is responsible for **peristalsis,** an intermittent, wavelike contraction that travels along the intestine at a rate of a few centimeters per second, advancing the intestinal contents. There are also segmental movements, consisting of alternate constriction and relaxation of short segments. These result in to-and-fro movements that agitate and mix the intestinal contents. In the terminal portion of the ileum, the muscularis is locally thickened, forming the **ileocecal sphincter** which normally remains partially contract-

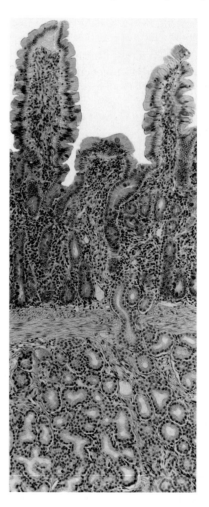

Fig. 17-11 Photomicrograph of the duodenal mucosa of a macaque. The villi, crypts, and Brunner's glands are clearly shown. A duct of Bunner's gland is seen traversing the muscularis mucosae to empty into a crypt.

ed. Some time after the last meal, there is reflex activation of ileal peristalsis and relaxation of this sphincter, permitting the small intestinal contents to move into the colon. Between the layers of the muscularis is the **myenteric nerve plexus (Auerbach's plexus)** (Fig. 17-12). Its efferent fibers are largely responsible for the motility of the intestine.

Serosa

The **serosa** of the intestinal tract consists of a continuous layer of squamous epithelium, commonly called **mesothelium.** This is separated from the underlying muscularis by a very thin layer of loose connective tissue. The small intestine is suspended from the dorsal wall of the abdomen by a **mesentery** consisting of two layers of mesothelium on either side of a thin layer of connective tissue, through which the blood vessels reach the intestine. At the posterior wall of the abdominal cavity, the two layers of mesothelium of the mesentery are continuous with a layer of mesothelium that lines the peritoneal cavity. Thus, the inner aspect of the abdominal wall and the surface of the organs suspended from it are covered by a continuous layer of mesothelium usually referred to as the **peritoneum.** The portion lining the cavity is called the **parietal peritoneum** and that covering the organs is the **visceral peritoneum.**

LARGE INTESTINE

The large intestine is about 1.5 m in length. It has a greater caliber and is more fixed in position than the small intestine. Different descriptive terms are applied to its several successive segments: the **caecum,** the **ascending colon,** the **transverse colon,** the **descending colon,** the **sigmoid flexure of the colon,** the **rectum,** and the **anus.** These terms are more useful to the surgeon than to the histologist, for the microscopic structure of the large intestine is much the same throughout its length. Its lumenal surface is devoid of any folds, comparable to the plicae circulares of the small intestine. There are no villi and the surface is quite smooth (Fig. 17-13 [see Plate 26]). The mucosa contains closely spaced, tubular glands. These are straight and 0.5 mm in length, considerably longer than glands of the small intestine. The epithelium consists of columnar **absorptive cells,** many **goblet cells,** and widely scattered **enteroendocrine cells.** The absorptive cells are abundant at the surface of the mucosa and in the upper third of the glands (Figs. 17-14 and 17-15 [see Plate 27]). Most of the absorption of nutrients takes place in the small intestine, but if lipid is not completely absorbed in the jejunum and ileum and enters the large intestine, the absorptive cells of the ascending colon are capable of taking it up and forming cylomicrons. However, the principal function of the absorptive cells throughout the large intestine is to absorb water and salts and to concentrate the feces. Sodium and chloride are absorbed, and potassium and bicarbonate are released from the cells into the lumen. Uptake of water follows the absorption of sodium and choride, resulting in concentration of the feces.

In the lower two-thirds of the glands, the epithelium consists almost entirely of goblet cells. They secrete the abundant mucus that facilitates onward movement of the intestinal contents and protects the epithelium against abrasion by the increasingly concentrated feces. The life span of cells of the colonic epithelium is about 6 days. Stem cells are located in the depths of the glands, and their progeny divide and differentiate as they migrate upward to replace cells lost at **extrusion zones** on the surface, midway between the openings of neighboring glands. At intervals throughout the length of the colon, there are lymphoid nodules in the lamina propria, some large enough to extend into the submucosa.

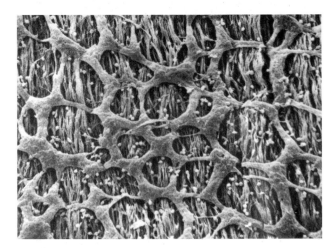

Fig. 17-12 Scanning electron micrograph of the myenteric plexus of rat intestine. The overlying longitudinal muscle and connective tissue have been removed by dissection and enzymatic digestion. (Courtesy of T. Fujiwara and Y. Uehara, Journal of Electron Microscopy 29:397, 1980.)

*Ulcerative colitis is an inflammatory disease of the colon of unknown etiology. The mucosa and submucosa are extensively infiltrated with leukocytes, and there are areas of ulceration. The major symptoms are fever, abdominal pain, and frequent liquid stools containing blood and pus. Late in the disease, fibrosis of the wall may lead to bowel obstruction. A similar disease, **regional enteritis** (Crohn's disease), may involve either the small intestine or the colon. The symptoms include fever, abdominal pain, and diarrhea usually without blood. The chronic inflammatory reaction extends through all layers of the wall, which may become greatly thickened, narrowing the lumen.*

In the distal portion of the rectum, the mucosa and lamina propria form several stable longitudinal folds, called the **columns of Morgagni.** In this terminal segment of the intestine, the glands become progressively shorter, and they cease along a line about 2 cm above the anal orifice. Along this line, there is an abrupt transition from columnar epithelium to stratified squamous epithelium. At the anus, this epithelium has a structure typical of skin, including associated sebaceous glands and large apocrine glands.

Muscularis Externa

The inner circular layer of the muscularis is relatively thin in the colon. The outer longitudinal layer differs from that of the small intestine in that it is not of uniform thickness. The majority of its smooth-muscle fibers are aggregated into three, evenly spaced, longitudinal bands called the **taeniae coli.** Between these bands, the outer smooth-muscle layer is very thin or lacking. The taeniae coli are normally in a state of partial contraction, resulting in a bulging of the intervening portions of the wall of the colon to form sacculations, called the **haustrae.** These are not observed in the rectum, where taeniae are absent and the outer layer of the muscularis forms a continuous layer of uniform thickness. At the level of the anus, the circular smooth muscle is thickened, forming the **internal anal sphincter.** Distal to this, there is a circumferential annulus of striated muscle forming the **external anal sphincter.**

In the connective tisue beneath the serosa of the entire colon, with the exception of the caecum, there are aggregations of adipose cells, covered by the peritoneum. These form slender pendulous lobules called the **appendices epiploicae.**

APPENDIX

The **vermiform appendix** is a tubular rudimentary organ with no significant function. It arises from the blind end of the caecum about 1 cm below the termination of the ileum and is 2–8 cm long and 0.5 cm in diameter. Its wall contains all of the layers typical of the intestinal tract. It is thickened by many small and large lymphoid nodules that form a nearly continuous layer in the lamina propria, and extending into the submucosa. The epithelium consists mainly of absorptive cells, and M cells overlying the lymphoid nodules. There are relatively few goblet cells. Occasional enteroendocrine cells may be found in the very short glands. The lamina propria between lymphoid nodules is crowded with lymphocytes, macrophages, and plasma calls. The lumen of the organ is small and angular in cross section and is often filled with dead cells and detritus.

QUESTIONS*

1. Which of the following is **incorrect** concerning intestinal villi?

   A. They are composed of epithelium and lamina propria.
   B. They are found in the large intestine.
   C. They contain a striated border.
   D. They contain lacteals.
   E. They contain smooth muscle.

2. Paneth cells are associated with which of the following glands?

   A. pyloric
   B. gastric
   C. esophageal
   D. Brunner's
   E. intestinal

3. The organelle which plays an important role in the absorption of lipids is the

   A. lysosome
   B. endoplasmic reticulum
   C. Golgi apparatus
   D. mitochondrion
   E. ribosome

4. Lacteals function in the absorption of which of the following?

   A. amino acids
   B. glucose
   C. VLDL particles
   D. chylomicrons
   E. none of the above

5. Cell turnover in the small intestine occurs every

   A. 6 hours
   B. 24 hours
   C. 2 days
   D. 4–6 days
   E. none of the above

6. Which of the following statements about Paneth cells is **false?**

   A. They are formed at the base of the intestinal glands.
   B. They contain elevated levels of lysozyme.
   C. They secrete peptide hormones.
   D. They exhibit large eosinophilic granules.
   E. They secrete cryptins.

7. Peristalsis is a function of the

   A. muscularis mucosae
   B. serosa
   C. lamina propria
   D. muscularis externa
   E. mucosa

8. M cells are found in the

   A. colon
   B. pyloric stomach
   C. ileum
   D. esophagus
   E. gastric glands of the body of stomach

9. In the small intestine, Auerbach's myenteric plexus is located in

   A. submucosa
   B. lamina propria
   C. between layers of muscularis externa
   D. serosa
   E. muscularis mucosae

10. About the large intestine,

    A. it is composed of well-developed villus structures
    B. it is responsible for absorption of most nutrients
    C. it is unable to absorb lipids
    D. it has easily observed plicae circulares
    E. its principal function is absorption of water and salts

11. Which pairing is **incorrect?**

    A. duodenum/Brunner's glands
    B. columns of Morgagni/appendix
    C. somatostatin/enteroendocrine cells
    D. taeniae coli/large intestine
    E. Peyer's patches/ileum

12. The longitudinal muscle of the muscularis externa is concentrated into three bands in the

    A. stomach
    B. jejunum
    C. appendix
    D. colon
    E. none of the above

*Answers on page 307.

18

LIVER AND GALL BLADDER

CHAPTER OUTLINE

Liver
    Organization
    Blood Supply
    Hepatocytes
    The Duct System
    Histophysiology
Gallbladder
    Histophysiology

KEY WORDS

Ampulla of Vater
Bile
Bilirubin
Canals of Hering
Central Vein
Cholecystokinin
Cystic Duct
Glisson's Capsule
Hepatic Acinus
Hepatic Artery
Hepatic Duct
Hepatic Sinusoid

Hepatocyte
Inlet Venule
Ito Cells
Kupffer Cells
Portal Lobule
Portal Triad
Portal Vein
Space of Disse
Sphincter of Oddi
Terminal Hepatic
    Venule

The **liver** is the largest gland in the body, weighing about 1.5 kg. Located in the right upper quadrant of the abdominal cavity, its rounded upper surface conforms to the left dome of the diaphragm. Its function as an accessory gland of the alimentary tract is the continuous production of **bile,** a fluid that is stored between meals in the **gallbladder,** which is attached to the under surface of the liver. Bile released into the small intestine emulsifies dietary fats and facilitates their absorption by the intestinal epithelium. The liver has many other functions in addition to its role in digestion. It stores carbohydrates in the form of glycogen and releases glucose as needed to maintain the normal concentration of this important energy source in the blood. It synthesizes the proteins of the blood plasma and releases them directly into the blood passing through the organ. It also takes up drugs and other potentially harmful substances from the blood and detoxifies them by oxidation or by forming harmless conjugates that are excreted, in the bile, back into the intestines.

Organization

The liver is covered by a thin film of connective tissue called **Glisson's capsule.** Unlike other glands that are separated into lobes by connective-tissue partitions, the liver contains relatively little connective tissue and its parenchyma is remarkably uniform in appearance throughout. It is possible, however, to detect a repeating pattern of roughly hexagonal subunits made up of fenestrated plates of the parenchymal cells **(hepatocytes)** arranged radially around a central vein. These units were traditionally designated **liver lobules.** In the pig and certain other species, they are enveloped by a very thin layer of connective tissue (Fig. 18-1 [see Plate 27]). In the human, they are not outlined by connective tissue. However, at the corners of these hexagonal units, there are small triangular areas of fibroblasts and collagen fibers enclosing a small **bile duct,** a branch of the **hepatic artery,** and a branch of the **portal vein.** These are referred to as the **portal triads** (Fig. 18-2). Bile is continually secreted into a network of minute **canaliculi** within the plates of hepatocytes, and flows outward to the bile ductules in the portal triads. At the periphery of each lobule, lateral branches of the small artery and venule of the triads are confluent with **hepatic sinusoids,** which occupy the spaces between the radially arranged plates of hepatic cells. Blood flows from the triads, through the sinusoids, to a **central vein** in the axis of each classical lobule (Fig. 18-3). The hepatic cells are thus exposed, on two sides, to a large volume of blood flowing centripetally in the system of sinusoids. These are lined by a discontinuous layer of fenestrated endothelial cells. The endothelium is separated from the plates of hepatic cells by a narrow perisinusoidal space, the **space of Disse** (Fig. 18-4). A network of reticular fibers in this space supports the plates of parenchymal cells (Fig. 18-5).

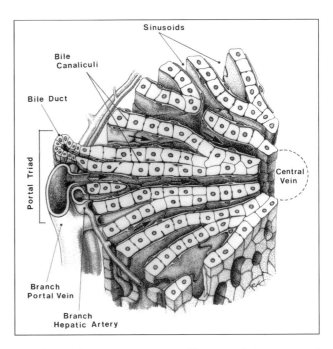

Fig. 18-2 Schematic representation of hepatic cell plates arranged radially around the central vein. The centripetal flow of blood and centrifugal flow of bile are indicated by arrows. (Modified from A.W. Ham, *Textbook of Histology,* 5th ed., J.B. Lippincott Co., Philadelphia, 1965.)

Blood plasma freely enters the space of Disse and directly bathes the surface of the hepatic cells. A population of phagocytic cells, called **Kuppfer cells,** adhere to the endothelium and extend processes through its fenestrations, into the space of Disse. These belong to the mononuclear phagocyte system of the body, referred to earlier (Chap. 4). They serve as tissue macrophages ingesting particulate foreign matter, and they are able to recognize and phagocytize aged or damaged erythrocytes. These cells are derived from bone marrow stem cells, as are other cells of the mononuclear phagocyte system. As long-lived antigen-presenting phagocytes, they can be considered one of the cell types of the immune system. The space of Disse also contains a few stellate **fat-storing cells (Ito cells)** that contain many lipid droplets. Their function is poorly understood.

The classical hepatic lobule, described above, was long the most widely accepted unit of structural organization of the liver, but over the years, two alternative interpretations have been proposed. In one of these, a triangular area of parenchyma around each portal triad, including all cells secreting into its bile ductule, was called a **portal lobule** (Fig. 18-6). It included sectors of three neighboring classical lobules. Its proponents argued that this unit was more consistent with lobules of other glands, having its blood supply radiating from axial vessels, and its secretory product draining into a central duct. However, this interpretation was not widely accepted. In the past 40 years, the preferred structural and functional unit of the liver has been the **hepatic acinus.** This is an elliptical unit that includes a sector of two neighboring classical lobules

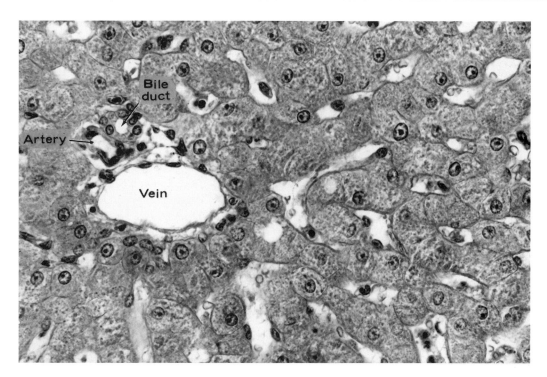

Fig. 18-3 Photomicrograph of the portal triad at the periphery of classical hepatic lobule, containing branches of the hepatic artery, portal vein, and a small bile duct.

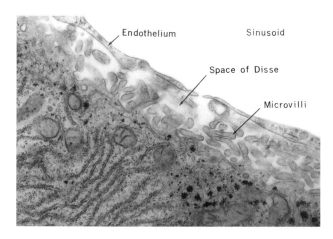

Fig. 18-4 Electron micrograph of a portion of a liver cell bordering on a sinusoid. Numerous microvilli project into the space of Disse between the hepatocyte and the endothelium of the sinusoid. (Courtesy of K.R. Porter and G. Millonig.)

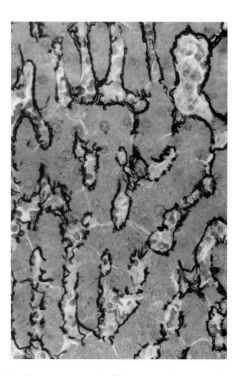

Fig. 18-5 Photomicrograph of liver stained with a silver method for reticular fibers. These fibers are in the space of Disse.

(Fig. 18-6). Traversing its center are branches of the terminal arteriole, and the portal venule that extend laterally from the portal triad. At either end of the acinus is a **terminal hepatic venule** (central vein of the classical lobule). The acinus is commonly considered to have three zones, with zone I closest to its axial vessels and hence first to be exposed to the incoming blood (Fig. 18-7). Zone II, in the middle, and zone III, at either end of the acinus, receive blood already depleted of some of its solutes by the cells in zone I. Support for the validity of this interpretation comes from the observation that, after a meal, the cells of zone I are first to receive glucose and

store it as glycogen, whereas glycogen appears later in zones II and III. In fasting, the cells of zone I are first to respond to a low circulating blood-glucose level by depolymerizing their glycogen to add glucose to the blood. The acinus has also been adopted as the functional unit of the liver because it facilitates an explanation of the pattern of cell degeneration seen in hypoxic or toxic damage to the liver.

Blood Supply

The liver receives blood from two sources: the general circulation and the portal vascular system. Its processing and metabolism of absorbed nutrients depends on its unique position between these two systems. About 75% of

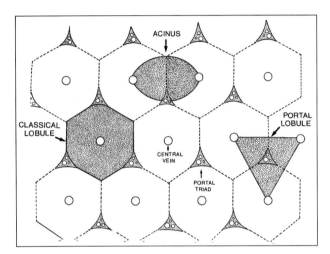

Fig. 18-6 Schematic depiction of the differing interpretations of the functional unit of the liver. The portal lobule is no longer in favor.

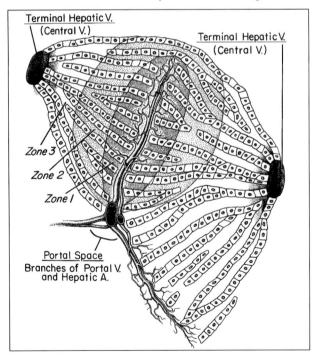

Fig. 18-7 Diagram of the acinus, consisting of parenchyma centered around the terminal branches of the hepatic artery and portal vein. The cells of zone 1 have first call upon the incoming oxygen and nutrients. The cells of zone 2 are less favored, and those of zone 3 are least favorably situated. (Redrawn from A.M. Rappaport, Z.J. Barroury, W.M. Lockheed and W.N. Lotto, Anatomy Record 119:11, 1954.)

its 15 ml/min blood flow is supplied by the **hepatic portal vein** which carries poorly oxygenated blood that has already circulated through the intestines, and is rich in absorbed nutrients. Entering the liver at the **porta hepatis,** the portal vein undergoes several orders of branching: **interlobar veins, conducting veins,** and **interlobular veins.** The latter give rise to **portal venules,** branches that accompany small branches of the hepatic artery in the portal triads. Small terminal branches of these veins course around the periphery of the classical hepatic lobule as **perilobular veins** and give off branches, called **inlet venules,** that empty into the sinusoids at the periphery of the classical lobule. The sinusoids, in turn, converge upon the **central vein** in the axis of the classical lobule. The wall of the central vein is thin, consisting of endothelium supported only by a loose network of reticular fibers. At the base of the classical lobules, their central veins joins **sublobular veins** that are confluent with **collecting veins.** These join to form large **hepatic veins** that empty into the inferior vena cava, the major vein of the general circulation that conducts blood back to the heart from all regions of the body below the diaphragm.

The **hepatic artery** enters the porta hepatis and branches into **interlobar** and **interlobular arteries.** The blood that these carry is distributed mainly to the connective tissue of the organ, but a small volume continues into the **hepatic arterioles** of the portal triads, whose lateral branches conduct oxygenated blood into the sinusoids. The sinusoids thus receive poorly oxygenated blood from the portal system and well-oxygenated blood from the general circulation. The cells at the periphery of the classical lobule, zone I of the acini, therefore receive oxygenated blood in higher concentrations that those more centrally situated.

Hepatocytes

Hepatocytes make up 80% of the cell population of the liver. In histological sections, they have one, or occasionally two, spherical nuclei with prominent nucleoli. The cytoplasm is acidophilic but contains conspicuous **basophilic bodies.** In electron micrographs, these are found to consist of parallel arrays of cisternae of the rough endoplasmic reticulum (Fig. 18-8). They are important sites for synthesis of albumen, prothrombin, fibrinogen, and lipoprotein of the blood plasma. In some areas, the rough endoplasmic reticulum is continuous with a network of tubules of smooth endoplasmic reticulum (Fig. 18-9). This organelle has an important role in carbohydrate metabolism, bile formation and the catabolism of drugs, and other potentially toxic compounds. It is also the site of synthesis of the very-low-density serum lipoprotein (VLDL) that is released into the blood as a carrier for cholesterol. Small (30–40 nm), dense globules of VLDL can often be seen in the lumen of the smooth reticulum (Fig. 18-9).

Hepatocytes have multiple, small Golgi complexes located at their periphery near the bile canaliculi (Fig. 18-

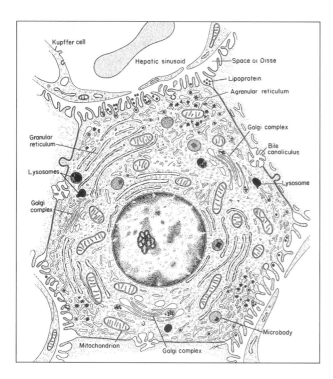

Fig. 18-8 Drawing depicting the ultrastructure of an hepatic cell and its relationship to the sinusoids. (Drawing by Sylvia Keene.)

10). Mitochondria are very numerous and there are many lysosomes and peroxisomes. The peroxisomes participate in oxidative activity in the metabolism of lipids, purines, and alcohol, and in gluconeogenesis (the formation of glu-

cose from molecules other than carbohydrates). The cytoplasm may also contain many small, dense granules of glycogen, which is the storage form of carbohydrate. (Figs. 18-11 [see Plate 28] and 18-12)

The ultrastructure of the hepatocytes differs significantly in the three zones of the hepatic acinus, reflecting differences in their functions. Gluconeogenesis occurs primarily in zone I, and glycolysis in zones II and III. The smooth endoplasmic reticulum is sparse in zone I but is well developed in zone III, which is more active in lipid metabolism. The mitochondria of zone III are very numerous but quite small. Those in the periportal region, zone I, are nearly twice the size of those of zone III. Glycogen is usually most abundant in zones I and II (the periphery of the clasical lobule).

Owing to the arrangement of hepatic cells in plates one cell thick, they have no surface that can appropriately be described as apical or basal. The sides of the cell exposed to the sinusoids are referred to as the **sinusoidal domain** of the plasmalemma, and the sides in contact with neighboring hepatocytes are the **lateral domain.** Midway along the lateral domain of adjoining hepatic cells, the opposing membranes diverge to bound a small intercellular channel 0.5–1.5 µm in diameter, the **bile canaliculus** (Fig. 18-10). Along either side of its lumen, the closely apposed cell membranes form a junction comparable to the tight junctions of other epithelial cells. These junctions isolate the lumen and prevent intercellular escape of bile secreted into the canaliculi. These minute channels form a network

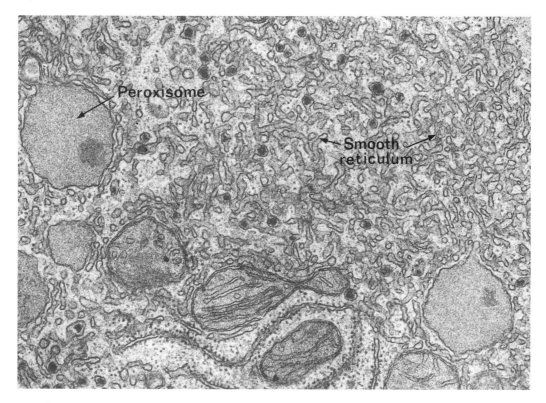

Fig. 18-9 Electron micrograph of an area of cytoplasm rich in smooth endoplasmic reticulum. Some of the tubnular elements of this organelle contain small dense droplets of newly synthesized very-low-density lipoprotein. Also present in this field are two peroxisomes. (Courtesy of R. Bolender.)

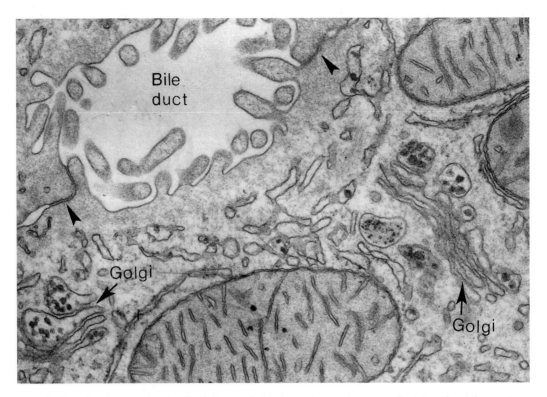

Fig. 18-10 Electron micrograph of a bile canaliculus between two hepatic cells. Note the tight junctions, indicated by arrows, at either side of the canaliculus. Two small Golgi complexes near the canaliculus contain particles of very-low-density lipoprotein. (Micrograph courtesy of R. Bolender.)

within the cell plates, with a single hepatocyte in each of its polygonal meshes. Although the membrane of the hepatocytes is similar in appearance throughout, cytochemical methods reveal regional functional differences. In the sinusoidal domain, the membrane contains receptors for sialoglycoproteins, mannose-6-phosphate, and other substances taken up from the blood by receptor-mediated endocytosis. The membrane of the lateral domain contains aminopeptidase, phosphatases, and three glycoproteins not found elsewhere on the cell surface. Adenyl cyclase and Na+, K+-ATPase are found in both the sinusoidal and lateral domains.

The Duct System

At the periphery of the classical lobule (axis of the acinus) the bile canaliculi are confluent with short bile ductules **(canals of Hering)** that drain into **interlobular bile ducts** of the portal triads (Fig. 18-2). These ducts, lined by cuboidal epithelium, continue into a system of progressively larger ducts that converge to form the **right** and **left hepatic bile ducts** from the corresponding lobes of the liver. These converge to form the **common bile duct,** which, in turn, is joined by the **cystic duct** from the gallbladder. The larger duct thus formed is joined in the wall of the duodenum by the pancreatic duct. These ducts are lined by columnar epithelium and have a thin submucosa, muscu-

laris, and adventitia. Where they traverse the wall of the duodenum, their intermingling circular muscle is thickened to form the **sphincter of Oddi** (hepatopancreatic sphincter). Between meals, when this sphincter is closed, the bile secreted by the liver refluxes into the gallbladder where it is stored and concentrated.

Histophysiology

The liver has a greater variety of functions than any other organ. Its principal contribution to the digestive process is the secretion of 500–100 ml of **bile** a day. Bile is a greenish solution containing cholesterol, neutral fats, phospholipids, lecithin, and bile salts. Of these, the bile salts (cholic acid and other derivatives of cholesterol) are the most important. They emulsify dietary fats, reducing them to micelles that are readily absorbed by the intestinal epithelium. An excretory function of the bile is the elimination of **bilirubin,** a toxic, greenish pigment formed in the Kupffer cell's degradation of the hemoglobin of senescent erythrocytes. Bilirubin is taken up by the hepatocytes, conjugated with glucuronide in the smooth endoplasmic reticulum, and excreted in the bile. In severe liver disease, interference with this function results in jaundice, a yellowing of the skin and mucous membranes. Determination of the relative amounts of conjugated and unconjugated bilirubin is a clinically useful measure of liver function.

*The liver is able to break down and render harmless many drugs and toxins, but daily consumption of a pint or more of whiskey or a volume of beer having an equivalent content of alcohol, over a period of 10 years may lead to **cirrhosis**. In its initial phase, fatty liver, there is impaired fatty acid oxidation and the cells become distended with lipid. This progresses to necrosis of hepatocytes and their replacement by increasing amounts of fibrous tissue. The patient gradually becomes emaciated, weak, and chronically jaundiced due to increasing amounts of circulating bilirubin.*

During the postprandial elevation of blood glucose, hepatocytes take it up from the blood and polymerize and store it as **glycogen** (Figs. 18-11 [see Plate 28] and 18-12). Between meals, glycogen is depolymerized to glucose which is returned to the blood, as needed. The liver is also capable of gluconeogenesis, the synthesis of glucose from compounds such as lactic acid, glycerol, and pyruvic acid. Fatty acids taken up by the hepatocytes are either used by the smooth endoplasmic reticulum to generate triglycerides that are stored in lipid droplets, or they are transformed into **very-low-density lipoprotein (VLDL)** that is released into the blood as a carrier for cholesterol. The liver is also the site of synthesis of the plasma proteins and blood-clotting factors of the blood: **albumen, fibrinogen, thrombin,** and **factor III.**

The hepatocytes have an accessory role in the immune system of the intestines. A large portion of the IgA antibodies produced by plasma cells in the intestinal mucosa is carried in the lymph to the thoracic duct and then into the general circulation. An immunoglobulin receptor, **secretory component,** is continuously synthesized by the hepatocytes and incorporated into the sinusoidal domain of their surface membrane. IgA is taken up from the blood by receptor-mediated endocytosis and transported to the bile canaliculi, where the secretory component is cleaved off, releasing the IgA into the bile for transport to the gut lumen to defend against intestinal bacterial flora.

GALLBLADDER

The **gallbladder** is a pear-shaped hollow organ occupying a shallow fossa on the under surface of the liver. It normally measures 10 cm by 4 cm and has a capacity of 40–70 ml. It has a fundus, a body, and a narrower neck region that continues into the **cystic duct.** Its wall consists of a mucosa, a lamina propria, a thin fibromuscular layer, and a serosa which is continuous with that covering the liver. In the empty gallbladder, the mucosa is raised into convoluted folds of varying length that run mainly longi-

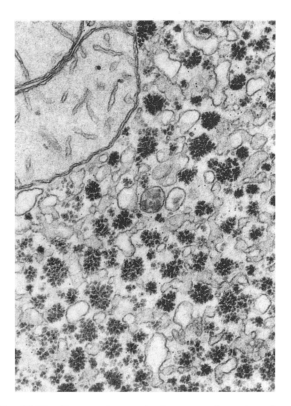

Fig. 18-12 Electron micrograph of an area of cytoplasm from a liver cell from zone I, showing many particles of glycogen.

tudinally. These are shorter and more widely spaced when the organ is distended.

The gallbladder epithelium is a single layer of tall columnar cells having an ovoid nucleus, and a faintly eosinophilic cytoplasm. There is a sparse population of short microvilli at the free surface of the cells. Their lateral surfaces are straight in the apical region but may be interdigitated in their lower portion. While bile is being concentrated by active transport of water across the epithelium, the lower portion of the intercellular clefts may be widened. In the neck region of the gallbladder, the epithelium is invaginated into the lamina propria to form short tubuloalveolar glands lined by mucus-secreting cuboidal cells. The cystic duct continues downward from the neck of the gallbladder and joins the common bile duct.

*The commonest disorder of the gallbladder is **cholelithiasis**, (gallstones). It is estimated that some 16 million people over 40 in this country have gallstones. These are concretions of cholesterol monohydrate, calcium salts, and phospholipid. They may cause painful inflammation of the gallbladder (**cholecystitis**). If they enter and obstruct the cystic duct, the gallbladder becomes distended and causes severe aching pain (biliary colic). The condition is treated by surgical removal of the gallbladder (cholecystectomy).*

Histophysiology

The main function of the gallbladder is to store and concentrate the bile by absorbing water. Active sodium transport across the epithelium creates an osmotic gradient that draws water out of the bile. Bile contains cholesterol, phospholipids, bile acids, and pigments, primarily bilirubin glucuronide. Release of bile into the duodenum is controlled by endocrine cells of the intestine epithelium. The presence of lipid in the lumen of the intestine stimulates enteroendocrine cells (I cells) in the mucosa to secrete a polypeptide hormone, **cholecystokinin** (CCK), also called pancreozymin. This induces contraction of the smooth muscle in the wall of the gallbladder, adding bile to the chyme to promote lipid absorption.

QUESTIONS*

1. All of the following are true about the liver **except**

   A. it can regenerate to some extent
   B. it functions as an exocrine gland
   C. it releases substances into the blood
   D. it stores glycogen in the smooth-surfaced endoplasmic reticulum
   E. it is rich in connective tissue

2. The space of Disse is

   A. in the portal triad area
   B. between Kupffer and endothelial cells
   C. surrounded by endothelium
   D. between the sinusoid and the hepatocyte
   E. none of the above

3. Which statement is correct about blood flow in the liver?

   A. central vein to hepatic artery
   B. portal vein to hepatic artery
   C. central vein to sinusoid
   D. hepatic artery to sinusoid
   E. central vein to portal vein

4. Which statement is correct concerning liver lobules?

   A. The peripheral landmarks of classical lobule are portal canals.
   B. The peripheral landmarks of portal lobule are portal canals.
   C. The peripheral landmarks of liver acinus are portal canals.
   D. The central axis of a portal lobule is the central vein.
   E. The central axis of a classical lobule is the portal canal.

5. Kupffer cells of the liver

   A. are located within sinusoids
   B. are located within the space of Disse
   C. are located along bile canaliculi
   D. are located in portal canals
   E. none of the above

6. The epithelium lining the gallbladder is

   A. pseudostratified columnar
   B. stratified squamous nonkeratinized
   C. simple columnar
   D. contains goblet cells
   E. none of the above

7. Glycogen synthesis is associated with which of the following in the hepatocyte?

   A. peroxisomes
   B. Golgi apparatus
   C. smooth endoplasmic reticulum
   D. rough endoplasmic reticulum
   E. none of the above

8. Detoxification of drugs in hepatocytes is associated with

   A. peroxisomes
   B. lysosomes
   C. smooth-surfaced endoplasmic reticulum
   D. rough-surfaced endoplasmic reticulum
   E. none of the above

9. A potential site of phagocytosis of drugs delivered in liposomes is

   A. the hepatocyte
   B. the Kupffer cell
   C. the space of Disse
   D. the fibroblasts lining the space of Disse
   E. the lipocytes found in the space of Disse

10. Hepatocytes are involved in

    A. synthesis and secretion of fibrinogen
    B. bile formation
    C. synthesis and secretion of lipoproteins
    D. formation of urea
    E. all of the above

11. The portal triad (of the liver) consists of

    A. the portal vein, the portal artery, and the portal lymphatic
    B. the portal vein, the portal nerve, and the portal lymphatic
    C. the confluens of the portal vein, the bile duct, and the pancreatic duct
    D. the portal vein, the hepatic artery, and the bile duct
    E. none of the above

12. The bile canaliculus

   A. is formed by specialized fibroblasts
   B. is formed by specialized endothelial cells
   C. develops from an outgrowth of the cystic duct
   D. is continuous with the heaptic duct
   E. is formed by grooves in two apposing hepato-
      cytes

*Answers on page 307.

19

PANCREAS

CHAPTER OUTLINE

KEY WORDS

A Cell	Intercalated Duct
Amylase	Interlobular Duct
B Cell	Intralobular Duct
Cholecystokinin	Lipase
Chymotrypsinogen	Pancreatic Duct
D Cell	Pancreatic
Elastase	Polypeptide
F Cell	Procarboxypeptidase
Glucagon	Secretin
Glucose Permease	Somatostatin
Hepatopancreatic	Trypsinogen
Ampulla	Vagus Nerve
Insulin	Zymogen

The **pancreas** is the second largest of the glands associated with the digestive tract. It is situated on the posterior wall of abdomen with its widest portion, the head, partially surrounded by the C-shaped curve of the duodenum, and its narrower neck and tail coursing transversely across the second or third lumbar vertebrae, toward the spleen. The gland consists of an **exocrine** portion and an **endocrine** portion. The exocrine portion secretes daily, into the duodenum, 1500–3000 ml of enzyme-rich fluid that is necessary for the digestion of dietary fats, carbohydrates, and proteins. The endocrine portion secretes hormones essential for controlling the metabolism of carbohydrates.

EXOCRINE PANCREAS

Pancreatic Acini

The pancreas is a compound gland made up of many small lobules bound together by loose connective tissue. Its secretory subunits, the **acini**, are round, or slightly elongate, and are made up of 40–50 pyramidal epithelial cells around a small lumen (Fig. 19-1). The acinar cells have a round nucleus with a prominent nucleolus, and an intensely basophilic cytoplasm. A less basophilic supranuclear region varies in size in different phases of the secretory cycle. This is filled with secretory granules, called **zymogen granules,** containing the precursors of several digestive enzymes (Figs. 19-2 and 19-3). In electron micro-

graphs, the basal cytoplasm is crowded with closely spaced cisternae of rough endoplasmic reticulum and many free polyribosomes (Fig. 19-3). Numerous small vesicles are clustered around the cis-face of the prominent Golgi complex, and developing zymogen granules are associated with its trans-face. Occasional lipid droplets and lysosomes may also be found in this region of the cell. The acini are surrounded by rich networks of unfenestrated capillaries.

Pancreatic Ducts

The pancreas is unique among compound acinous glands in having **intercalated ducts** that extend into the acini. The portion within the acinus is made up of pale-staining, low-cuboidal to squamous **centroacinar cells** that have few cytoplasmic organelles (Figs. 19-2 and 19-4). Outside of the acini, the duct cells are cuboidal. The slender intercalated ducts emerging from several acini converge to form **intralobular ducts,** and these join to form **interlobular ducts** in the connective tissue between the lobules of the gland. These ducts, lined by low-columnar epithelium, are not simply conduits for the secretory product, they also make a major contribution to the total volume of pancreatic secretion by actively transporting bicarbonate and water into their lumen. The interlobular ducts join a **main pancreatic duct** that runs longitudinally throughout the length of the gland. In the neck of the gland, the main pancreatic duct turns downward approaching the **bile duct** from the gall bladder. The two ducts then traverse the wall of the duodenum together

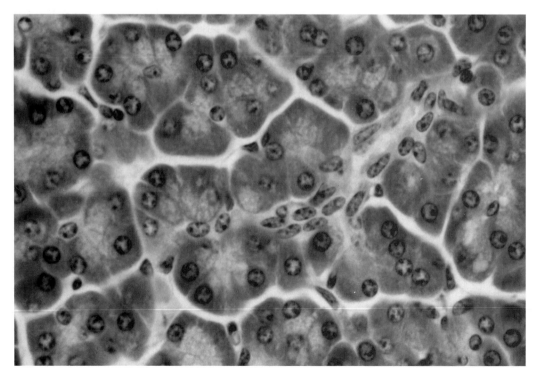

Fig. 19-1 Photomicrograph of the exocine pancreas, showing the glandular acini and one intercalated duct near the center of the field. Note the intense basophilic staining of the basal cytoplasm of the acinar cells.

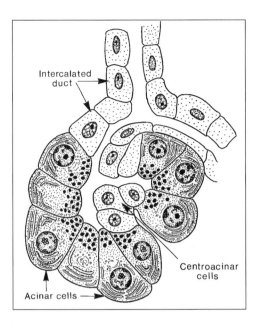

Fig. 19-2 Drawing of a pancreatic acinus, centroacinar cells, and intercalated duct.

and unite to form a single duct that opens into the duodenum at the tip of a projection called the **hepatopancreatic ampulla.**

Innervation

Small clusters of ganglion cells are located in the interlobular connective tissue of the gland. Small nerves can be observed penetrating the basal lamina of the acini and ending in intimate contact with the base of the acinar cells. These are believed to be postganglionic cholinergic fibers of the **vagus nerve** (10th cranial nerve). Electrical stimulation of the vagus nerve results in some secretion into the lumen of the acini and small ducts, but nervous control of pancreatic secretion is thought to be of less importance than its regulation by hormones released by the enteroendocrine cells of the duodenal mucosa. The membrane at the base of the acinar cells contains receptors for three or more of these hormones and their binding to the cells stimulates enzyme secretion.

Histophysiology

After a meal, the pancreas releases a large volume of alkaline fluid containing up to 20 enzymes that are necessary for digestion of food in the small intestine. The presence of food and gastric acid in the duodenum causes the enteroendocrine **I-cells** to release the hormone **cholecystokinin** which is carried in the blood to the pancreas. Its binding to receptors on the acinar cells triggers release of the highly concentrated proenzymes stored in the zymogen granules. The enteroendocrine **S-cells** release the hormone **secretin** stimulating the cells lining the smaller ducts of the gland to secrete a large volume of fluid rich in bicarbonate as a vehicle for the enzymes released by the acinar cells. Upon reaching the duodenum, this fluid creates an alkaline environment necessary for maximal activity of the digestive enzymes.

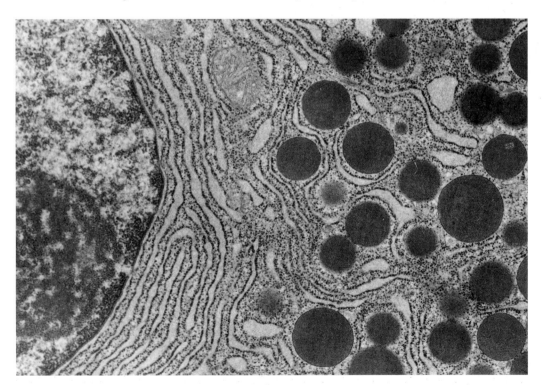

Fig. 19-3 Electron micrograph of a portion of a human pancreatic acinar cell showing the large nucleolus, abundant rough endoplasmic reticulum, and zymogen granules.

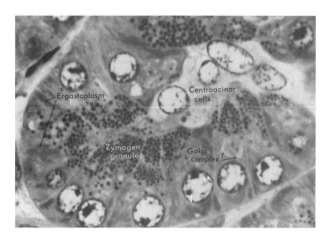

Fig. 19-4 Photomicrograph of an acinus of the human pancreas. Several centroacinar cells are seen at the upper right. (Courtesy of S. Ito.)

Few cells in the body produce as great a variety of secretory proteins as the acinar cells of the pancreas. Translation of many m-RNAs results in synthesis of the proenzymes of **trypsin, chymotrypsin, ribonuclease, carboxypeptidase, decarboxylase, lipase, elastase, amylase** and other enzymes. To protect the gland itself from digestion, the acinar cells contain protease inhibitors and the enzymes are secreted as proenzymes that are activated only after they have reached the duodenum.

> *A serious and potentially fatal disease of the pancreas is **acute pancreatitis**. The pancreas synthesizes proenzymes that are normally not activated until they reach the duodenum. However, drugs, viral infections, or unidentified trauma may activate trypsin and other proteolytic enzymes within the pancreas, resulting in digestion of cells, periacinar connective tissue, and blood vessels. The disease is often local and self-limiting, subsiding in a week or two, with adequate treatment. More severe cases may be fatal.*

ENDOCRINE PANCREAS

The endocrine component of the pancreas consists of **islets of Langerhans** that are widely scattered among the acini of the exocrine pancreas (Fig. 19-5 [see Plate 28]). These are aggregations of a few thousand cells enclosed in a thin layer of reticular fibers. They are most numerous in the body and tail of the gland. Although they are estimated to number over a million in the human pancreas, they make up only 1–2% of its volume. Each islet is a compact mass of epithelial cells permeated by a rich network of fenestrated capillaries.

The islets of Langerhans contain four types of cells:

A-cells, (α-cells) secreting **glucagon; B-cells** (β-cells) secreting **insulin; D-cells** secreting **somatostatin;** and **F-cells** (PP-cells) secreting **pancreatic polypeptide.** These cell types cannot be distinguished from one another in routine histological sections, but they can be identified by selective staining techniques (Fig. 19-6 [see Plate 28]), or by use of fluorescein-conjugated antibodies to their respective products (Fig. 19-7). The only distinctive features that permit their identification in electron micrographs are differences in cell size, location in the islet, and internal structure of the secretory granules. The majority of the A-cells are at the periphery of the islet but occasional isolated cells may be found in its interior (Fig. 19-7A). The B-cells are the predominant cell type, occupying the central region of the islet and accounting for 70% of its volume. The D-cells and F-cells are few in number and variable in location (Fig. 19-7B). In electron micrographs, the granules of the 4 types of cells are subject to great interspecific variation. In the human pancreas, the granules of the A-cells have a dense center surrounded by a narrow clear zone (Fig. 19-8B), and the B-cell granules contain one or more dense crystals of zinc insulin in a matrix of low density (Fig. 19-8A). Upon release, the contents of the granules diffuse into the lumen of the neighboring fenestrated capillaries.

Ganglion cells are occasionally found adjacent to a few of the islets and both cholinergic and adrenergic nerves can be found terminating on a very small number of the islet cells, but the autonomic nervous system is believed to play a relatively minor role in islet cell function.

Histophysiology

The major product of the digestion of carbohydrates is **glucose** which is an important energy source for cells throughout the body. The hormones of the islets of Langerhans control the level of glucose circulating in the blood. Following a meal, the elevation of blood glucose stimulates B-cells to secrete insulin which acts to reduce the level of blood glucose. Binding to receptors in the membrane of many cell types in the body, insulin induces a rapid increase in the concentration of an enzyme **glucose permease** in the cell membranes and causes a change in molecular configuration that permits passage of glucose into the cytoplasm. In the fasting state, the relatively low level of blood glucose activates the A-cells to secrete glucagon, which stimulates the liver to mobilize glucose from its intracellular stores of glycogen, thus increasing the level of blood glucose.

The D-cells of the islets, producing the hormone somatostatin, are believed to be involved in the inhibition of release of glucagon by the A-cells during periods of high blood glucose. To date, little is known about the function of the F-cells secreting pancreatic polypeptide.

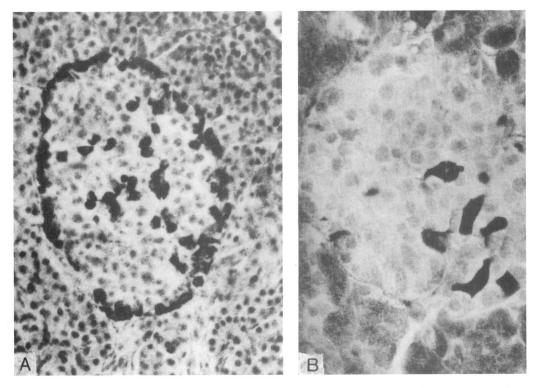

Fig. 19-7 (A) Human pancreatic islet stained with a technique that selectively stains the glucagon-secreting alpha cells. Note that these are preferentially located at the periphery near the capillaries. (B) An islet stained to reveal the somatotrophin-secreting delta cells. These are few and irregular in shape. (Courtesy of C. Hellerstrom, Acta Paediatrica Scandinavica (Suppl.) 270:7, 1977.)

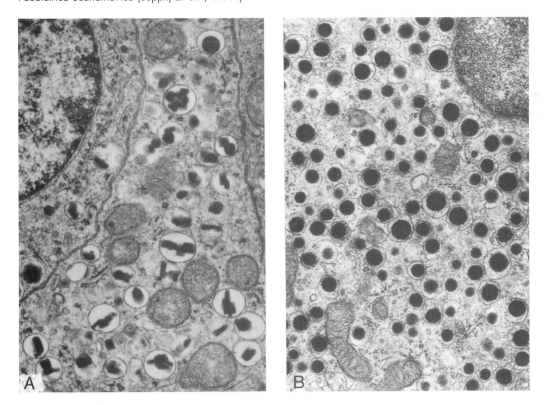

Fig. 19-8 (A) Electron micrograph of an area of cytoplasm of a beta cell. In man and certain other species, the granules contain crystals of varying size. (B) A juxtanuclear area of cytoplasm of an alpha cell. The granules have a dense core and a less dense periphery.

The most common endocrine disease of humans is **diabetes** in which there is impaired function of the beta cells of the islets of Langerhans, resulting in high blood levels of glucose and excretion of glucose in the urine. In genetically susceptible individuals, the disease may be triggered by a viral infection that renders the B cells no longer recognizable as self. T lymphocytes then invade the islets and the B cells are destroyed in a cell-mediated immune response. In the absence of insulin, certain acids may be produced faster than they can be metabolized (ketoacidosis). This may affect the central nervous system resulting in diabetic coma. The disease is successfully treated by diet and daily insulin injections. Late complications include accelerated atherosclerosis and partial blindness from degenerative changes in the retina.

QUESTIONS*

1. Which of the following matched pairs is **incorrect?**

   A. glucagon/beta cells
   B. insulin/beta cells
   C. somatostatin/delta cells
   D. alpha cells/glucagon
   E. PP cells/pancreatic polypeptide

2. Which of the following statements is true about the pancreas?

   A. The alpha cells are located primarily at the center of islets.
   B. Delta cells are the primary cell type in islets.
   C. The alpha cells produce insulin.
   D. The pancreas contains striated ducts.
   E. Intercalated ducts are present in the pancreas.

3. Which of the following statements is **false** about the pancreas?

   A. The beta cells secrete insulin.
   B. The granules of the beta cells contain crystals in electron micrographs.
   C. The alpha cells produce glucagon.
   D. Its delta cells produce somatostatin.
   E. None of the above

4. Which is **incorrect** about the exocrine pancreas?

   A. contains acinar cells
   B. contains zymogen granules
   C. contains striated ducts
   D. contains intercalated ducts
   E. none of the above

5. Beta cells of the islet of Langerhans produce which of the following?

   A. glucagon
   B. carbonic anhydrase
   C. insulin
   D. trypsinogen
   E. somatostatin

6. Which is **incorrect** about the acinar cells of the pancreas?

   A. contain a well-developed rough-surfaced endoplasmic reticulum
   B. are serous cells
   C. are basophilic in staining
   D. contain many free ribosomes
   E. are stimulated by gastrin

7. The exocrine pancreas produces

   A. trypsinogen
   B. lipase
   C. elastase
   D. amylase
   E. none of the above

8. Insulin is produced in the pancreas by

   A. the acinar cells
   B. the delta cells
   C. the beta cells
   D. the alpha cells
   E. none of the above

9. An increase in concentration of glucose permease is related to all but one of the following. Which one is unrelated?

   A. insulin
   B. decreased blood lipid
   C. elevated blood glucose
   D. a change in the structure of cell membranes
   E. a good meal

10. The presence of food in the duodenum is related to all of the following **except**

    A. release of proenzymes from acinar cells
    B. secretion of fluid rich in bicarbonate
    C. an increase in duodenal pH
    D. production of cholecystokinin
    E. release of glucagon

*Answers on page 307.

20

RESPIRATORY SYSTEM

CHAPTER OUTLINE

KEY WORDS

Alveolar Duct
Alveolar Pore
   (of Kohn)
Alveoli
Arytenoid Cartilage
Basal Cell
Bowman's Gland
Bronchi
Bronchial Tree
Bronchiole Nasal
   Septum
Bronchopulmonary
   Segment
Clara Cell
Conchae
Cribriform Plate
Cricoid Cartilage
Dipalmitoyl
   Phosphatidyl-
   choline
Elastic Recoil
Epiglottis
Ethmoid Bone
Expiration
False Vocal Cord
Frontal Bone

Hemosiderin
Hilum
Hyoid Cartilage
Inspiration
Interalveolar Septum
Kulchitsky Cell
Larynx
Lobar
Maxillary Bone
Nares
Nasopharynx
Olfactory Cell
Olfactory Epithelium
Pharynx
Pneumocyte
Surfactant
Sustentacular Cell
Thyroarytenoid
   Muscle
Thyroid cartilage
Trachea
True Vocal Cord
Vestibular Fold
Vocal Ligament
Vocalis Muscle

The respiratory system consists of the **lungs** and the passages that conduct air to and from them. The **conducting portion** of the system includes the **nose, pharynx, larynx, trachea,** and the **bronchi** that enter the lungs and undergo several orders of branching. The **respiratory portion** of the system, where gas exchange takes place between the blood and the inspired air, includes **respiratory bronchioles,** the terminal branches of the bronchi, **alveolar ducts,** and myriad **alveoli,** the thin-walled, air-filled sacs that make up the greater part of the parenchyma of the lungs. The alveoli, each surrounded by a dense network of capillaries, are structural units admirably constructed to facilitate diffusion of oxygen from the inspired air into the blood, and diffusion of carbon dioxide from the blood into their lumen for elimination upon expiration. Carbon dioxide, formed as a by-product of tissue metabolism throughout the body, is carried to the lungs in the blood pumped to them by the right ventricle of the heart, and oxygen is carried away in the blood returning to the left ventricle for distribution to all the other tissues of the body.

NOSE

The **nose** consists of a framework of bone and cartilage covered by skin and subcutaneous connective tissue. Its interior is divided, by a thin, cartilaginous **nasal septum,** into right and left **nasal cavities** that open anteriorly, at the **nares,** and posteriorly into the **nasopharynx.** The surface area of each nasal cavity is increased by three scroll-like projections from its lateral walls, called the **nasal conchae.** The nasal cavities are lined by four types of epithelium. Stratified squamous epithelium continues from the skin into the **vestibule,** a slight dilation just inside the nares. This epithelium bears a few stiff hairs that project into the airway and help to filter out any large foreign particles that may be in the inspired air. A few millimeters into the vestibule, stratified squamous epithelium gives way to a narrow zone of nonciliated cuboidal or columnar epithelium. Beyond this, the greater part of the nasal cavity is lined by ciliated pseudostratified columnar epithelium containing goblet cells that increase in number from anterior to posterior. On the lower and middle conchae, the lamina propria is richly vascularized and the flow of arterial blood warms the inspired air as it passes through the nose. Here, the air also takes up water that prevents dessication of the delicate alveoli of the lung. There is an extensive venous plexus on the lower part of the septum and on the lower two conchae. Under certain environmental conditions these thin-walled veins becomes engorged, periodically occluding the airway, first on one side of the septum and then on the other. This intermittent occlusion is thought to enable the nasal mucosa on the closed side to recover from desiccation caused by the airflow. These vessels are also a common site of nosebleed.

The roof of the nasal cavity and a small area of the septum and superior concha are lined by **olfactory epithelium,** an unusually thick pseudostratified epithelium (60–100 μm) containing the receptor cells for the sense of smell. It is composed of three kinds of cells: **sustentacular cells, olfactory cells,** and **basal cells** (Fig. 20-1 [see Plate 29]). The sustentacular cells are tall columnar cells with a striated border and a conspicuous terminal web. Their apical cytoplasm contains smooth endoplasmic reticulum, a supranuclear Golgi complex, mitochondria, and a few pigment granules that give the olfactory epithelium a pale yellowish-brown color.

Between the sustentacular cells are the olfactory cells, the neurosensory elements (neurons) of the epithelium. Their nuclei are aligned in the epithelium at a level below those of the supporting cells (Fig. 20-2A). Their apical portion is narrowed to a thin cylindrical process that terminates in a small, rounded expansion, called the **olfactory bulb,** or **knob,** that projects somewhat above the apices of the surrounding sustentacular cells (Fig. 20-2B). It contains the

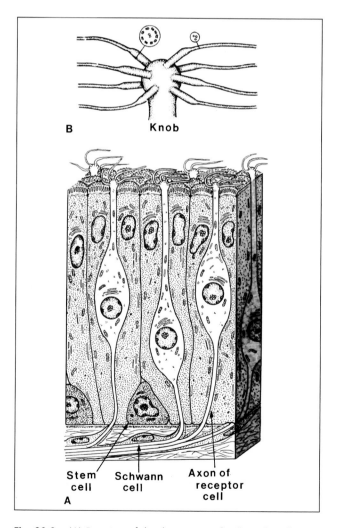

Fig. 20-2 (A) Drawing of the three types of cells in the olfactory epithelium and the Schwann cells around the axons of the receptors. (B) Drawing of the knob at the end of the receptor cell dendrite.

basal bodies of six to eight nonmotile **olfactory cilia** that radiate from it parallel to the surface of the epithelium. These are very long, attaining a length of 70 μm. In their initial portion, the axoneme contains the usual "9 + 2" arrangement of doublet microtubules. A short distance from the basal body, there is an abrupt narrowing of the cilia, and in this slender distal portion, the axoneme consists of a variable number of single microtubules, instead of the usual doublets. Toward its base, the body of the olfactory cell tapers down to form an axon about 0.5 μm in diameter. The axon passes through the basal lamina into the lamina propria, where it joins those of other olfactory cells in fascicles of unmyelinated axons surrounded by Schwann cells. These pass through the **cribriform plate** of the skull and synapse in the **olfactory lobe** of the brain. At the base of the olfactory epithelium, there are small deeply basophilic **basal cells,** considered to be stem cells, that can divide and differentiate into either sustentacular cells or olfactory cells. The olfactory cells have a limited life span and are continually replaced by differentiation from stem cells. This ability of the olfactory epithelium to regenerate its primary sensory neurons is unique in the nervous system.

In the lamina propria of the epithelium, there are branched tubuloalveolar glands, the **glands of Bowman,** made up of pyramidal cells with apical secretory granules. Their secretion creates a fluid environment around the olfactory cilia that may facilitate access of odors from the air to the sensory receptors on the olfactory cilia.

Histophysiology

In passing through the nose, the inspired air is warmed and humidified to prevent desiccation of the delicate alveoli of the lung. A moving blanket of mucus on the surface of the nasal epithelium entraps dust particles and moves them to the pharynx, where they are swallowed. Immunological defense of the nasal mucosa depends on numerous plasma cells in the lamina propria, secreting IgA that binds to the secretory component on the base of cells of submucous glands. The complex thus formed is interiorized and transported, with the secretion of the glands, onto the surface of the mucosa. Blood-borne immunoglobulins also diffuse from fenestrated capillaries around the glands and reach the surface of the epithelium to participate in the defense against inhaled bacteria.

Olfactory reception employs a very great number of receptors located in the membrane of the nonmotile olfactory cilia. The human genome contains about 1000 genes that encode 1000 different odor receptors. Each type of receptor is expressed on a great many olfactory cells, but only one type is expressed on any one cell. Humans can distinguish about 10,000 odors. An "odor" probably consists of several different chemical groups that activate those olfactory cells (neurons) bearing receptors for each of those chemical groups. To identify an odor, the brain evidently analyzes the particular combination of receptors that have been activated. The continuous secretion and transport of mucus over the epithelium may serve to remove residues of odorants to which the epithelium is exposed and thus keep the receptors accessible to new chemical stimuli.

Most mammals have a second smaller olfactory epithelium on the nasal septum, the **vomeronasal organ.** Its cells lack sensory cilia but have many microvilli containing receptors for the pheromones that govern the reproductive activity of the animal. If this epithelium is destroyed, the animal never mates. The vomeronasal organ is vestigial in humans.

Paranasal Sinuses

The paranasal sinuses are cavities in the frontal, maxillary, and ethmoid bones, lined by a relatively thin mucosa with a ciliated columnar epithelium similar to that lining the nose. Goblet cells and submucosal glands secrete a blanket of mucus. The beating of the cilia normally moves this mucus toward the opening of the sinuses into the nasal cavity. The normal function of the sinuses is obscure. The maxillary sinuses are often the site of painful infections, and the inflammatory process may destroy the cilia, resulting in poor drainage and accumulation of pus in the cavity.

LARYNX

Between the oropharynx and the trachea is the larynx, a hollow organ with two principal functions: (1) to produce sound and (2) to close the airway during swallowing to prevent food and saliva from passing down the trachea to the lungs. The wall of the larynx is supported by the **thyroid and cricoid cartilages.** These are joined to one another and suspended from the **hyoid bone** by sheets of dense connective tissue. Two folds of the mucosa lining the larynx project inward from its wall, on either side. The upper pair are called the **vestibular folds** (so-called **false vocal cords**) and the lower pair are the **vocal folds (true vocal cords).** In the latter, there is a dense marginal band of elastic tissue, the **vocal ligament.** Lateral to this, is the **vocalis muscle (thyroarytenoid muscle)** originating, anteriorly, from the inner surface of the **thyroid cartilage,** and inserting posteriorly, into an **arytenoid cartilage.** This cartilage articulates with the upper rim of the cricoid cartilage (Fig. 20-3A). In phonation, the arytenoid cartilages are adducted (moved toward the medial plane) and sound is produced by vibration of the approximated vocal cords as air is forced through the narrow space between them. Contraction of a muscle joining the thyroid and cricoid cartilages, changes the tension on the vocal cords and thus influences the pitch of the sound produced. During inspiration, the vocal folds are abducted (moved away from the

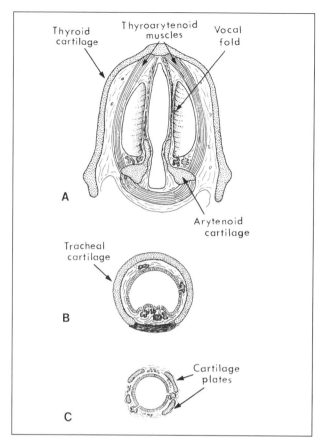

Fig. 20-3 (A) Cross section of larynx at the level of the margin of the vocal folds; (B, C) cross sections of the trachea and a bronchus.

medial plane), widening the interspace between them for passage of air to the lungs.

The vocal folds are covered by nonkeratinized stratified squamous epithelium, but all the rest of the larynx is lined by ciliated pseudostratified columnar epithelium. The direction of ciliary beat is upward, toward the pharynx. Goblet cells are found in the epithelium, and tubuloacinar mucus-secreting glands, with crescents of serous cells, are present in limited number in the lamina propria.

A thin leaf of fibroelastic cartilage, **the epiglottis,** is attached by its narrow stem to the inner surface of the thyroid cartilage and projects upward and backward over the opening from the pharynx into the larynx. On its upper, or lingual, surface it is covered by stratified squamous epithelium. During swallowing, the epiglottis is pressed downward by the base of the tongue, closing the opening into the larynx and presenting a smooth upper surface over which the bolus of food slides into the esophagus.

TRACHEA

From the larynx, the conducting portion of the respiratory tract continues as the **trachea,** a flexible tube about 11 cm long and 2 cm in diameter. Its wall is reinforced by

16–20 C-shaped hyaline cartilages separated by interspaces that are bridged by fibroelastic connective tissue (Figs. 20-3B and 20-4 [see Plate 29]). This arrangement gives the trachea great flexibility, while the cartilaginous rings in its wall enable it to resist external forces that might otherwise constrict the airway. External to the cartilages is a layer of connective tissue rich in elastic fibers. The rings of cartilage are incomplete posteriorly and the gap between their ends is bridged by a fibroelastic ligament and a thick band of smooth muscle that mingles, at either end, with the surrounding layer of connective tissue. During the cough reflex, contraction of this muscle can slightly decrease the diameter of the lumen to accelerate the airflow.

The trachea is lined by ciliated, pseudostratified columnar epithelium that has an unusually thick basal lamina. Ciliated cells comprise about 30% of the total cell population, goblet cells 28%, and basal cells 29%. From the upper to the lower trachea, the percentage of ciliated cells increases at the expense of the other cell types. Sparsely distributed at the base of the epithelium are small cells containing dense, secretory granules that accumulate between the nucleus and the cell base and discharge their content in response to hypoxia. These small granule cells (**Kulchitsky cells**) occur in both trachea and bronchi and are believed to be endocrine cells comparable to the enteroendocrine cells of the intestine, but they have been less studied. In addition, there are occasional **brush cells,** slender cells with microvilli up to 2 μm in length with an actin filament core extending down into the cytoplasm. These cells contain no secretory granules and their function remains unknown. The occasional observation of nerve endings at their base has led to the speculation that they might have a sensory function, but physiological validation of this suggestion is lacking. A row of small pyramidal **basal cells** are stem cells that can divide and differentiate to replace other cell types damaged or lost in the normal turnover of the epithelium.

At the boundary of the lamina propria and the submucosa, there is a dense layer of elastic fibers. The submucosa contains numerous mucosa glands that have serous demilunes. Their ducts ascend through the elastic lamina to open onto the surface of the epithelium.

LUNGS

The lungs occupy the right and left sides of the thoracic cavity, separated by the heart and mediastinum. Their shape conforms to that of the cavity, but they are separated from its wall by a thin film of fluid that permits sliding movement between the two. The left lung has two lobes and the right lung three lobes, separated by fissures. The filling of the lungs at each **inspiration** depends on enlargement of the thoracic cavity. This is accomplished by descent of the diaphragm due to contraction of its intrinsic muscle, and expansion of the rib cage by contraction of the intercostal muscles. Expiration, due to **elastic recoil,** follows upon relaxation of the intercostal and diaphragmatic muscles.

Bronchi

In the mediastinum, the trachea branches into right and left **primary bronchi** that enter the lungs through an opening on the medial surface of each lung, called the **hilum.** The primary bronchi branch into **lobar bronchi** to the two lobes of the left lung and the three lobes of the right lung. These divide into **segmental bronchi** to the several **bronchopulmonary segments** of each lobe. Each of these, in turn, branches into several **small bronchi.** The numerous branches of the small bronchi, called **bronchioles,** are the 12th to 15th orders of branching of the airway. Each bronchiole branches into five to seven **terminal bronchioles,** which are the terminal segments of the conducting portion of the respiratory tract. Their total number is about 65,000. Collectively, this arborization of the tract is referred to as the **bronchial tree.**

The structure of the primary bronchi is similar to that of the trachea up to their point of entry into the lungs. Thereafter, the cartilaginous rings are replaced by small irregularly shaped plates of cartilage that are distributed around their circumference (Fig. 20-3C). These decrease in number and disappear distal to the segmental bronchi. They are replaced in the smaller bronchi by two thin layers of spirally oriented bundles of smooth muscle. The pitch of the spiral differs in the two layers, so that the bundles cross one another at an angle (Fig. 20-6A). The mucosa of the bronchi is not significantly different from that of the trachea, but the submucosal glands gradually decrease in number and end at the level of the bronchioles.

Bronchioles

The bronchioles are tubules 5 mm or less in diameter with no cartilage or glands in their wall (Fig. 20-5 [see Plate 29]). The epithelium is columnar and consists of ciliated cells and nonciliated cells that replace the mucus-secreting cells found in more proximal segments of the bronchial tree. The nonciliated bronchiolar cells, called **Clara cells,** have a rounded apical end that protrudes into the lumen and bears numerous microvilli. These cells first appear in small bronchi but greatly increase in number in the bronchioles. Their basal cytoplasm contains long mitochondria and cisternae of rough endoplasmic reticulum. In some species, the apical cytoplasm contains an abundance of smooth endoplasmic reticulum, but in primates, this organelle is less developed. Also present are conspicuous apical secretory granules of low electron density. The function of the Clara cells is a subject of dispute, but there

is some evidence that they secrete a glycoprotein that contributes to a protective layer of surfactant that coats the epithelium throughout the lower respiratory tract.

The smooth muscle present in the wall of the smaller bronchi continues into the bronchioles, but here some of the fascicles of smooth muscle course circularly and others obliquely so that they appear to form a loose network (Fig. 20-6A). They are innervated by parasympathetic nerve fibers that stimulate bronchiolar constriction, and by sympathetic nerve fibers that relax the smooth muscle and permit the bronchioles to return to their full diameter. In persons suffering from asthma, there is excessive bronchiolar constriction, which makes it difficult to empty the lungs during expiration. Sympathomimetic (imitating the action of the sympathic nervous system) drugs are administered to relax the smooth muscle and open the airway.

Branching of each bronchiole gives rise to five to seven smaller **terminal bronchioles.** The epithelium, which was pseudostratified columnar in the larger bronchi, is gradually reduced in height to simple columnar epithelium in the bronchioles and is further reduced in the terminal bronchioles to cuboidal epithelium. The thin intersecting fascicles of smooth-muscle cells outline sizable polygonal areas of the wall that are free of muscle.

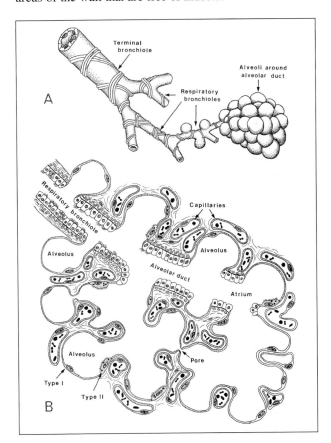

Fig. 20-6 (A) Drawing of a terminal bronchiole, three generations of respiratory bronchioles, and an alveolar duct surrounded by alveoli. (B) Drawing of a section of the respiratory unit of the lung. (Redrawn and modified from Gray's Anatomy, 38th Brit. edi., W. B. Saunders Co., Philadelphia.)

Asthma *is hyperirritability of the respiratory passages, expressed in contraction of the bronchial smooth muscle (bronchospasm), edema of the mucosa, and increased mucus secretion. It may be transient, following a viral upper respiratory infection. More commonly, the sensitization has an immunological basis and the symptoms are episodic. Reexposure to an airborne allergen (viz. pollen) causes release of histamine and other mediators from subepithelial mast cells and eosinophils, precipitating immediate bronchoconstriction, increased airway resistance, and labored breathing. Various drugs are helpful in minimizing the severity of the attacks.*

Respiratory Bronchioles

The transition from the conducting portion of the tract to its respiratory portion occurs at the branching of the terminal bronchioles into the **respiratory bronchioles.** In the human, there are three further orders of branching of the respiratory bronchioles. Their epithelium is initially cuboidal but becomes nonciliated low cuboidal in subsequent branches. Their wall is interrupted at intervals by **alveoli,** saccular outpocketings of the wall, lined by squamous epithelial cells thin enough to permit gas exchange,

hence the name respiratory bronchiole (Fig. 20-6B). With each branching of the respiratory bronchioles, the number of alveoli in their wall increases.

The terminal branches of the respiratory bronchioles are continuous with **alveolar ducts** (Fig. 20-6B), in which, alveoli are so numerous and so closely spaced that the limits of the duct proper are discernible only as thickenings of the edges of narrow septa between alveoli. On their lumenal surface, these thickenings have a few low cuboidal epithelial cells (Fig. 20-6B). Alveolar ducts terminate in small spaces, called **atria,** outlined by the edges of the several interalveolar septa within a cluster of alveoli.

Pulmonary Alveoli

The alveoli (Figs. 20-6B and 20-7) are where most of the gas exchange takes place between the blood and the inspired air. In the human lung, they number about 300 million, presenting to the inspired air a total surface of about 140 m² (two-thirds the area of a tennis court). In histological sections, they are round or polygonal in shape and about 200 µm in diameter (Figs. 20-8 and 20-9). All of the alveoli distal to those of the respiratory bronchioles are separated from one another by thin interalveolar septa only. These contain occasional fibroblasts and macrophages and a network of capillaries, supported by delicate reticular and elastic fibers (Fig. 20-11 [see Plate 29]).

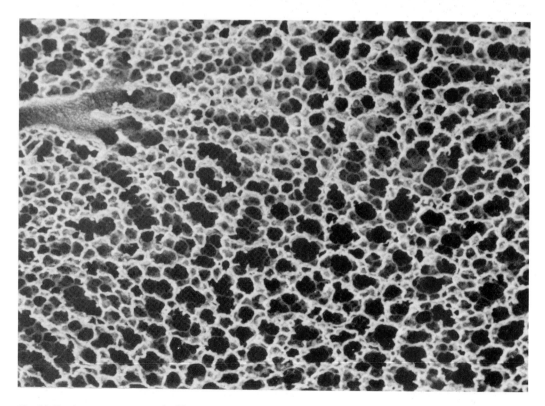

Fig. 20-7 Scanning micrograph of lung prepared by instillation of fixative into the bronchi to prevent collapse of the alveolar ducts and alveoli that usually occurs with simple immersion fixation. A terminal bronchiole can be identified at the upper left. (Courtesy of P. Gehr.)

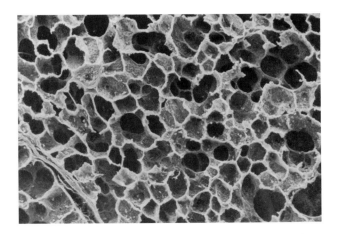

Fig. 20-8 Scanning micrograph of the cut surface of the human lung illustrating the saccular form of the alveoli and the very thin alveolar septa (Courtesy of P. Gehr.)

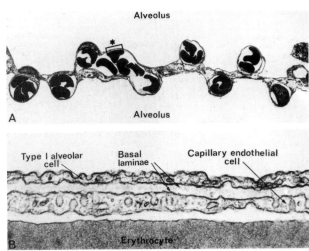

Fig. 20-10 Electron micrograph of the septum between two alveoli of rabbit lung. Capillaries covered by very thin type I alveolar cells bulge into the lumen, exposing a large surface to the inspired air. (B) A higher magnification of an area like that in the rectangle at the asterisk in (A), showing the layers making up the diffusion barrier to gas exchange. (Courtesy of P. Gehr.)

Collectively, the interalveolar septa constitute the major part of the pulmonary interstitium. The septa are traversed by occasional openings, called **alveolar pores (pores of Kohn),** that permit movement of air between adjacent alveoli if normal access to one becomes obstructed (Fig. 20-12). No connective tissue intervenes between the alveolar epithelium and the endothelium of the capillaries. The air in the alveolus is separated from the blood only by (1) the unfenestrated endothelium of the capillaries, (2) the alveolar epithelium, and (3) their shared basal lamina. These layers form a blood–air barrier only 1.5–2.0 μm thick, which offers little resistance to diffusion of oxygen and carbon dioxide.

The alveolar epithelium contains two types of cells: type I alveolar cells (squamous epithelial cells) and type II alveolar cells (great alveolar cells). Some histologists prefer the terms **pneumocytes** I and II for these cells. The type I cells occupy 95% of the surface area, and the type II cells occur singly or in small groups, accounting for the remaining 5%. The rounded adlumenal surface of the type II cells, covered with short microvilli, projects slightly

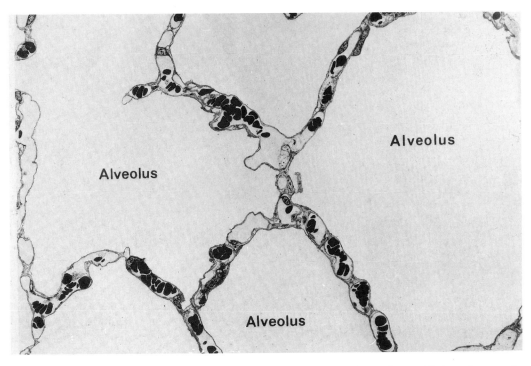

Fig. 20-9 Electron micrograph of several alveoli of equine lung, showing the erythrocyte-filled capillaries in the interalveolar septa. (Courtesy of P. Gehr.)

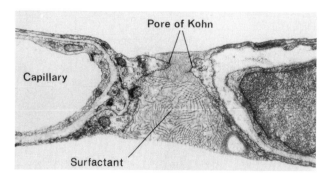

Fig. 20-12 Electron micrograph of a small segment of an alveolar septum. Occasional small openings (pores of Kohn) traverse the thin wall between neighboring alveoli. The pore shown here is partially obstructed by a local accumulation of surfactant. (Courtesy of P. Gehr.)

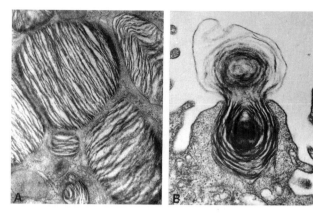

Fig. 20-15 (A) Micrograph of lamellar bodies in a type II alveolar cell. (B) Lamellar body being released by exocytosis into the lumen of the alveolus. (Courtesy of M. C. Williams.)

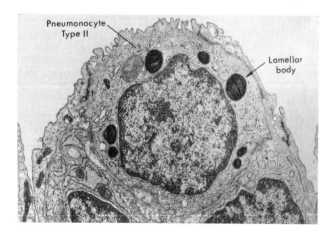

Fig. 20-13 Scanning micrograph of a small area of the interior of a human pulmonary alveolus showing a type II alveolar cell, with very short microvilli at the periphery of its bulging free surface. (Courtesy of P. Gehr.)

above the surrounding type I cells (Fig. 20-13). In addition to the usual cell organelles, they contain dense **lamellar bodies** that are unusual secretory granules with a content composed of closely spaced, membranelike lamellae (Fig. 20-15). The secretion of the type II alveolar cells, **pulmonary surfactant**, consists mainly of **dipalmitoyl phosphatidylcholine**. It spreads as a monomolecular layer over the thin film of fluid that normally coats the surface of the alveolar epithelium. It serves to reduce surface tension and facilitate expansion of the alveoli by lowering intermolecular forces in the surface film of fluid.

> *Pneumonia* is an infectious disease of the lungs affecting some 3 million people a year in this country. Its cause is inhalation of bacteria or aspiration of secretions from the nasopharynx which always contains infectious microorganism. The ability of alveolar macrophages to ingest and destroy the bacteria is overwhelmed, and inflammatory exudate accumulates, filling the alveoli and excluding inspired air. This consolidation of one or more lobes of the lung is accompanied by fever, cough, and difficulty in breathing. Timely use of antibiotics usually prevents a fatal outcome.

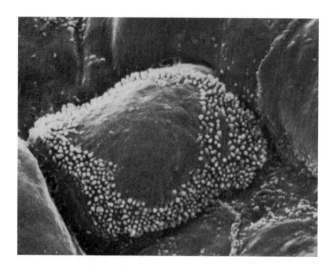

Fig. 20-14 Electron micrograph of a type II alveolar cell, illustrating the characteristic lamellar bodies in the cytoplasm. (Courtesy of M. C. Williams.)

Alveolar Macrophages

Macrophages are found in the **interalveolar septa.** Some of these migrate into the lumen of the alveolae and adhere to the epithelial cells (Fig. 20-16A). There, they phagocytize dust particles and other particulates that have escaped entrapment by the layer of mucous in the upper respiratory tract. In cigarette smokers, these cells are blackened by large accumulations of ingested carbon and

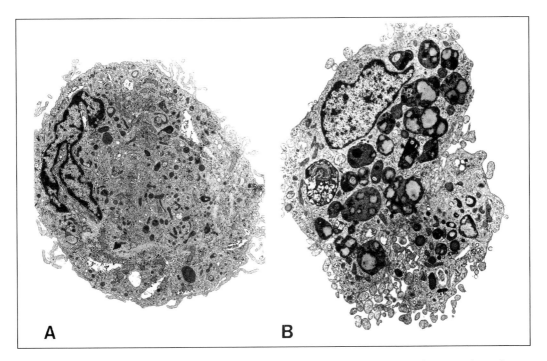

Fig. 20-16 (A) Micrograph of an alveolar macrophage from a nonsmoker. (B) Alveolar macrophage from a smoker, crowded with lipochrome pigment, representing undigestible residues of materials phagocytized from the lumen of the alveoli. (Courtesy of S. Pratt and A. J. Ladman.)

tars from inhaled smoke (Fig. 20-16B). The alveolar macrophages are the first line of defense against pulmonary infections. They have surface receptors for IgG and the C3b component of complement and their ability to ingest bacteria is enhanced in the presence of specific antibody. When stimulated by the metabolic products of bacteria, they secrete chemoattractants that induce transendothelial migration of polymorphonuclear leukocytes to join them in combating the invading bacteria. Erythrocytes may accumulate in the alveoli of patients with heart failure and are phagocytized by the alveolar macrophages. These can be identified in the sputum by their content of **hemosiderin,** a product of hemoglobin degradation. Therefore, such cells are sometimes referred to as **heart-failure cells.** They are also often called **dust cells** due to the accumulation of phagocytized particles from inspired air. Alveolar macrophages are continually carried upward in the respiratory tract in the moving surface film and are swallowed upon reaching the pharynx. The rate of clearance of alveolar macrophages from the lungs is estimated to be in excess of 2×10^6/h.

*In **emphysema,** there is an enlargement of many of the air spaces beyond the terminal bronchioles due to destruction of interalveolar septa. Reduction in the total surface area available for gas exchange results in inefficient respiration. Cigarette smoking is usually a contributing factor. Smoke inhibits ciliary motility and alveolar macrophage function. There is a mild chronic inflammation, and proteolytic enzymes released by the polymorphonuclear leukocytes damage the alveolar septa.*

Pleura

The thoracic cavity is lined by a serous membrane, the **parietal pleura** that is reflected onto the surface of the lung as the **visceral pleura.** The superficial layer of both is a mesothelium similar to peritoneum that lines the abdominal cavity and covers its viscera. The visceral and parietal pleura are normally separated only by a thin film of fluid, which permits them to slide smoothly over one another in the movements of the lung during respiration. Beneath the mesothelium is a thin layer of connective tissue containing many capillaries and lymphatics.

Blood Supply

The lungs receive deoxygenated blood from the right ventricle via the **pulmonary trunk** which divides into **right and left pulmonary arteries** that enter the hila of corresponding lungs. These vessels, in turn, branch into arteries of progressively diminishing caliber that follow the branches of the intersegmental bronchi as far as the respiratory bronchioles. Branches to the alveolar ducts then give rise to capillary networks in the interalveolar septa. The lung also receives blood and nutrients from **bronchial arteries** that arise from the **aorta** and **upper intercostal arteries.** These supply the pleura, interlobular connective tissue, and the wall of the bronchial tree as far as the respiratory bronchioles, where they anastomose with the small branches of the pulmonary artery. Oxygenated blood from the alveolar capillaries is carried by venules in the interlobular septa. These converge to form veins of increasing diameter that run parallel to the arteries. They course along branches of the bronchi and join to form a single large vein draining each lobe of the lung. These, in turn, join to form two **pulmonary veins** from each lung that emerge at the hila and open into the left atrium of the heart.

Lymphatics

There are two systems of lymphatics in the lungs. Lymph, in an extensive network of lymphatics in the pleura, is drained by several main trunks into lymph nodes in the hilum of the lungs. Parenchymal lymphatics originate in the walls of the bronchioles and are drained by a submucosal network of lymphatics and by peribronchial lymphatics to larger vessels that converge upon the hilar lymph nodes. The efferent trunks from the hilar nodes join to form the right lymphatic duct, which is the principal pathway of drainage from both right and left lungs.

Nerves

The lungs receive parasympathetic innervation from the vagus nerve, and sympathetic innervation via nerves from the second to the fourth thoracic sympathetic ganglia. Nerves from these two sources form a plexus around the hilum from which intrapulmonary nerves accompany the ramifications of the bronchial tree and pulmonary artery. These nerves include **parasympathetic bronchoconstrictor** fibers from the vagus and **sympathetic bronchodilator** fibers from the **thoracic sympathetic ganglia.**

Histophysiology

The primary life-sustaining functions of the respiratory tract are the uptake of oxygen from the inspired air and the elimination of carbon dioxide from the blood. These functions require expansion of the lungs on inspiration and their recoil on expiration. The abundant elastic fibers in the pulmonary interstitium (Fig. 20-11 [see Plate 29]) permit expansion of the alveoli and provide for their recoil. A major additional factor in their recoil in expiration is the surface tension in the thin film of fluid coating the walls of the alveoli.

Several mechanisms have evolved to remove foreign matter taken in with the inspired air. The continual secretion of surfactant in the alveoli creates a gradient that results in movement of the surface film into the bronchioles and upward to join the blanket of mucus in the upper respiratory tract. This mucus layer is moved upward at a rate of about 2 cm/min by the cilia of the lining epithelium. The cilia beat constantly at about 14 cycles/s, carrying dust, cellular debris, bacteria, and chemical pollutants to the pharynx where they are swallowed. Another device for removal of particulate matter is the cough reflex, which depends on sensory nerve endings in the mucosa of the upper respiratory tract. Any irritant in the tract sends afferent impulses to the brain, which trigger an involuntary sequence of events that involves deep inspiration, closure of the glottis, and forceful contraction of abdominal and intercostal muscles. This raises pressure on the air impounded in the lung. The epiglottis is then suddenly opened and the air bursts out, attaining velocities as high as 100 mph. The rush of air carries with it the irritant foreign matter. The sneeze reflex involves a similar train of events intended to clear the nasal passages.

QUESTIONS*

1. The true vocal cords usually contain all of the following **except**

   A. collagenous fibers
   B. elastic fibers
   C. metaplastic squamous cells
   D. diffuse lymph nodules
   E. skeletal muscle

2. What cell is **not** found in the alveolar wall?

   A. fibroblast
   B. pneumocyte II
   C. endothelial cell
   D. pneumocyte I
   E. Clara cell

3. The respiratory division of the respiratory system includes all **except**

   A. respiratory bronchioles
   B. alveolar sacs
   C. alveolar ducts
   D. secondary bronchioles
   E. alveoli

4. Type II pneumocytes

   A. are squamous
   B. have microvilli
   C. line terminal bronchioles
   D. contain secretion granules
   E. produce mucus

5. The recoil capacity of the whole lung, including the alveoli, is best served by

   A. collagenous fibers
   B. reticular fibers
   C. elastic fibers
   D. smooth muscle
   E. hyaline cartilage

6. Alveolar macrophages are

   A. also called dust cells
   B. often found in the alveolar walls
   C. often found in the interior of alveoli
   D. also called cardiac (heart) failure cells under certain circumstances
   E. all of the above

7. The respiratory bronchiole

   A. contains cartilagenous rings
   B. contains primarily ciliated columnar cells
   C. has submucosal glands
   D. has direct contact with alveoli
   E. has no elastic fibers

8. Which cell is normally found **only** in bronchioles?

   A. ciliated cells
   B. pneumocyte II cells
   C. Clara cells
   D. fibroblasts
   E. macrophages

9. The olfactory region contains all of the following **except**

   A. basal cells
   B. bipolar neurons
   C. sustentacular cells
   D. serous gland cells
   E. Kulchitsky cells

10. Cells of the alveolar septum include

    A. fibroblasts
    B. epithelial cells
    C. endothelial cells
    D. reticular fibers
    E. all of the above

11. Functions of the conducting subdivision of the respiratory system include all of the following **except**

    A. transport of gases
    B. gaseous exchange across membranes
    C. temperature regulation of gases
    D. filtration
    E. humidification

12. The primary role of elastin (elastic fibers) in the respiratory system is to

    A. facilitate expiration
    B. increase lung capacity
    C. aid in inspiration
    D. augment bronchiolar dilatation
    E. decrease the tracheal diameter

*Answers on page 307.

21

URINARY SYSTEM

CHAPTER OUTLINE

KEY WORDS

Afferent Arteriole
Aldosterone
Angiotensin
Antidiuretic Hormone
    (ADH)
Arcuate Vessels
Bowman's Capsule
Brush-Border
Bulbourethral Gland
Colliculus Seminalis
Cortex
Cortical Intertubular
    Capillary
    Network
Cortical Nephron
Efferent Arteriole
Ejaculatory Duct
Erythropoietin
External Sphincter
Filtration Slit
Fossa Navicularis
Glands of Littre
Glomerulus
Hilum
Intercalated Cell
Interlobar Vessels
Intralobular Vessels
Internal Sphincter
Juxtamedullary
    Nephron
Lobar Vessels

Macula Densa
Major Calyx
Medulla
Mesangial Cell
Mesangium
Minor Calyx
Papillary Duct
    (Bellini)
Pedicel
Penile Urethra
Peritubular Capillary
Podocyte
Principal Cell
Prostate Gland
Prostatic Utricle
Prostatic Urethra
Renal Column
Renal Lobule
Renal Pyramid
Renal Vessels
Renin
Slit Diaphragm
Stellate Vein
Urea
Uric Acid
Urinary Pole
Urine
Urogenital
    Diaphragm
Vasa Recta
Verumontanum

The urinary system consists of two **kidneys,** two **ureters,** the **urinary bladder,** and the **urethra.** In producing urine, the kidneys control the acid–base balance, eliminate waste products of metabolism, and maintain the normal volume of extracellular fluid by excreting excess water. The urine is transported through the ureters to the bladder for temporary storage and is later voided via the urethra. The urethra of the female is solely a duct for urine, but in the male it also serves as a pathway for ejaculation of semen. The kidneys also have an endocrine function, releasing two hormones, **erythropoietin,** which stimulates production of erythrocytes by the bone marrow, and **renin** which plays an important role in the control of blood pressure.

KIDNEYS

The kidneys are located retroperitoneally on the posterior wall of the abdominal cavity on either side of the vertebral column. They are 10–12 cm in length, 5–6 cm in width, and 3–4 cm in anteroposterior thickness. The medial border of the kidney is concave, and in its center there is a cleft, called the **hilum,** which leads inward to the **renal sinus,** a deep recess in the interior of the organ that contains **renal arteries** and **veins,** some adipose tissue, and a funnel-shaped expansion of the upper end of the ureter, called the **renal pelvis.** The renal pelvis bifurcates into two branches, the **major calyces,** and each of these, in turn, has short branches, the **minor calyces** (Fig. 21-1). In the hemisected kidney, viewed with the naked eye, a dark reddish-brown **cortex** is readily distinguishable from a paler **medulla.** The latter includes 6–10 conical regions called the **renal pyramids.** The broad base of each pyramid is continuous with the cortex, and its apex, called a **renal papilla,** projects into the lumen of a minor calyx of the renal pelvis. The pyramids are bounded laterally by darker inward extensions of the cortex, called the **renal columns.** One renal pyramid and its bounding renal columns constitute a **renal lobule.**

The cortex of the kidney is made up 1.5–3 million tubu-

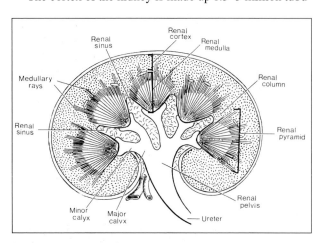

Fig. 21-1 Drawing of the structural components identifiable with the naked eye in the hemisected kidney.

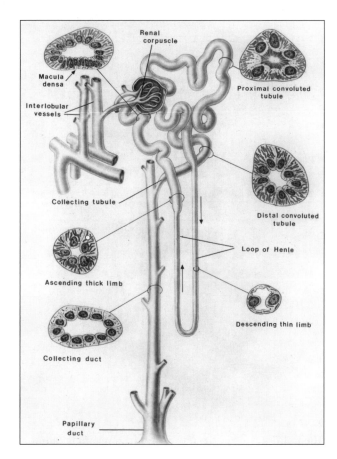

Fig. 21-2 Drawing of the several segments of a juxtamedullary uriniferous tublule, and their appearance in cross section. The length of the loop of Henle and collecting duct are longer than illustrated here.

lar subunits called **nephrons** (Fig. 21-2). Each has several segments that differ in histological structure and function. These are the **renal corpuscle,** the **proximal convoluted tubule,** the **loop of Henle,** and the **distal convoluted tubule.** Each nephron is continuous with a tubule of different embryological origin, the **collecting tubule** which, in turn, joins a **collecting duct** (Fig. 21-2). A nephron, its collecting tubule, and the collecting duct, together, constitute a unit called the **uriniferous tubule.** The kidney cortex contains the renal corpuscles, proximal and distal convoluted tubules, and the collecting tubules. The loops of Henle and greater part of the length of the collecting ducts are in the medulla.

The renal corpuscle collects a filtrate of the blood passing through its capillaries (Fig. 21-3 [see Plate 30]). As the filtrate passes through the nephron, its composition is altered by the addition of metabolic wastes and by selective reabsorption of components that need to be conserved. At various levels in the cortex, the distal convoluted tubules of several nephrons are joined via collecting tubules to a straight collecting duct. In these two collecting segments of the uriniferous tubule, water is absorbed from the filtrate to concentrate the urine. The collecting ducts gradually increase in diameter along their course through the pyramid, and their terminations,

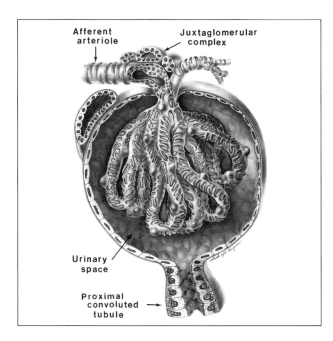

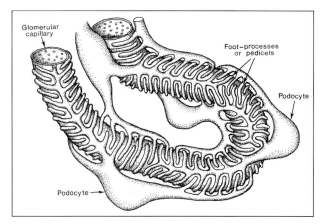

Fig. 21-5 A greatly simplified drawing of a capillary loop of the glomerulus, to show the disposition of podocytes and the alternating interdigitation of their secondary processes. The filtration slits are much narrower than depicted, and the secondary processes are actually highly branched and elaborately interdigitated. See Fig. 21-7.

Fig. 21-4 A drawing of the renal corpuscle. Although the glomerulus was traditionally described as a cluster of capillary loops, as shown here, it is now known to be a complex network of capillaries. (Redrawn and modified from Bargmann, Zeitschr. fur Zell forsch. 8:765, 1929.)

the papillary ducts (**ducts of Bellini**), open into a minor calyx of the renal pelvis.

The Nephron

Renal Corpuscle

At the blind proximal end of each nephron, there is a thin-walled expansion of the proximal tubule, which is deeply invaginated to form a cup-shaped hollow structure called **Bowman's capsule.** The concavity of this capsule is occupied by a globular tuft of convoluted capillaries called the **glomerulus.** The glomerulus and its double-walled epithelial capsule together constitute a renal corpuscle (Fig. 21-3 [see Plate 30] and Fig. 21-4). It has a **vascular pole,** where **afferent and efferent arterioles** are continuous with the capillaries of the glomerulus, and a **urinary pole,** where the capsular space between the outer, **parietal layer,** and the inner **visceral layer** of Bowman's capsule is continuous with the lumen of the proximal convoluted tubule (Fig. 21-4). At the vascular pole of the renal corpuscle, the visceral layer of Bowman's capsule covering the vessels is continuous with the **parietal layer** of the capsule. At the urinary pole of the renal corpuscle, the squamous epithelium of the parietal layer is continuous with the cuboidal epithelium of the proximal convoluted tubule (Fig. 21-4).

In the development of the renal corpuscle, the shape of the cells in the visceral layer of Bowman's capsule becomes so modified that they bear little resemblance to

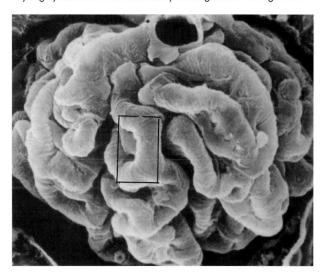

Fig. 21-6 A scanning micrograph of a glomerulus. The area enclosed in the rectangle is shown at higher magnification in Fig. 21-7. (Courtesy of P. Andrews, Journal of Electron Microscope Techniques 9:115, 1988.)

those of any other epithelium. The individual cells, called **podocytes,** have several radiating primary processes that embrace the underlying capillaries and give rise to very numerous secondary branches, called foot processes or **pedicels** (Fig. 21-5). These interdigitate with corresponding processes of neighboring podocytes but are separated from them by narrow intercellular spaces, about 25 nm wide, that permit the plasma filtrate escaping from the glomerular capillaries to enter the capsular space. These are referred to as the **filtration slits.** Although the secondary processes of the podocyte are closely applied to the basal lamina of the underlying capillary, the cell body is usually separated from it by 1–3 μm. This permits nearly the entire surface of the capillary loop to be carpeted with the elaborately interdigitated foot processes. This arrangement maximizes the total area of intercellular clefts available for passage of the filtrate (Fig. 21-6 and 21-7).

The cytoplasm of a podocyte contains a small Golgi complex, a moderate amount of rough endoplasmic reticulum, and abundant free ribosomes. Microtubules and intermediate filaments are plentiful only in the cell body and in its primary processes. In thin sections of a glomerulus, cross sections of foot processes are seen to be aligned on an unusually thick basal lamina, which is a product of both the capillary endothelium and the podocytes (Fig. 21-8). On the basal lamina, the space between adjacent foot processes is traversed by the **slit diaphragm,** a membrane 4–6 nm in thickness that has a porous substructure. The pores are believed to be small enough to prevent the passage of albumin and larger molecules from the blood to the glomerular filtrate. Three layers are distinguishable in the underlying basal lamina: a **lamina rara interna** adjacent to the endothelium; an intermediate **lamina densa;** and a **lamina rara externa** adjacent to the podocyte processes. The lamina densa consists of a meshwork of type IV collagen fibrils and laminin. The laminae rarae are rich in heparan sulfate proteoglycan and fibronectin. These compounds may serve to anchor the endothelium and podocytes to the basal lamina. The glomerular basal lamina and the slit diaphragms form a selective physical barrier that excludes molecules greater than 10 nm in diameter from the filtrate. Its negatively charged proteoglycans may contribute an additional electrostatic barrier.

The thin squamous cells of the capillary endothelium have numerous 70–90-nm pores. Unlike those of fenestrated capillaries elsewhere, the pores are not spanned by a pore diaphragm. The thicker portion of the endothelial cell, containing the nucleus and organelles, is usually on the side of the capillary away from the capsular space. The spaces between the glomerular capillaries is occupied by the **mesangium,** a connective tissue consisting of **mesangial cells** in an extracellular matrix that is largely devoid of fibrous elements other than fibronectin. The mesangial cells correspond to the pericytes of other capillaries but have special properties that set them apart. They are phagocytic and may dispose of filtration residues that might otherwise clog the filter. It is speculated that they may also participate in a continual turnover of the basal lamina. They are contractile and have receptors for **angiotensin-II** and other vasoconstrictors and may mediate the effects of these on glomerular filtration rates.

*The kidneys excrete some substances that have relatively low solubility, and they resorb water from the glomerular filtrate to concentrate the urine. A disturbance of the delicate balance between these two functions may lead to **nephrolithiasis (kidney stones**). Concretions that form in the renal pelvis may consist of calcium oxalate, calcium phosphate, or uric acid. Passage of a small stone down the ureter is attended by very severe pain in the flank and hematuria (bloody urine). If passage is not complete, blockage of the ureter may result in progressive loss of kidney function.*

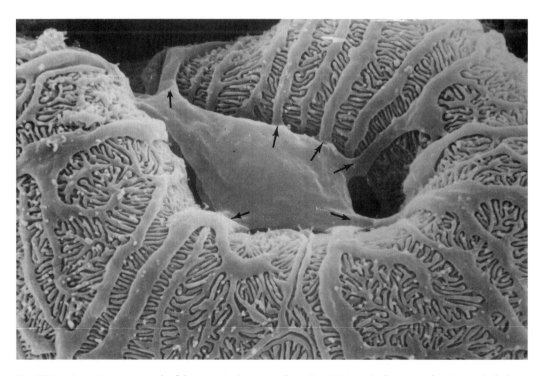

Fig. 21-7 Scanning micrograph of the area in the rectangle in Fig. 21-6, at higher magnification. Included are a capillary loop, a podocyte cell body, and its primary processes (at arrows). The elaborate branching and interdigitation of its secondary processes with those of other podocytes is clearly revealed. (Courtesy of P. Andrews, Journal of Electron Microscope Techniques 9:115, 1988.)

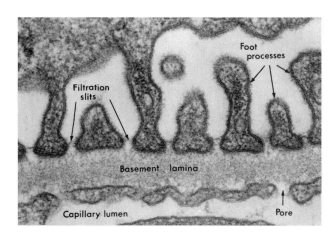

Fig. 21-8 Electron micrograph of a portion of the wall of a glomerular capillary (below) and cross sections of podocyte foot processes on the outer surface of the thick basal lamina. (Courtesy of D. Friend.)

Proximal Convoluted Tubule

Near its origin from the urinary pole of the renal corpuscle, the initial segment of the uriniferous tubule is highly tortuous. In this so-called **proximal convoluted tubule,** the cells are cuboidal, or low columnar, and have a spherical nucleus in an eosinophilic cytoplasm. On their free surface, there is a conspicuous **brush-border** that results in a 20-fold increase in the area of cell membrane exposed to the glomerular filtrate in the lumen (Fig. 21-9). The tips of the microvilli have a prominent glycocalyx. Opening

into the spaces between the microvilli are tubular invaginations of the plasmalemma called the **apical canaliculi.** Numerous small vesicles are found around their ends, suggesting that the canaliculi are involved in endocytosis of macromolecules from the lumen. These vesicles subsequently fuse with lysosomes, where the macromolecules are degraded. The lateral cell boundaries are poorly resolved by the light microscope, due in part to their elaborate interdigitation with neighboring cells. Their complex shape can only be fully appreciated in three-dimensional reconstructions from serial sections (Fig. 21-10). Alternating ridges and grooves extend the full length of the cell, becoming increasingly prominent toward the base, where they divide into slender processes that undermine adjacent cells. In electron micrographs, paired membranes course inward from the cell base, dividing the basal cytoplasm into a number of narrow compartments. These are occupied by long mitochondria oriented in the long axis of the cell. Some of these basal compartments that are not open to the overlying cytoplasm are obviously cross sections of undermining processes of neighboring cells. The elaborate fluting of the lateral cell surfaces can be seen in scanning micrographs of a cross section of a proximal tubule (Fig. 21-11). These specializations greatly increase the area of the basal and lateral cell membranes which are rich in Na^+K^+-ATPase, an enzyme involved in the pumping of sodium out of these cells to create an electrochemical gradient that moves water from the lumen, across the cell to the peritubular capillaries, thus concentrating the urine. The proximal convoluted tubule absorbs about 85% of the

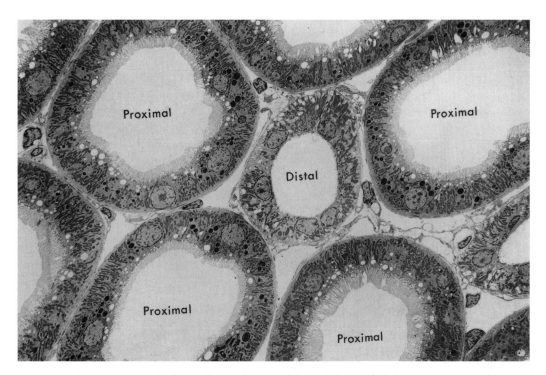

Fig. 21-9 Electron micrograph of a small area of cortex of the rat kidney. Included are cross sections of proximal convoluted tubules and one distal tubule. The initial portion of the proximal tubule (lower right) has a thicker brush-border than the three other cross sections. A brush border is lacking in the distal tubule. (From A. Maunsbach, Journal of Ultrastructure Research 15:252, 1966.)

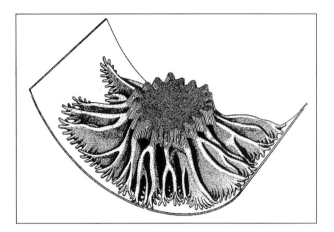

Fig. 21-10 Three-dimensional model of a proximal convoluted tubule cell showing the long finlike radiating processes and their smaller branches at the cell base. (From A. P. Evans, D. A. Hay, and W. G. Dail, 191:397, 1976.)

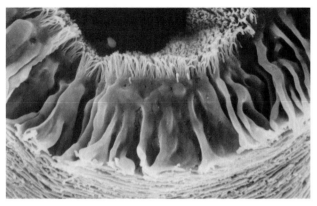

Fig. 21-11 Scanning electron micrograph of the ridges on the lateral cell surfaces of the epithelium in a proximal convoluted tubule. (From Cells and Tissues. A Three-dimensional Approach, Alan R. Liss, Inc., New York, 1989; courtesy of H. Takahashi-Iwanaga.)

water and salt of the glomerular filtrate. It also absorbs glucose and amino acids and excretes creatinine and certain drugs into the urine.

Loop of Henle

From its convoluted juxtaglomerular portion, the proximal tubule continues downward into the medulla, forming the long **loop of Henle.** Its initial segment, called the **descending thick limb** of the loop is similar to the proximal convoluted tubule in diameter, but in the outer part of the medulla, it abruptly narrows from 60 μm in diameter to about 15 μm and continues as the **descending thin limb** of the loop of Henle. At this junction, the brush-border ends and the cuboidal epithelium abruptly gives way to a squamous epithelium bearing a few short microvilli (Fig. 21-12). Due to its small diameter and squamous epithelium, the thin limb resembles a venule in cross section (Figs. 21-3 and 21-13 [see Plate 30]). The thin limb of the loop pumps Na+ and Cl− out of the lumen and reabsorbs about 5% of the water of the glomerular filtrate.

> *After an infection of the throat or skin with certain strains of streptococcus, the infection may spread to the kidneys, resulting in **glomerulonephritis.** The inflammatory response is largely confined to the glomeruli, with accumulation of neutrophils and lymphocytes around the capillaries. There is proliferation of mesangial cells and perivascular deposits of immunoglobulins. The capillaries and basal lamina are damaged and proteins and erythrocytes appear in the urine. The disease usually subsides without specific therapy, but there may be residual impairment of kidney function.*

Two categories of nephrons are distinguished on the basis of the length of their loop of Henle. The **cortical nephrons** have a relatively short loop, in which the

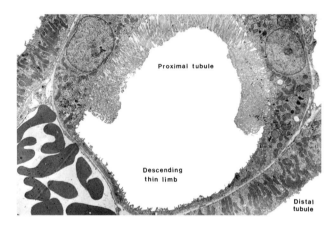

Fig. 21-12 Electron micrograph of a slightly oblique section of the abrupt transition from the descending thick limb of the proximal tubule to the thin limb of the loop of Henle. (From J. Osvaldo and H. Latta, Journal of Ultrastructure Research 15:144, 1966.)

descending thin limb is continuous at the bend of the loop with the ascending limb of the distal tubule. The **juxtamedullary nephrons,** which make up a relatively small fraction of the total number, have a very long loop of Henle (Fig. 21-14). In these, the loop extends deep into the pyramid, and the transition of its **thin ascending limb** to the **ascending thick limb** of the distal tubule is in the upper medulla. In short-looped nephrons, the squamous cells of the thin segment are polygonal in outline throughout its length. In long-looped nephrons, the cells of the descending limb have long interdigitating lateral processes (Fig. 21-15). These decrease in number and length toward the bend, and increase again in the ascending thin limb. These changes in cell outline along the length of long loops have no known physiological significance.

Distal Convoluted Tubule

The initial portion of the distal tubule, in the outer medulla, is called the **ascending thick limb** of the loop of Henle. Continuing into the cortex, it returns to the vascu-

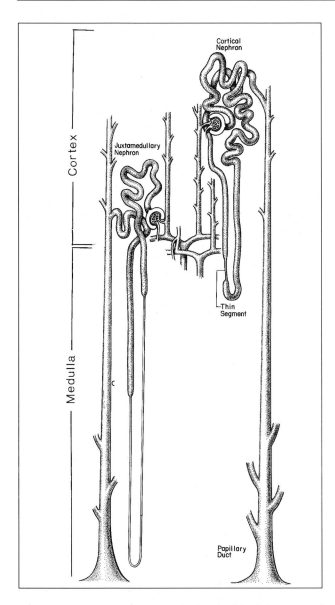

Fig. 21-14 A drawing comparing the length of the thin segment of a cortical nephron having a short loop of Henle with that of a juxtamedullary nephron with a long loop.

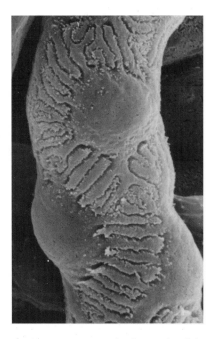

Fig. 21-15 A scanning micrograph of an isolated thin limb of a long-looped nephron showing the interdigitation of the radiating processes of the squamous cells. (From Cells and Tissues, A Three Dimensional Approach, Alan Liss, Inc., 1987, New York, courtesy of H. Takahashi-Iwanaga.)

lar pole of the renal corpuscle of same nephron, where it contacts the afferent arteriole of the glomerulus. On the side adjacent to the arteriole, its cells are narrower and the closer spacing of their nuclei results in a darker-staining sector of the wall that histologists called the **macula densa.** Beyond this landmark, the tubule pursues a tortuous course as the **distal convoluted tubule.** The cells of the ascending thick limb are cuboidal and 7–8 μm in height, gradually diminishing to about 5 μm in the distal convoluted tubule. A brush-border is lacking, but there may be a few short microvilli. A single, short flagellum, arising from a pair of centrioles in the apical cytoplasm, projects into the lumen. There are small vesicles near the cell apex but no apical canaliculi. There are a few cisternae of rough endoplasmic reticulum, a small Golgi complex, and abundant mitochondria, generally oriented parallel to the long axis of the cell. The nucleus tends to be displaced toward

the lumen by deep infoldings of the basal plasmalemma that bound narrow compartments containing long mitochondria. Closed basal compartments that represent undermining processes of neighboring cells are less common in the epithelium of the distal convolution than they are in the proximal convoluted tubule. The thick ascending limb of the loop actively transports Cl^- out of the tubule, followed by Na^+. The distal convoluted tubule is under control of **antidiuretic hormone** and absorbs Na^+ and secretes K^+. This segment absorbs about 8% of the water of the filtrate.

Collecting Tubule and Collecting Duct

Each distal convoluted tubule is joined by a short transitional segment, the **collecting tubule** to a **collecting duct.** The collecting tubules of a number of nephrons join the same collecting duct. As these ducts course deeper into the medulla, their epithelium becomes low columnar with wider cells (Fig. 21-13 [see Plate 30]). At least two cell types are distinguishable in the epithelium of the collecting tubules and collecting ducts. The **principal cells** have short microvilli and a centrally located single flagellum. The nucleus is ovoid and the cytoplasm contains randomly oriented small mitochondria. There are many short invaginations of the basal plasmalemma, but these do not bound basal alcoves containing mitochondria. A darker-staining cell type, the **intercalated cell,** is identified by the presence of numerous small folds, or **microplicae,** on their free surface. The apical cytoplasm contains very large numbers of vesicles ranging from 50 to 200 nm in diameter. Short, plump mitochondria are distributed throughout

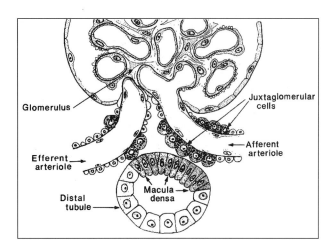

Fig. 21-16 Drawing of the juxtaglomerular complex. It consists of specialized cells in a short segment of the distal convoluted tubule, and modified smooth-muscle cells in the afferent arteriole (and rarely in the efferent arteriole) of the glomerulus.

the cytoplasm. In laboratory rodents, intercalated cells make up 35% of the cells in the ducts of the outer medulla but diminish in number to 10% toward the papilla. None have been reported in the inner medulla of the human kidney. These cells participate in acid–base balance by resorption of bicarbonate. In animals subjected to chronic bicarbonate loading, their number increases dramatically. The collecting duct is controlled by antidiuretic hormone and absorbs about 4% of the water in the filtrate.

Juxtaglomerular Complex

The **juxtaglomerular complex** has three components: (1) the specialized cells of the **macula densa** in the distal tubule; (2) **juxtaglomerular cells** in the wall of the adjacent afferent arteriole of the glomerulus; and (3) pale-staining **mesangial cells** in the angle between the diverging afferent and efferent arterioles of the glomerulus (Fig. 21-16). The juxtaglomerular cells are modified smooth-muscle cells in the media of the afferent arteriole. Rarely, they may be found in the efferent arteriole as well. Some retain myofilaments typical of smooth-muscle cells and have relatively few dense secretory granules. Others contain many secretory granules and no myofilaments. In the macula densa, the polarity of the epithelial cells is reversed, with the Golgi complex between the nucleus and the cell base, suggesting that they may have a secretory function influencing the activity of the juxtaglomerular cells. The secretory granules of the juxtaglomerular cells contain the hormone **renin,** a protease that cleaves **angiotensinogen** in the blood plasma to **angiotensin-I.** In its subsequent passage through the circulation, an enzyme on the surface of the endothelial cells of lung capillaries transforms angiotensin-I to **angiotensin-II.** This is a potent vasoconstrictor that raises blood pressure and indirectly influences the rate of renal blood flow.

Renal Interstitium

The content of the spaces between the renal tubules constitutes the **renal interstitium.** Its volume in the cortex is small, but it increases in the medulla. It includes small bundles of collagen fibers, cells resembling fibroblasts, and cells of the monocyte–macrophage lineage in a matrix of highly hydrated proteoglycans. In the interstitium of the medulla, there are pleomorphic **interstitial cells** that differ from the fibroblastlike cells of the cortex. They are often oriented transversely with respect to the surrounding tubules, with the tips of their long processes adherent to tubules and blood vessels. They contain lipid droplets that vary in abundance in various states of salt and water balance. They were formerly thought to produce prostaglandins, but this is now questioned. There is some evidence that they have an endocrine function in the regulation of systemic blood pressure, but this awaits verification.

Renal Circulation

The kidneys have a very large blood flow, averaging about 1200 ml/min. The **renal artery,** entering the hilum, divides into two main branches, one supplying the anterior and the other the posterior half of the kidney. Arising segmentally from the primary branches of the renal artery are short **lobar arteries** that branch into **interlobar arteries.** These course between the pyramids to the corticomedullary boundary, where they divide into **arcuate arteries** that run parallel to the surface of the kidney. **Interlobular arteries,** arising from the arcuate arteries, course radially toward the kidney surface. Along their course they give rise to **intralobular arteries** that give off the **afferent arterioles** to the juxtamedullary, midcortical, and superficial renal glomeruli. **Efferent arterioles** from the cortical glomeruli ramify to form a cortical intertubular capillary network. Efferent arterioles of the juxtamedullary glomeruli course into the medulla, forming vessels somewhat larger than capillaries, called the **vasa recta.** Deep in the medulla, these turn back toward the cortex. These slightly larger, thin-walled, recurrent vessels intermingle with the descending vasa recta, forming **vascular bundles** or **rete** (Fig. 21-17). These constitute an efficient countercurrent system that facilitates diffusion of ions between the blood and the loops of Henle, thereby conserving the osmotic gradient established in the interstitium.

The venous drainage parallels the course of the arteries. Blood from the capsular and cortical capillaries is drained via **stellate veins** into **interlobular veins,** then to **arcuate veins,** and then to **interlobar veins** that converge to form the **renal vein.**

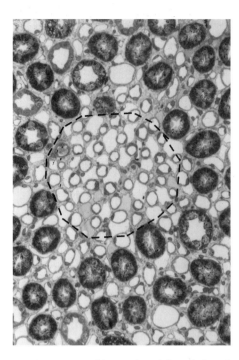

Fig. 21-17 Cross section of the renal medulla including descending thin limbs and ascending thick limbs of the loops of Henle. Outlined in the center is a vascular rete with its juxtaposed thicker-walled descending and thinner-walled ascending portions of the loops.

Histophysiology

While **excreting** waste products of metabolism, the kidneys **conserve** water, electrolytes, and nutrients in the amounts needed by the body. They carry out this dual mission by a combination of filtration, passive diffusion, active secretion, and selective reabsorption. Blood circulates through the glomeruli with a hydrostatic pressure that forces the fluid constituents of the plasma through the endothelium, the basal lamina, the filtration slits between podocytes, and into Bowman's capsule. With blood flowing through the glomeruli of both kidneys at a rate of about 1300 ml/min, glomerular filtrate is produced at a rate of 125 ml/min. From this large volume of filtrate, urine is produced at a rate of only 1 ml/min. The other 124 ml of water is reabsorbed during passage through the renal tubules. The composition of the filtrate is modified by the addition of some substances through active secretion and the removal of others by osmotic forces or active transport.

The glomerular capillaries are fenestrated and freely permeable, but the principal physical barrier, the basal lamina, is size-selective, excluding plasma constituents of molecular weight greater than 70,000. The filtrate therefore normally contains no large protein and only traces of albumin. The filter is also charge-selective. The heparan sulfate proteoglycan, the type IV collagen of the basal lamina, and the sialoglycoprotein of the surface coat of the podocyte processes are all negatively charged. Electrostatic repulsion prevents other negatively charged molecules from passing through the barrier.

In the proximal convoluted tubule, 70–85% of the water and the Na$^+$ ions are reabsorbed, together with chloride, calcium, phosphate, glucose, and amino acids. Sodium enters the cell by facilitated diffusion through the plasmalemma of the brush-border and is actively pumped out through the basolateral membranes into the interstitial flu-

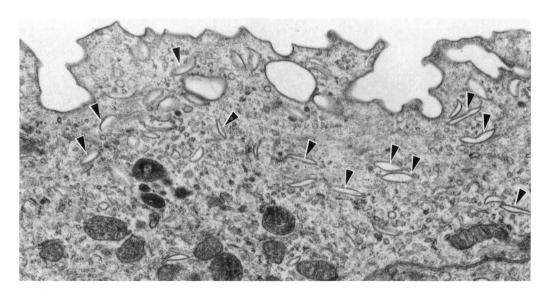

Fig. 21-18 Electron micrograph of a superficial cell of the transitional epithelium of the bladder. The lumenal membrane has an unusual angular contour, owing to its content of relatively stiff plaques connected by more flexible unspecialized regions of the membrane. The arrows indicate elliptical vesicles consisting of pairs of plaques that can be inserted into the membrane during distension of the bladder. (From M. Hicks and B. Ketterer, 45:452, 1970.)

id. In the electrochemical gradient thus created, water and chloride follow to maintain osmotic equilibrium. Glucose and amino acids diffuse through the luminal membrane with the sodium and are cotransported through the basolateral membranes and into the peritubular capillaries. The brush-border and the remarkable shape of the proximal tubule cells are specializations to increase the efficiency of these processes. Urea, uric acid, and other waste products remain in the tubular fluid and are voided in the urine.

The ability of the kidney to excrete a hypertonic urine depends on the loop of Henle. The thin descending limb of the loop is permeable to water but not to salt; the thin ascending limb is permeable to salt but not to water. Diffusion of water from the descending limb increases the intratubular concentration of salt and other solutes. The permeability of the ascending limb to salt permits it to diffuse into the interstitium, contributing passively to the high osmolarity of the inner medulla.

The thick ascending limb of the loop is relatively impermeable to diffusion, but it actively transports chloride out of the tubule, accompanied by passive movement of sodium, thus diluting the tubule fluid and rendering the interstitium hyperosmotic. This osmotic gradient draws water from the distal tubules and collecting ducts, increasing intratubular concentration of the waste product urea. Its concentration is increased nearly 100-fold during passage through the renal tubules.

The blood flow through the medulla is less than 2% of the total flow. If it were greater, it would wash out solutes in the interstitium, and the high osmolarity of the medulla could not be maintained. The countercurrent arrangement of blood vessels around the loops of Henle further reduces solute extraction. The conservation of water and electrolytes by the kidney is strongly influenced by the adrenal hormone **aldosterone.** It binds to receptors on the cells and affects sodium transport across the basolateral membranes. The permeability of the collecting tubules and ducts to water is regulated by **antidiuretic hormone** from the pars nervosa of the pituitary.

Renal Pelvis and Ureters

The renal pelvis is lined by a thin transitional epithelium that becomes somewhat thicker in the ureters. Beneath the epithelium is a lamina propria rich in elastic fibers. The lamina propria is surrounded by smooth muscle that does not form distinct longitudinal and circular layers but is made up of bundles of smooth-muscle fibers of varying orientation. The thickness of the wall gradually increases, and in the lower third of the ureter, an additional layer of predominantly longitudinal smooth muscle is added. Muscle contraction, in the renal pelvis and ureter, creates peristaltic waves that slowly progress toward the urinary bladder.

URINARY BLADDER

The wall of the urinary bladder is covered by pelvic peritoneum which constitutes it **serosa.** The **muscularis** is made up of three layers of smooth muscle that intermingle to such an extent that their boundaries are indistinct. In the outer layer, smooth-muscle bundles are oriented longitudinally along its sides and then transversely over its dome. The thin middle layer is discontinuous and its scattered bundles are predominantly circular or oblique. The fibers of the thin inner layer are again primarily longitudinal.

The **mucosa** lining the bladder is loosely attached to the muscularis and has a **transitional epithelium** which is thin in the full bladder but thicker when the wall is contracted. In the latter state, the epithelium may be six to eight cells thick and the superficial cells are much larger than those more deeply situated, and their rounded free surface bulges into the lumen. In the full bladder, the epithelium is reduced to three or four cells in thickness and the cells are flattened. In electron micrographs, the luminal surface of the cells has a peculiar scalloped appearance (Fig. 21-18). This irregularity is due to the presence of thicker plaques within the plasmalemma that are connected by thinner and more flexible interplaque regions. In freeze-fracture preparations, the plaques appear as rounded areas of closely spaced intramembrane particles (Fig. 21-19). In negatively stained preparations of isolated plaques viewed at high magnification, the plaques are made up of hexagonally arranged particulate subunits, each of which appears to be a hexamer of smaller subunits.

The apical cytoplasm of the superficial cells contains unique discoid vesicles that are lenticular in section (Fig. 21-18). These are made up of pairs of the plaques. They appear to be formed by interiorization of adjoining plaques of the surface membrane when the bladder empties. They are subsequently reinserted into the membrane to provide

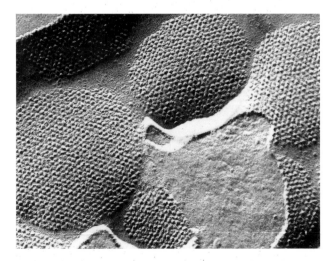

Fig. 21-19 Micrograph of a freeze-fracture preparation of lumenal membrane of the transitional epithelium of the bladder, showing the plaques within the membrane. (Courtesy of M. Hicks and B. Ketterer.)

for its rapid expansion during bladder distension.

The superficial cells are joined by juxtalumenal tight junctions, and there are desmosomes between cells throughout the epithelium. The occluding junctions and the special properties of the thick lumenal membrane are thought to create a permeability barrier that prevents dilution of the hypertonic urine by movement of water through the epithelium.

URETHRA

The urethra of the male is the terminal portion of both the urinary tract and the reproductive tracts. Its initial segment, the **prostatic urethra,** passes through the prostate. On its posterior wall, there is a slight elevation, the **verumontanum (colliculus seminalis).** In its midline is the opening of the **prostatic utricle,** a small blind pouch of unknown function extending into the substance of the prostate. On either side of the verumontanum are the openings of the **ejaculatory ducts.** On the posterior wall of the urethra in this region are numerous small openings of the multiple ducts of the prostate gland. Distal to the ejaculatory ducts, the epithelium lining the urethra changes from transitional to pseudostratified or stratified columnar epithelium. There is no change in the epithelium in the **membranous urethra,** the portion that passes through the urogenital diaphragm below the pubic symphysis. In this short segment, the urethra is surrounded by striated muscle of the **external urethral sphincter.** The **penile urethra** is lined by stratified columnar epithelium, but this changes in its slightly dilated terminal portion, called the **fossa navicularis,** to stratified squamous epithelium which continues onto the glans penis.

On the upper surface of the urogenital diaphragm, on either side of the urethra are two **bulbourethral glands** about 1 cm in diameter. Scattered in the lamina propria along the entire length of the urethra are small **glands of Littré.** These glands are unrelated to the excretory function of the urinary tract and will be considered in Chapter 22.

The short female urethra is lined by stratified squamous epithelium interrupted by areas of pseudostratified columnar epithelium. There are shallow invaginations along its length that are lined by mucous cells resembling those of the glands of Littré. The female urethra is enveloped by smooth muscle which is thickened below the bladder neck, forming an involuntary **internal urethral sphincter,** and immediately above the urogenital diaphragm, there is a voluntary **external urethral sphincter** of striated muscle.

QUESTIONS*

1. The renal corpuscle does **not** contain

   A. mesangial cells
   B. filtration slits
   C. visceral epithelium of Bowman
   D. cells of the macula densa
   E. glomerulus

2. Podocytes are

   A. glomerular endothelial cells
   B. parietal epithelial cells of Bowman
   C. mesangial cells
   D. juxtaglomerular cells
   E. visceral epithelial cells of Bowman's capsule

3. Which of the following statements is **incorrect?**

   A. Endothelial cells of a glomerulus possess fenestrations.
   B. The macula densa is part of the juxtaglomerular apparatus.
   C. An intertubular capillary network is found in the cortex of the kidney.
   D. Cells of the efferent artery belong to the juxtaglomerular apparatus.
   E. Podocytes touch the basement membrane (basal lamina) of the glomerulus.

4. Which of the following statements is **incorrect** about kidney circulation?

   A. Blood flows from interlobal artery to arcuate artery to interlobular artery.
   B. Blood flows from glomerulus to efferent arteriole to peritubular capillary.
   C. Plexus blood flows from interlobular vein to arcuate vein to interlobar vein.
   D. Vasa recta are found in the medulla of the kidney.
   E. Afferent arterioles give origin to vasa recta.

5. The urinary bladder

   A. has two layers of muscle
   B. has two urethras entering it
   C. contains hypertonic urine
   D. is lined by simple columnar epithelium
   E. none of the above

6. Which of the matched pairs is **incorrect?**

   A. collecting tubule/medullary ray
   B. fenestrations/glomerulus
   C. renin/collecting tubule
   D. glomerulus/renal corpuscle
   E. none of the above

7. Which matched pair is **incorrect?**

   A. macula densa/distal convoluted tubule
   B. glomeruli/cortex of kidney
   C. renin/efferent arteriole of glomerulus
   D. fenestrated capillaries/glomerulus
   E. many mitochondria/proximal convoluted tubule cells

8. Which statement is correct about kidney circulation?

   A. Blood flows from the arcuate artery to the interlobar artery.
   B. Blood flows from the arcuate vein to the interlobular vein.
   C. Vasa recta are found in the cortex of the kidney.
   D. Afferent arteriole connects with a glomerulus.
   E. None of the above are correct.

9. A brush border is present in the

   A. glomerulus
   B. proximal convoluted tubule
   C. loop of Henle
   D. distal convoluted tubule
   E. collecting tubule

10. Blood in route to glomeruli flows through which sequence of arteries?

    A. interlobar–interlobular–arcuate
    B. renal–interlobar–interlobular
    C. renal–interlobular–arcuate
    D. renal–interlobar–arcuate
    E. none of the above

11. An apical brush border is associated with which of the following cells?

    A. distal convoluted tubule
    B. proximal convoluted tubule
    C. Henle's loop
    D. macula densa
    E. none of the above

12. The calyx of the kidney, the ureter, and the
urinary bladder

A. are all invested by skeletal muscle
B. are all lined by transitional epithelium
C. all share a distinct and continuous submucosa
D. do not have any properties in common
E. none of the above

*Answers on page 307.

22

MALE REPRODUCTIVE SYSTEM

CHAPTER OUTLINE

The Testis
    Seminiferous Tubules
    Blood–Testis Barrier
    Spermatogenesis
    Spermiogenesis
    Spermiation
    The Spermatozoon
    Cycle of the Seminiferous Epithelium
    Interstitial Tissue
    Blood Vessels and Lymphatics
    Histophysiology
    Ducts of the Testis
        Tubuli Recti and Rete
        Ductuli Efferentes
Epididymis
Ductus Deferens
Ejaculatory Duct
Accessory Glands
    Seminal Vesicles
    Prostate Gland
    Bulbourethral Glands
Penis

KEY WORDS

Acrosomal Vesicle
Acrosome
Ampulla
Annulus
Axoneme
Bartholin's Gland
Capacitation
Corpora Amylacea
Corpus Cavernosum
Corpus Spongiosum
Cowper's Gland
Cremaster Muscle
Crystals of Reinke
Deep Dorsal Vein
Ductus Epididymidis
Ejaculate
Ejaculation
Flagellum
Foreskin
Glands of Littre
Glans Penis
Helicine Artery
Inguinal Canal

Leydig Cell
Lobuli Testis
Manchette
Mediastinum
Meiosis
Myoid Cell
Pampiniform Plexus
Prepuce
Scrotum
Semen
Septula Testis
Sertoli Cell
Spermatic Cord
Spermatid
Spermatocyte
Spermatogonia
Stereocilium
Synapsis
Testosterone
Tunica Albuginea
Tunica Vaginalis
Urethra

The external genitalia of the male include a copulatory organ, the **penis,** and two **testes** that are suspended in a skin-covered fibroelastic sac, the **scrotum.** The excurrent ducts from the testes, the **ductuli efferentes,** join a long convoluted duct that forms the **epididymis,** an elongated organ on the posterior surface of each testis. The coiled duct of the epididymis is continuous with a long, uncoiled **ductus deferens** that ascends from the scrotum and passes through the **inguinal canal** to enter the pelvis. Its terminal segment, the **ejaculatory duct,** empties into the **urethra.** Associated with the intrapelvic portion of the duct system are three accessory glands of male reproduction, the **seminal vesicles,** the **prostate,** and the **bulbourethral glands** (Fig. 22-1). Spermatozoa developed in the testes are stored in the epididymis. The semen that is expelled at **ejaculation** consists of **spermatozoa** in a semifluid medium made up of the secretory products from the accessory glands.

THE TESTIS

The testes are ovoid in shape, 4–5 cm in length, 2.5 cm in width, and 3 cm in anteroposterior diameter. They develop early in embryonic life in the abdominal cavity and later descend into the scrotum. In their descent, they carry with them an outpocketing of the peritoneum, called the **tunica vaginalis propria testis,** which forms an independent serous cavity around the anterior and lateral surfaces of the testis. Like the peritoneum, this closed cavity is lined by mesothelium. The limited amount of mobility permitted within this cavity, and within the elastic scrotum, helps to prevent damage to the organ. Descent into

the scrotum provides a testicular environment with a temperature a few degrees lower than that of the abdominal cavity. This lower temperature is a necessary condition for development of the spermatozoa.

The testis is enclosed in a thick, fibrous capsule, the **tunica albuginea.** On its posterior surface, dense connective tissue extends inward from the capsule, forming the **mediastinum** of the testis, through which its blood vessels enter and its ducts leave the organ. Thin, fibrous **septula testis** radiate from the mediastinum to the tunica albuginea dividing the interior of the organ into about 250 pyramidal compartments, the **lobuli testis.** Each lobule contains from one to four tortuous **seminiferous tubules,** 150–200 µm in diameter and 30–70 cm in length (Fig. 22-2). The majority of these form highly convoluted loops that return to the mediastinum, but a few may end blindly. At the apex of each pyramidal lobule, there is an abrupt transition of its seminiferous tubules to the **tubuli recti.** These converge upon a plexus of epithelium-lined spaces within the mediastinum, called the **rete testis.** From the rete, a number of **ductuli efferentes** emerge from the testis. These conduct spermatozoa to the **ductus epididymidis.**

The interstices between the seminiferous tubules of the testes are occupied by a highly vascular reticular connective tissue, containing perivascular mesenchymal cells, fibroblasts, and a few macrophages. Within this loose stroma, there are clusters of **Leydig cells,** the so-called interstitial cells of the testis. These cells are the endocrine component of the testis, secreting the male sex hormone **testosterone.**

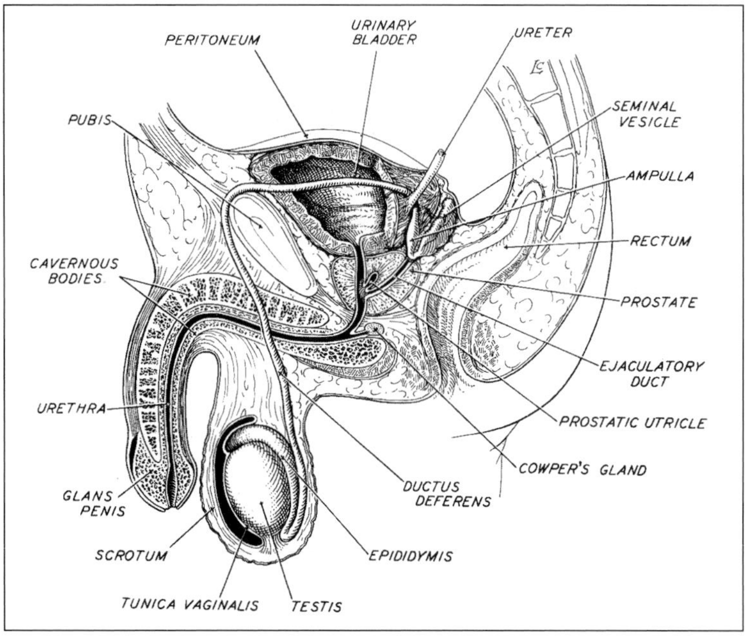

Seminiferous Tubules

The long, tortuous seminiferous tubules are 150–200 µm in diameter (Fig. 22-3). The total length of the seminiferous tubules of the testes is over 200 m. Each is ensheathed in a single epitheloid layer of flat polygonal cells, called **myoid cells.** These have the ultrastructural characteristic of smooth muscle, and they are responsible for rhythmic shallow contractions that can be observed in the seminiferous tubules of living laboratory rodents. In larger species, the tubules are ensheathed by multiple layers of fusiform cells, with the innermost layer consisting of myoid cells. In the human, all of the sheath cells appear to be fibroblasts. No myoid cells are identifiable and no contractility of the tubules has been observed. Each seminiferous tubule is surrounded by a dense capillary network.

The seminiferous tubules are lined by the seminiferous epithelium (Fig. 22-4), a very complex stratified epithelium made up of supporting cells, called **Sertoli cells:** stem cells,

Fig. 22-1 Diagram of the male reproductive system. Midline structures are shown in saggital section. Bilateral structures, such as the testis, are depicted in the round. (After C. D. Turner.)

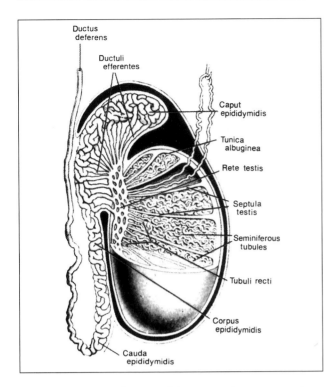

Fig. 22-2 Cut-away diagram of the testis and its excretory ducts. Septula divide the organ into compartments occupied by convoluted semeniferous tubules. (Modified from W. J. Hamilton, Textbook of Human Anatomy, London, McMillan & Co., 1927.)

called **spermatogonia,** at the base of the epithelium, and four cell types at progressively higher levels that represent successive stages in the differentiation of the male germ cells. These are **primary spermatocytes, secondary spermatocytes, spermatids,** and **spermatozoa.** The seminifer-

ous epithelium can be thought of as consisting of a population of nonproliferating Sertoli cells and a population of germ cells that divide near the base of the epithelium and slowly move upward toward the free surface as they differentiate into spermatozoa. The Sertoli cells provide nutritional and mechanical support, and by changes in their shape, they actively participate in the upward movement of the differentiating germ cells. They are also involved in the release of mature spermatozoa at the luminal surface of the epithelium.

The Sertoli cells extend from the basal lamina to the free surface of the epithelium, with the germ cells aligned vertically between them. Unlike the columnar cells of other epithelia which have straight sides, the Sertoli cells are deformed by the germ cells which occupy deep recesses in their sides. Slender lateral processes extend between the germ cells to contact neighboring Sertoli cells. They have an ovoid nucleus with a large nucleolus that is usually flanked by two rounded masses of heterochromatin. The Golgi complex is large but has no associated vesicles or secretory granules. Granular endoplasmic reticulum is sparse, but smooth reticulum is abundant near the cell base. A few lipid droplets and aggregations of lipochrome pigment are found in the basal cytoplasm. The cytoskeleton of the Sertoli cell is well developed. A meshwork of actin filaments forms a thin layer immediately beneath the plasmalemma, and fascicles of intermediate filaments are oriented more or less parallel to the cell axis. Microtubules of similar orientation are abundant at certain stages of the spermatogenic cycle. The actin filaments and microtubules are no doubt involved in the changes of Sertoli cell shape that move the germ cells toward the surface.

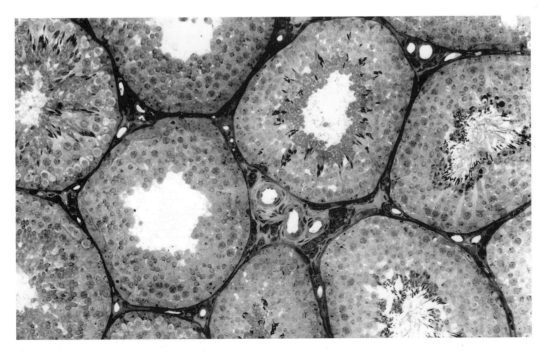

Fig. 22-3 Histological section of mammalian testis, showing cross sections of seminiferous tubules. Note that the associations of cells differ from tubule to tubule. Some have late spermatids near the lumen; others do not.

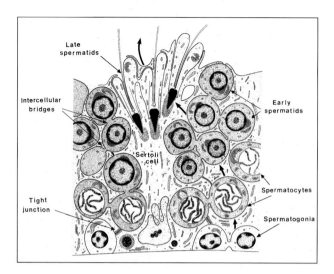

Fig. 22-4 Drawing of the seminiferous epithelium showing the groups of conjoined spermatocytes and spermatids occupying deep recesses in the sides of the tall Sertoli cells. Late spermatids are then moved to deep invaginations in the apical cytoplasm of the Sertoli cells.

Blood–Testis Barrier

Many epithelia have occluding junctions between the apices of the cells. The seminiferous epithelium is unusual in having occluding junctions nearer the cell base. They occur between lateral processes of the Sertoli cells that arch over the spermatogonia. Thus, they divide the epithelium into two compartments: a **basal compartment,** containing the stem cells, and an **adlumenal compartment,** containing the later stages of germ cell differentiation. These junctions constitute a **blood–testis barrier** that prevents large molecules from entering, or leaving, the adlumenal compartment. The barrier may be necessary for maintenance of a special environment for germ cell differentiation in that compartment.

Spermatogenesis

The term "spermatogenesis" encompasses the entire sequence of proliferative events and cytological changes undergone by the germ cells in their development from stem cells to mature spermatozoa. Stem cells with pale-staining nuclei, called **type A spermatogonia,** are situated on the basal lamina. In the initial phase of spermatogenesis, these undergo multiple mitotic divisions. Half of the daughter cell population goes on to differentiate into **type B spermatogonia,** and the others maintain the stem cell population. Division of each type B spermatogonium produces two **primary spermatocytes,** which are larger spherical cells located above the spermatogonia (Fig. 22-4). These immediately enter prophase of the first meiotic cell division. **Meiosis** occurs only in the development of the germ cells of both sexes and consists of two successive divisions that reduce

the normal somatic chromosome number from 46 (44+XY in the male) to 23 (22+X or 22+Y in spermatozoa). Five stages of **meiotic prophase** can be recognized by the appearance of the chromosomes in the nucleus of the primary spermatocytes. These are called **leptotene, zygotene, pachytene, diplotene,** and **diakinesis.** Prophase of the first meiotic division is a slow process extending over 20 days. Therefore, most of the spermatocytes seen in histological sections will be in one or another of the stages of meiotic prophase. In leptotene, the chromosomes appear as long, thin filaments. These later begin to shorten and thicken. In zygotene, homologous chromosomes come together in pairs, in register along their length; a process called **synapsis.** In pachytene, shortening of the chromosomes continues, and in diplotene, each of the paired chromosomes splits along its length into two chromatids, resulting in tetrads of four parallel **chromatids.** Adjacent chromatids of the paired chromosomes exchange segments; a process called **crossing-over.** In diakinesis, the homologous bivalent chromosomes shorten further and begin to separate, but they may adhere briefly at sites of crossing-over. Prophase ends with the dissolution of the nuclear envelope and migration of the chromosomes to the equatorial plate. In **metaphase,** the centrioles at opposite poles of the cell are connected to the chromosomes by microtubules of the spindle, and in **anaphase,** the pairs of chromosomes, each consisting of two chromatids, separate and migrate to the poles. In **telophase,** the cytoplasm constricts, separating two haploid (i.e., containing half the number of chromosomes found in the somatic cells) secondary spermatocytes. These proceed quickly through prophase of the second meiotic division. The chromosomes gather on the equatorial plate, and at anaphase, the two chromatids of each chromosome separate and migrate to opposite poles. At telophase, the second meiotic division is completed. The two meiotic divisions thus result in four haploid spermatids that develop into haploid spermatozoa. Because of the separation of the members of the XY pair during meiosis, half of the spermatozoa have a chromosome complement of 22+X, and the other half, 22+Y. The ova of the female are all 22+X. Their fertilization by an X-bearing spermatozoon results in a girl, and fertilization by a Y-bearing spermatozoon results in a baby boy.

*A failure of the chromosomes to separate normally during meiotic division in spermatogenesis or oogenesis may result in male offspring with one or more extra X-chromosomes (XXY, XXXY) (**Klinefelter's syndrome**). These men have long legs and small firm testes with no spermatogenesis. They may have enlarged mammary glands owing to a high level of follicle-stimulating hormone (FSH) and a low level of testosterone in their blood plasma.*

Telophase of the cell divisions in spermatogenesis is atypical in that the daughter cells do not completely separate but remain in continuity through a narrow intercellular bridge. Therefore, a pair of conjoined type B spermatogonia give rise to a group of four conjoined primary spermatocytes. The two following divisions produce chains of 8 secondary spermatocytes and 16 spermatids that differentiate without further division to yield 16 spermatozoa (Fig. 22-5).

Spermiogenesis

The term "spermiogenesis" refers to the sequence of postmeiotic changes by which spermatids are transformed into spermatozoa. For descriptive purposes, this process is divided into a **Golgi phase,** an **acrosome phase,** and a **maturational phase.** The spermatids are initially small closely spaced spherical cells, 7–8 μm in diameter, located above the spermatocytes. In the Golgi phase, small membrane-limited proacrosomal granules appear in their juxtanuclear Golgi complex. These coalesce into a large granule within a sizable **acrosomal vesicle** that adheres to the nuclear envelope (Fig. 22-6A). The Golgi complex remains closely applied to the outer aspect of the vesicle and continues to form condensing vacuoles that fuse with it, contributing to an increase in the volume of the vesicle and the size of the single acrosomal granule in its interior. The area of the limiting membrane of the vesicle adherent to the nucleus spreads laterally from the point of initial contact, and the vesicle assumes a hemispherical shape (Fig. 22-6B). This marks the end of the Golgi phase.

In the acrosome phase, the granule remains at the pole of the nucleus while the surrounding vesicle continues to expand, forming a thin fold that extends laterally and posteriorly until it forms a cap over the entire anterior half of the nucleus (Fig. 22-6C). The substance of the granule is then redistributed throughout the interior of the cap formed by the acrosomal vesicle. This completes the development of the **acrosome.** Concurrent with these changes, there is a condensation of the chromatin, and the ovoid nucleus takes on a narrower shape (Fig. 22-7). In the course of these events, the cell as a whole changes its orientation so that the acrosome is directed toward the basal lamina of the epithelium. The cell elongates and the centrioles move to the posterior pole of the nucleus and becomes fixed to the nuclear envelope. One member of the pair is oriented transversely; the other is parallel to the long axis of the nucleus. The triplet microtubules in the wall of this centriole serve as templates for assembly of tubulin to form nine doublet microtubules that rapidly elongate to form the

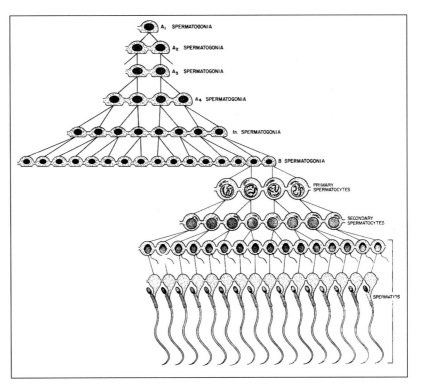

Fig. 22-5 Diagram of the clonal expansion of the developing male germ cells and their connection by intercellular bridges. Only the type A spermatogonia complete their division and give rise to separate daughter cells. The number of interconnected cells in the clones is greater than depicted here.

axoneme of the **sperm flagellum** (a very long cilium that serves as a locomotor organelle) (Fig. 22-8).

In the cytoplasm of the elongating spermatid, microtubules increase in number and become arranged in a cylindrical array, termed the **manchette.** This extends backward from the posterior rim of the acrosome. In the formation of the manchette, the bulk of the spermatid cytoplasm is shifted posteriorly and the plasma membrane at the anterior end becomes closely applied to the outer membrane of the acrosome. After this shape change, the tubules of the manchette depolymerize.

Where the plasma is continuous with the flagellar membrane, dense material accumulates on its cytoplasmic surface to form a dense ring, the **annulus.** As the flagellum continues to elongate, the annulus moves along it and the mitochondria of the spermatid assemble behind it and become arranged in a tight spiral around the initial portion of the axoneme, forming the **mitochondrial sheath** of the sperm flagellum. While these events are in progress, a longitudinal outer dense fiber is formed parallel to each of the nine doublets of the axoneme and peripheral to it (Fig. 22-9). Posterior to the annulus, semicircular riblike structures form in the thin layer of cytoplasm between the flagellar membrane and the outer dense fibers. These are joined together at their ends by their continuity with dorsal and ventral longitudinal columns. The circumferential ribs and the longitudinal columns together constitute the **fibrous sheath** of the developing sperm tail.

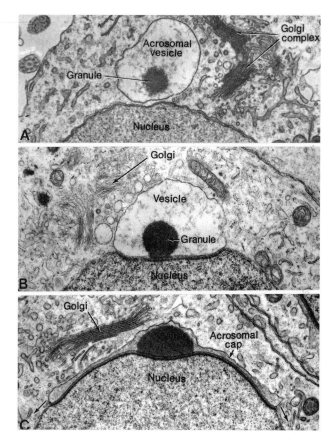

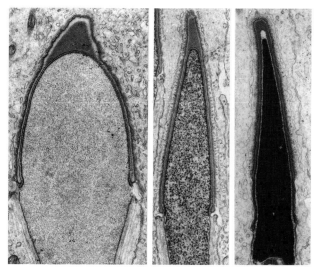

Fig. 22-7 Three later stages in acrosome formation and condensation of the nucleus.

Fig. 22-6 Electron micrographs of spermatids illustrating three stages in formation of the acrosome. (A) The acrosomal vesicle and granule develop in the Golgi complex, like a secretory granule. (B) The vesicle adheres to the nuclear envelope. (C) It then spreads laterally over the anterior pole of the nucleus, forming an acrosomal cap.

Spermiation

The term "spermiation" is applied to the release of spermatozoa from the seminiferous epithelium. In the course of spermatogenesis, the spermatids are slowly moved toward the surface of the epithelium by the Sertoli cells and by proliferation of the spermatocytes below them (Fig. 22-10B). When they have reached the stage described in the foregoing paragraph, they consist of a condensed nucleus capped by an acrosome, a flagellum with mitochondrial and fibrous sheaths, and a retort-shaped appendage of excess cytoplasm. At this stage, the heads of the spermatids occupy conforming recesses in the apical surface of the Sertoli cells, with their flagella projecting into the lumen of the serminiferous tubule. In the subsequent release of spermatozoa, the sperm heads are actively extruded from the Sertoli cell, and the slender connection with their residual cytoplasm is broken (see 22-10C and 22-10D). Thus each spermatozoon becomes free in the lumen while the residual cytoplasm of the spermatids is retained in the apical cytoplasm of the Sertoli cell and is subsequently degraded by lysosomal enzymes.

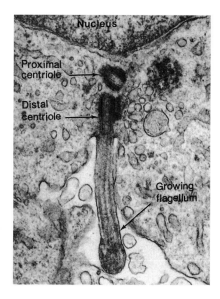

Fig. 22-8 Electron micrograph of an early stage in formation of the sperm flagellum. A short axoneme can be seen extending from the end of one of the centrioles.

The Spermatozoon

The mature spermatozoon is commonly considered to have a **head** and a **tail.** The head consists of the condensed nucleus capped by the acrosome. The tail includes (1) a **connecting piece** consisting of nine cross-striated fibers that are continuous distally with the outer dense fibers of the flagellum; (2) a **midpiece** 5–7 μm in length, made up of the axoneme surrounded by the mitochondrial sheath; (3) a **principal piece,** about 45 μm in length in which the axoneme is enclosed in the fibrous sheath; and (4) the **endpiece,** 5–7 μm long, consisting of the terminal part of the axoneme distal to the termination of the fibrous sheath (Fig. 22-11). It is enclosed throughout by the plasmalemma. The

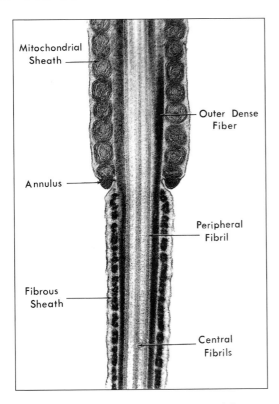

Fig. 22-9 A longitudinal section of a portion of the sperm tail showing the mitochondrial sheath of the midpiece, the fibrous sheath of the principal piece, and the annulus at the end of the mitochondrial sheath.

spermatozoon is motile in the female tract and undergoes chemical changes in the uterus and uterine tube that make it capable of fertilization. This is called **capacitation.**

Cycle of the Seminiferous Epithelium

At any one site in the seminiferous tubule, the development of the clusters of germ cells, joined by intercellular bridges, is synchronous, but from segment to segment along the tubule, different associations of cell types, representing different stages of germ cell differentiation, can be identified. Therefore, in cross sections of the testis, neighboring tubules will have a different appearance (Fig. 22-3). For each species, there is a specific number of recognizable cell associations. In the guinea pig, there are 12 and cells of the same stage are found around the entire circumference of the tubule. If cross sections of enough tubules are examined, all 12 associations can be found. At any point along the length of a seminiferous tubule, the cell types change with the passage of time, ultimately passing through all 12 stages and then repeating the sequence. The **cycle of the seminiferous epithelium** is defined as the series of changes occurring in a given area of epithelium between two successive appearances of the same cell association. In the human, there are only six different cell associations (Fig. 22-12). Unlike in rodents, these associations

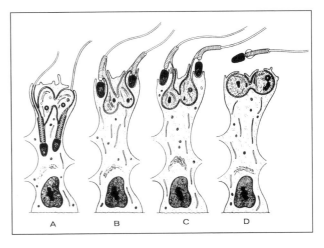

Fig. 22-10 Drawing of successive stages in release of the spermatozoa from the epithelium. (B) Sperm are moved to the apex of the Sertoli cells; (C) sperm are pushed into the lumen still connected to residual spermatid cytoplasm by a narrow stalk; (D) the stalk gives way, freeing the spermatozoa. The residual bodies are retained and degraded by lysosomes of the Sertoli cell.

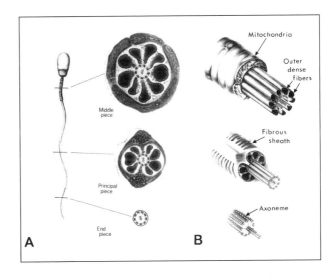

Fig. 22-11 (A) Micrographs of cross sections of the midpiece, principal piece and end-piece of the tail of a spermatozoon. (B) Drawings of the three-dimensional structure of the three segments of the tail.

do not extend around the entire circumference of the tubule but occupy small wedge-shaped areas of the epithelium. Thus, one may find three different associations of cells in the same cross section. The duration of one cycle in man is 16 days and the total duration of spermatogenesis is 64 days.

Interstitial Tissue

In the human testis, the angular spaces between seminiferous tubules are occupied by a loose connective tissue containing blood and lymphatic vessels, clusters of **Leydig cells,** occasional fibroblasts, macrophages, mast cells, and undifferentiated mesenchymal cells. Collagen

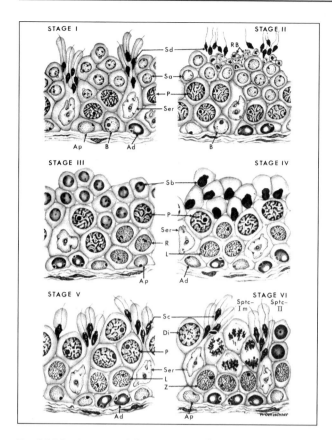

Fig. 22-12 Drawing of the six stages of spermatogenesis in the cycle of the human seminiferous epithelium: Sertoli cell (Ser); dark and pale type A spermatogonia (Ad and Ap; type B spermatogonia (B); resting spermatocyte (R); leptotene spermatocyte (L): pachytene spermatocyte (P); dividing primary spermatocyte (Sptc-Im); spermatids in various stages (Sa, Sb, Sc, Sd); residual bodies (RB). (From Y. Clermont, American Journal of Anatomy, 112:35, 1963.)

fibers are few (Fig. 22-13). In other mammals, notably the opposum, boar, and stallion, the Leydig cells are far more numerous, filling nearly all of the extravascular space of the interstitium.

The Leydig cells are the principal endocrine cell type of the testis, secreting the male sex hormone, **testosterone,** and other androgenic steroids. They appear in the interstitium at puberty and increase to a maximum by age 30 and then slowly decline in number with advancing age. Where they are closely packed, they are irregularly polyhedral and 14–20 µm across. Binucleate cells are common. There is a prominent Golgi complex but no secretory granules, as they secrete continuously without intracellular storage of their product. The cytoplasm contains abundant mitochondria and variable numbers of lipid droplets. There are occasional cisternae of rough endoplasmic reticulum, but the most conspicuous feature of these cells is an extensive smooth endoplasmic reticulum throughout the cytoplasm. Deposits of lipochrome pigment are common and increase with age. A feature unique to the human Leydig cell is the presence, in the cytoplasm, of conspicuous crystals 3 µm or more in diameter and up to 20 µm in length, called the **crystals of Reinke.** Such crystals occur in most men, from puberty to senility, but their number is highly variable. They have the solubility properties of protein. Their significance is unknown.

Blood Vessels and Lymphatics

The **testicular arteries,** arising from the aorta, pass through the inguinal canal and descend into the scrotum

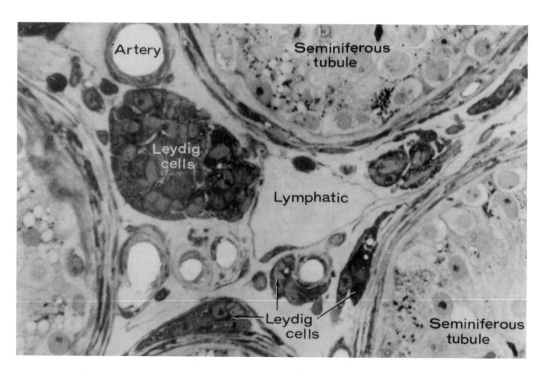

Fig. 22-13 Electron micrograph of interstitial tissue of a mammalian testis. Clusters of Leydig cells are found near blood vessels. Lymphatic vessels are also numerous in the interstitial tissue.

with other components of the **spermatic cord.** Branches in the tunica albuginea enter the parenchyma via the mediastinum and ramify in the interstitium. Each seminiferous tubule is surrounded by a very rich network of fenestrated capillaries. Unusually large sinusoid lymphatics are common in the interstitium (Fig. 22-13). The Leydig cells are not always intimately related to either blood or lymphatic vessels, but their hormone, released into the interstitial fluid, diffuses into both.

Histophysiology

The normal functioning of the testis depends on the maintenance of a temperature about 3°C below normal body temperature (37°C). Cooling of the testis depends, in part, on perspiration and evaporative heat loss from the scrotum. An equally important mechanism depends on a special arrangement of the blood vessels supplying the organ. In the upper scrotum and spermatic cord, a plexus of veins draining blood from the testis closely surrounds the testicular artery. A countercurrent heat-exchange system is thus created, in which the cooler venous blood returning from the testis precools the arterial blood flowing to the testis. In a cold environment, the **cremaster muscle** draws the testes up to a warmer site near the inguinal canal.

Spermatozoa can be thought of as a holocrine secretory product of the seminiferous epithelium. In the human, the number produced daily is very large, 5.6×10^6/g of testicular tissue. The normal **ejaculate** contains 20–40 million spermatozoa. However, these numbers are low compared to other species (viz. rabbit, 25×10^6/gram of testis; boar, 23×10^6 per gram of testis). Taking into account the weight of the boar testes, the daily production would be 16.2×10^9.

Spermatogenesis depends on gonadotrophic hormones secreted by the hypophysis. **Luteinizing hormone (LH)** binds to specific receptors on the Leydig cells. This stimulates production of cyclic AMP and activation of kinases. Cholesterol esterase releases free cholesterol from the lipid droplets in the cytoplasm of the Leydig cells. Mitochondrial enzymes cleave off the side chain of cholesterol to yield **pregnenolone,** and enzymes of the smooth endoplasmic reticulum carry out several steps in its transformation to testosterone. It is calculated that a single Leydig cell can produce 10,000 molecules of testosterone per second. **Follicle-stimulating hormone (FSH)** stimulates Sertoli cell synthesis of androgen-binding protein, which binds testosterone produced by the Leydig cells. There is a feedback control of hypophyseal FSH release by a hormone, **inhibin,** produced by the Sertoli cells.

Testosterone circulating in the blood is essential for maintenance of the function of the prostate, seminal vesicles, and bulbourethral glands. It is also responsible for establishment of the male secondary sex characteristics: pattern of pubic hair, growth of beard, low-pitched voice, and muscular body build.

DUCTS OF THE TESTIS

Tubuli Recti and Rete

The several seminiferous tubules in each lobule of the testis converge upon the **rete testis,** an epithelium-lined plexus in the mediastinum. As they approach the rete, they narrow and are joined to the rete by short **tubuli recti.** The tubuli recti and rete testis are lined by a cuboidal epithelium that does not appear to be secretory. There are microvilli on its free surface and many of the cells have a single long cilium.

Ductuli Efferentes

From the rete testis, 12 or more **ductuli efferentes** conduct the spermatozoa to the ductus epididymidis. They are highly coiled and coalesce to form the single ductus epididymidis. They are lined by an epithelium made up of clusters of columnar ciliated cells alternating with groups of shorter nonciliated cells. The latter have invaginations of their apical membrane, indicating that they take up fluid from the lumen by endocytosis. The action of the cilia on the taller cells moves fluid and spermatozoa toward the epididymis (Fig. 22-14).

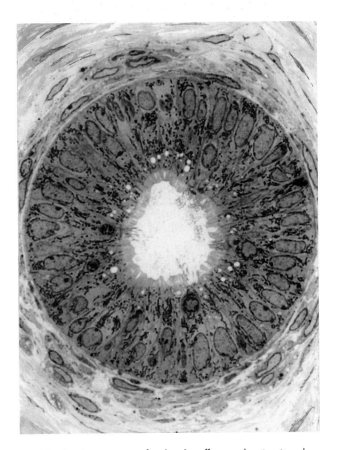

Fig. 22-14 Cross section of a ductulus efferens, showing its columnar epithelium and prominent brush border. (Courtesy of A. Hoffer.)

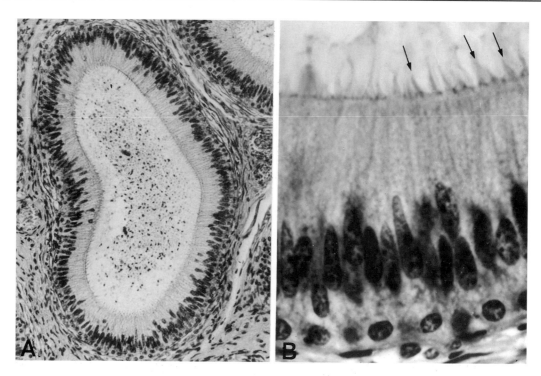

Fig. 22-15 (A) Photomicrograph of cross sections of the ductus epididymidis. The lumen is packed with spermatozoa. (B) Higher magnification of the epithelium of the epididymis. Note the long tufts of stereocilia (at arrows) and the basal cells near the basal lamina.

EPIDIDYMIS

The epididymis is an organ, about 7 cm long, running along the posterior surface of the testis from its upper to its lower pole. It consists of a single, highly convoluted tube, the **ductus epididymidis.** If freed of connective tissue and straightened out, it would be some 6 m in length. At its lower end, it is continuous with the ductus deferens.

The epididymis is the site of accumulation, maturation, and storage of spermatozoa. When the spermatozoa leave the testis, they are physiologically immature, but after 3–5 days in transit through the epididymis, they acquire motility. Products of the epididymal epithelium contribute to their maturation. The duct is lined by a pseudostratified columnar epithelium consisting of two types of cells: **principal cells** and **basal cells** (Fig. 22-15B). The principal cells are very tall in the first part of the duct but decrease in height along its length, becoming cuboidal at its lower end. Each cell has on its free surface a tuft of very long microvilli (Fig. 22-15B). Because they are as long as cilia, but immobile, they are commonly called **stereocilia.** There are numerous shallow invaginations of the membrane between sterocilia, and many vesicles and multivesicular bodies in the apical cytoplasm, indicating that the cells take up fluid from the lumen by pinocytosis. Ninety percent of the volume of fluid leaving the testis is absorbed in the ductuli efferentes and epididymis.

The nucleus of the principal cells, in the lower third of the cytoplasm, is highly irregular in outline. The supranuclear Golgi complex is exceptionally large, but there is no

cytological evidence of its involvement in concentration of a secretory product. However, it has been established that these cells do incorporate amino acids and carbohydrate into a glycoprotein that is released into the lumen and is believed to influence sperm maturation. Large granules throughout the cytoplasm were formerly considered to be secretory granules, but these have now been identified as lysosomes. The small rounded, or pyramidal, basal cells resemble the stem cells of renewing epithelia, but there is no evidence that they have such a role in this epithelium. Their function is unknown.

DUCTUS DEFERENS

In the transition from the ductus epididymidis to the **ductus deferens (vas deferens),** the lumen widens and the wall thickens. The pseudostratified epithelium and its lamina propria form longitudinal folds that give the lumen an irregular cross-sectional outline (Fig. 22-16). The surrounding muscular coat is about 1 mm in thickness and consists of inner and outer longitudinal layers separated by a middle layer of circular smooth muscle. The ductus deferens ascends to the pelvis in the **spermatic cord** that contains the testicular artery, nerves, and the pampiniform plexus of veins. There it expands into a fusiform **ampulla,** in which the mucosa has longer and highly branching folds. Outpocketings between the folds extend a short distance into the muscularis and are lined by pale-staining low-columnar secretory cells. The taper-

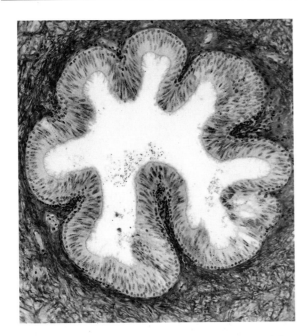

Fig. 22-16 Histological section of the human ductus deferens, showing its irregularly shaped lumen, pseudostratified epithelium, and the surrounding smooth muscle and reticular fibers. (Courtesy of A. Hoffer.)

ing distal portion of the ampulla is joined by the duct of the seminal vesicle. Their confluence forms the **ejaculatory duct,** a tube nearly 2 cm long that opens into the prostatic urethra.

EJACULATORY DUCTS

The mucosa of the ejaculatory ducts forms short folds projecting into the lumen. These are covered by a simple columnar epithelium, but near their termination, the epithelium becomes stratified, and resembles the transitional epithelium that lines the bladder and urethra.

ACCESSORY GLANDS

Seminal Vesicles

The seminal vesicles are a pair of glands about 5 cm long situated behind the neck of the urinary bladder and lateral to the ampulla of the ductus deferens. They have an external layer of connective tissue investing a muscularis that is thinner than that of the ductus deferens and consists of outer longitudinal and inner circular smooth muscle. Each vesicle is a convoluted tube with numerous diverticula along its length that result in a lumen of labyrinthine complexity (Fig. 22-17 [see Plate 30]). In histological sections, thin folds of the mucosa branch into secondary and tertiary folds that bound narrow compartments. These open into a wider central portion of the lumen. They are

lined by pseudostratified epithelium. The cells have sparse microvilli and some have a single cilium. They have a well-developed rough endoplasmic reticulum and abundant secretory granules that resemble those of goblet cells. The secretion of the seminal vesicles, discharged at orgasm, makes up a large fraction of the volume of the ejaculate. It contains fructose that serves as an energy source for the spermatozoa.

Prostate Gland

The prostate is the largest of the accessory glands of the male reproductive tract. It surrounds the urethra at its origin from the urinary bladder. It has a fibrous capsule from which fibroelastic septa extend deep into the gland. Its parenchyma consists of 30 or more highly branched tubuloalveolar glands. Their ducts empty separately into the prostatic urethra. The epithelium is simple columnar but may be cuboidal in the cystic dilatations of the glands (Fig. 22-18 [see Plate 30]). The cells have abundant granular endoplasmic reticulum, a large Golgi complex, and numerous secretory granules. In older individuals, ovoid dense bodies of glycoprotein, called **corpora amylacea (prostatic concretions),** are often found in the lumen of the glands (Fig. 22-19 [see Plate 31]). Their significance is not known. The stroma of the prostate contains smooth-muscle cells that contract during ejaculation, adding its secretory product to the semen. The prostatic secretion contains **acid phosphatase, amylase,** and **fibrinolysin.** It appears to promote sperm motility.

*The cells of the prostate often begin to proliferate slowly in men over 45, leading to **prostatic hyperplasia.** The new nodules of hyperplastic glandular tissue, stroma, and smooth-muscle constrict the urethra running through the center of the gland. There is difficulty in starting to urinate, dribbling after voiding, and incomplete emptying of the bladder. Eighty percent of men in their seventies have this condition. It is treated surgically by transurethral prostatectomy. The third most common cancer of men in this age group is **adenocarcinoma of the prostate** which requires radical prostatectomy.*

Bulbourethral Glands

The paired **bulbourethral glands (Cowper's glands)** (Fig. 22-20 [see Plate 31]) are distal to the prostate and partially embedded in the muscle of the urogenital diaphragm. They are compound tubuloalveolar glands less than 1 cm in diameter, each opening via a single duct into the beginning of the penile urethra. The capsule and the septa within the gland contain both smooth and striated muscle. The nuclei of the cuboidal epithelium are irregular in outline and displaced to the cell base by large numbers of secretory granules. The ducts are lined by epithelium resembling that of the urethra. The secretion is a clear viscous fluid that is thought to have a lubricating function. The bulbourethral glands are the first to be activated during sexual arousal, resulting in the appearance of clear droplets at the urethral meatus of the erect penis.

PENIS

The penis is made up of three cylindrical bodies of erectile tissue: two **corpora cavernosa** dorsally, and a single **corpus spongiosum** ventrally (Fig. 22-21). The corpus spongiosum is expanded at its distal end into the acorn-shaped **glans penis,** which forms a cap over the ends of the two corpora cavernosa. The glans is covered with a fold of skin, the **prepuce** or **foreskin.** The penile urethra runs through the center of the corpus spongiosum for its entire length. In the shaft of the penis, the three corpora are enclosed in a thick connective-tissue sheath called the tunica albuginea, which also forms a partition between the two corpora cavernosa. The tunica is separated from the skin by a layer of loose connective tissue.

The erectile tissue of the corpora is a spongelike mass of endothelium-lined vascular spaces that are fed by **afferent arteries** and drained by **efferent veins.** Dense fibrous trabeculae, containing smooth-muscle cells, extend inward from the tunica albuginea, branching and rejoining to form an elaborate framework around the vascular spaces. A **central artery** in each corpus gives off multiple **helicine arteries** that course in the trabeculae and open into the vascular spaces. These are drained by a number of veins on the inner aspect of the tunica albuginea that penetrate the tunica to join branches of the **deep dorsal vein** of the penis. In the flaccid state, the vascular spaces contain little blood and appear as narrow clefts. During erection, they

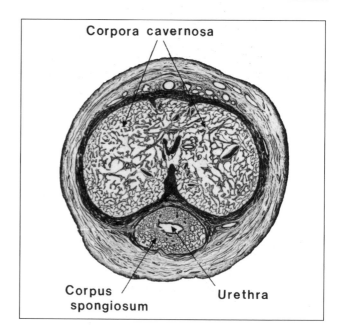

Fig. 22-21 Drawing of a cross section of the penis. The septum between the corpora cavernosa is incomplete in this figure from the distal part of the organ. (Modified from H. Stieve, Männliche Genitalorgane, Handbuch der mikroscopische Anatomie des Menschen, part 2, (von Möllendorff), Julius Springer, Berlin, 1930.)

expand as they become engorged with blood under pressure. Psychic and afferent sensory input cause vasodilation of arteries to the vascular spaces, resulting in their distention. Compression of the peripheral veins against the inner surface of the tunica albuginea retards the outflow from the vascular spaces, contributing to erection. The vascular spaces in the erectile tissue of the corpus spongiosum are much smaller than those of the corpora cavernosa. They communicate with a venous plexus beneath the urethral mucosa.

Scattered along the length of the urethra are small mucous **glands of Littré.** They secrete under the same conditions that activate the bulbourethral glands, and like them, their secretion is thought to have a lubricating function.

QUESTIONS*

1. Very well-developed stereocilia occur in which one, if any, of the following?

   A. seminiferous tubules
   B. straight tubules
   C. epididymis
   D. seminal vesicle
   E. rete testis

2. "Concretions" are found in which of the following?

   A. testis
   B. epididymis
   C. seminal gland
   D. prostate gland
   E. Cowper's gland

3. In the aging male, hypertrophy is common in which one, if any, of the following?

   A. mediastinum
   B. epididymis
   C. Cowper's glands
   D. prostate
   E. none of the above

4. Concerning the ejaculatory duct, which one, if any, of the following is correct?

   A. is part of the urethra
   B. connects the testes with the epididymis
   C. passes through Cowper's gland
   D. drains the seminal vesicles
   E. is located between the epididymis and ductus deferens

5. Concerning the glans penis, which one, if any, of the following is correct?

   A. secretes large quantities of fructose
   B. hypertrophies in old age
   C. is traversed by the ejaculatory duct
   D. appears at puberty
   E. none of the above

6. Concerning the rete testis, which one, if any, of the following is correct?

   A. site of capacitation of the spermatozoa
   B. site of maturation of the spermatozoa
   C. connects with the efferent tubules
   D. connects with the epididymis
   E. none of the above

7. Concerning myoid cells, which one, if any of the following is correct?

   A. control the movements of the epididymis
   B. are common in the prostate
   C. are common in the testis
   D. control the blood flow in the corpora cavernosa
   E. none of the above

8. Spermiogenesis is the process by which

   A. spermatogonia differentiate into spermatids
   B. spermatozoa begin to function
   C. germ cells migrate to the primitive male gonad
   D. spermatids differentiate into spermatozoa
   E. none of the above

9. Capacitation

   A. occurs in the testis
   B. occurs in the epididymis
   C. occurs in the female genital system
   D. involves mitotic activity
   E. occurs in the rete testis

10. Spermatogenesis

   A. begins at birth
   B. begins at puberty
   C. normally ceases at the age of 50
   D. refers to the formation of spermatocytes
   E. refers to change in morphology of spermatozoa

*Answers on page 307.

23

FEMALE REPRODUCTIVE SYSTEM

CHAPTER OUTLINE

KEY WORDS

Amniotic Cavity
Ampulla
Antral Follicle
Antrum
Arcuate Artery
Bartholin's Gland
Broad Ligament
Capacitation
Casein
Cervix
Chorion Frondosum
Chorionic
     Gonadotrophin
Chorion Laeve
Chorionic Villi
Chorion Laeve
Clitoris
Corpus Albicans
Cumulus Oophorus
Cytotrophoblast
Decidua Basalis
Decidua Capsularis
Decidua Functionalis
Decidua Parietalis
Ectoderm
Endoderm
Endometrial Gland
Estradiol
Estrone
Exocoelom
Fimbria
Germinal Epithelium
Glans Clitoridis
Graafian Follicle
Granulosa Cell
Granulosa Lutein Cell
Hymen
Infundibulum

Inner Cell Mass
Interstitial Segment
Isthmus
Labia Majora
Labia Minora
Lactiferous Duct
Lactose
Langerhans Cell
Liquor Folliculi
Menarche
Menopause
Mesovarium
Oocyte
Oogenesis
Oolemma
Ovarian Follicle
Ovary
Oviduct
Placental Lactogen
Polar Body
Primary Oocyte
Primordial Follicle
Progesterone
Prolactin
Stigma
Straight Artery
Syncytiotrophoblast
Theca Externa
Theca Folliculi
Theca Interna
Theca Lutein Cell
Tunica Albuginea
Umbilical Cord
Uterus
Vagina
Yolk Sac
Zona Pellucida

The female reproductive system includes the **ovaries,** the **oviducts,** the **uterus,** the **vagina,** and the **external genitalia** (Fig. 23-1). The uterus and ovaries arise early in embryonic life, but their development is not completed until gonadotrophic hormones of the hypophysis initiate puberty. In the female, puberty involves widespread changes in the body, including increased muscle mass, a increase in adipose tissue over the hips and buttocks, development of the breasts, appearance of axillary and pubic hair, and further growth and differentiation of the ovaries and uterus. The changes in these organs lead to the first menstrual flow, **menarche,** at about age 13. Thereafter, the ovaries and uterus undergo cyclic changes, about 28 days in length throughout a woman's reproductive life. At 50–55 years of age, she enters **menopause,** a period in which the menstrual cycles become irregular and then cease several years later.

OVARY

Each ovary is a slightly flattened ovoid organ, 3 cm in length, 1.5 cm in width and 1 cm in thickness, suspended from the broad ligament of the uterus in a fold of peritoneum called the **mesovarium.** The organ is covered by a low-cuboidal **germinal epithelium,** supported by a pale-staining layer of connective tissue called the **tunica albuginea.** Beneath this is the cortex of the ovary, a highly cellular zone that contains the germ cells (**oocytes**) in **ovarian follicles** in various stages of development (Fig. 23-2). Deep to the cortex is the medulla, the connective-tissue core of the ovary, made up of collagen fibers, fibroblasts, occasional smooth-muscle cells, and numerous tortuous arteries and veins, from which branches radiate into the cortex. The cortex and medulla grade into one another without a clear line of demarcation.

The Oocytes

Oocytes arise in the early embryo from precursors called **oogonia** (primordial germ cells) that first appear in

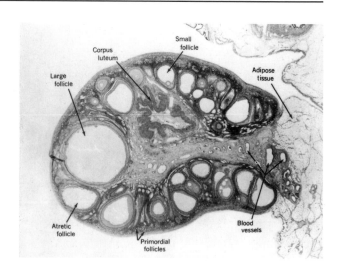

Fig. 23-2 Photomicrograph of a longitudinal section of a monkey ovary, showing its fibrous medulla and a cortex containing numerous follicles in various stages of development. (Courtesy of H. Mizoguti.)

the yolk sac and later migrate into the germinal ridge from which the ovaries develop. There they proliferate by mitotic division until they number in the millions. They then enter prophase of the first meiotic division, but proceed no further. At this stage they are called **primary oocytes.** Although great numbers of these later undergo atresia (degeneration and resorption) both before and after birth, as many as 400,000 are present in the ovaries of a young woman, where they form a conspicuous layer immediately beneath the tunica albuginea (Fig. 23-3).

In the postnatal ovary, the primary oocytes are large, spherical cells, about 25 μm in diameter, each enveloped by a single layer of squamous epithelial cells. An oocyte and its cellular investment constitute a **primordial follicle** (Fig. 23-4). The nucleus of the oocyte has a prominent nucleolus, and with appropriate stains, the meiotic chromosomes can be seen as thin meandering threads in the nucleoplasm. A large number of mitochondria are aggregated near the nucleus. There is a small Golgi complex and the endoplasmic reticulum is represented by tubular profiles with relatively few associated ribosomes.

Development of Follicles

In the years approaching puberty, some of the primordial follicles undergo further development to become **primary follicles** in which the oocyte is surrounded by two or more layers of cuboidal cells (Fig. 23-5B). In each menstrual cycle, after puberty, several primary follicles enter a phase of rapid growth, with further enlargement of the oocyte and proliferation of the surrounding follicular cells, now called **granulosa cells** (Fig. 23-5C). Proliferation of the granulosa cells results in a rapid increase in diameter of the follicle. Glycoprotein is secreted into the space between the oocyte and the innermost granulosa cells and condenses to form a highly refractile layer, called the **zona**

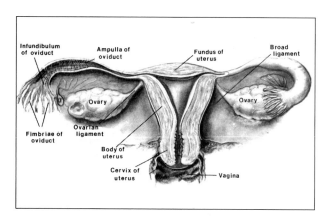

Fig. 23-1 Drawing of the human female reproductive organs.

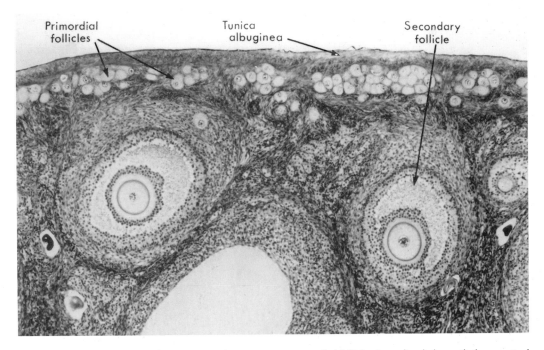

Fig. 23-3 Photomicrograph of a cat ovary showing many primordial follicles immediately beneath the germinal epithelium and antral follicles deeper in the cortex.

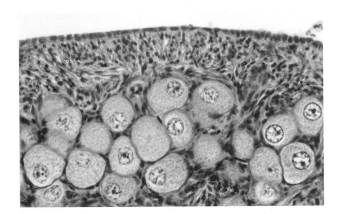

Fig. 23-4 Photomicrograph of a portion of the cortex of a cat ovary containing numerous oocytes in primordial follicles.

pellucida (Fig. 23-6). The granulosa cells and the oocyte are in communication via gap junctions between filiform processes that each extend into the zona pellucida.

Small fluid-filled spaces appear among the proliferating granulosa cells, and when the growing follicle reaches a diameter of about 200 μm, they coalesce to form the **antrum**, a single, fluid-filled cavity of larger size that displaces the oocyte to one side. The oocyte is located in the **cumulus oophorus**, a thickening of the granulosa cell layer that projects into the antrum. At this stage of development the follicle is called an **antral** or **secondary follicle** (Fig. 23-4C). The clear **liquor folliculi** within the antrum is a transudate of blood plasma, but it contains a much higher concentration of steroids and gonadotrophic hormones.

While these events are occurring within the follicle, stromal cells gather around it to form a highly cellular lay-

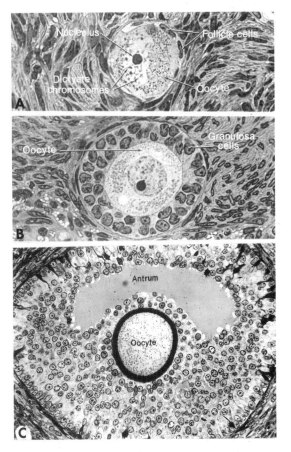

Fig. 23-5 Photomicrographs of early stages of follicular development: (A) a primordial follicle; (B) a primary follicle with two rows of granulosa cells; (C) a secondary follicle. The oocyte and surrounding granulosa cells form its cumulus oophorus projecting into a fluid-filled antrum.

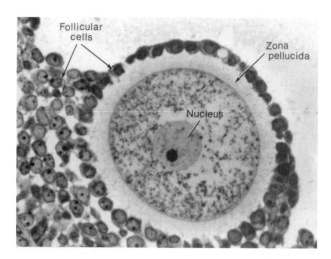

Fig. 23-6 Photomicrograph of a human oocyte in an antral folli-cle. Where is projects into the antrum, it is covered by a single lay-er of granulosa cells with processes embedded in the zona pellucida. Note the great number of mitochondria in the oocyte. (Courtesy of L. Zamboni.)

er with ill-defined outer limits, called the **theca folliculi.** This layer is separated from the granulosa cells by a thick basal lamina. As development progresses, two zones become distinguishable in the theca, a richly vascularized **theca interna** and a less vascular **theca externa.** In their differentiation, the cells of the theca interna acquire an extensive smooth endoplasmic reticulum and other charac-teristics of steroid-secreting cells. They synthesize andro-genic steroids that diffuse into the follicle and are converted to **estradiol** by the granulosa cells. The fibroblastlike cells of the theca externa do not synthesize steroids.

The ovary of a woman of reproductive age contains a very large reserve of primordial follicles, many quiescent primary follicles, and five or six developing antral follicles (Fig. 23-2). In each menstrual cycle, one member of the cohort of follicles that have reached the antral stage becomes dominant and continues to enlarge. Continuing its growth and accumulation of liquor folliculi, the domi-nant follicle attains a diameter of up to 20 mm and bulges from the surface of the ovary. The other members of the cohort of antral follicles undergo **follicular atresia**, a nor-mal process of regression and ultimate degeneration. Of the hundreds of thousands of primordial and primary folli-cles in the ovary of a young woman, fewer than 500 will complete their maturation and release an ovum during her reproductive life span.

> *Exhaustion of the supply of ovarian follicles and loss of the hormones they produce leads to* **menopause** *at about age 50, with cessation of men-strual bleeding, vasomotor instability (hot flashes), and a variety of associated somatic and emotional problems.*

At midcycle (days 13–14) the dominant follicle, now 15–20 mm in diameter, bulges 1 cm or more above the sur-face of the ovary. At this stage of follicular development, the oocyte that began meiotic division during embryonic life but was arrested in prophase resumes division. The nucleus moves near the oolemma and the chromosomes

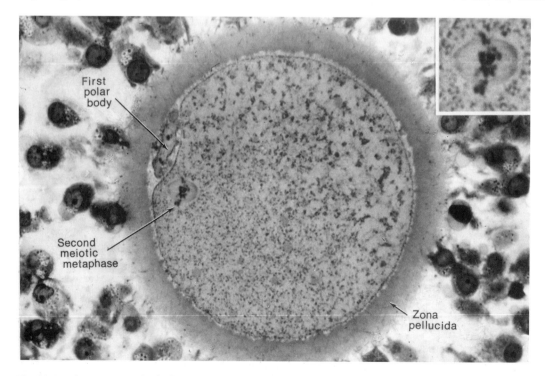

Fig. 23-7 Photomicrograph of a human oocyte at the completion of the first meiotic division. The first polar body can be seen between the oocyte and the zona pellucida, and the chromosomes and spindle of the second meiot-ic division are visible. These are shown at higher magnification in the inset. (Courtesy of L. Zamboni.)

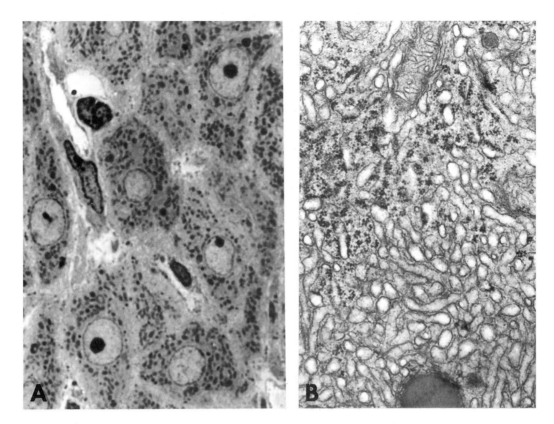

Fig. 23-8 (A) Photomicrograph of cells of the corpus luteum. Note the euchromatic nucleus with large nucleolus, and the large number of mitochondria in the cytoplasm. (B) Electron micrograph of a small area of cytoplasm showing the abundant smooth endoplasmic reticulum.

assemble on the metaphase plate of a spindle oriented tangential to the cell surface. The spindle then rotates 90°, and at anaphase, a small rounded mass of protoplasm around its outer pole projects above the surface of the oocyte. Telophase of this division results in two daughter cells of vastly unequal size—a tiny spherical cell with little cytoplasm, called the **first polar body**, and the huge **secondary oocyte**, which proceeds quickly to metaphase of the second meiotic division (Fig. 23-7), where it is again arrested. While these events are occurring, fluid-filled spaces appear among the granulosa cells at the base of the cumulus oophorus and their coalescence results in detachment of the oocyte. The oocyte now floats free in the liquor folliculi, with a few granulosa cells still adhering to its zona pellucida (Fig. 23-7).

Ovulation

Ovulation has been observed directly in anaesthetized animals and humans. A pale, translucent, oval area, called the **stigma** or **macula pellucida**, appears on the bulging surface of the mature follicle. Its blanching is due to local cessation of blood flow in the capillaries of the theca interna. This is followed by a further thinning of the theca and the overlying tunica albuginea. The thinning is believed to result from a rearrangement of the cells and enzymatic digestion of the collagen fibrils of the theca and tunica

albuginea. Through this thin area, a small translucent vesicle then bulges outward. With a minute or two of its formation, it ruptures and the ovum and adherent cumulus cells pass through the opening, followed by a gush of follicular fluid. The ovum then passes into the oviduct for transport to the uterus.

Corpus Luteum

After ovulation, the wall of the follicle collapses and becomes extensively infolded. Blood vessels and stromal cells invade the previously avascular layer of granulosa cells. The granulosa cells, and those of the theca interna, then hypertrophy (enlarge). They develop smooth reticulum, accumulate lipid droplets, and become plump, pale-staining **lutein cells** that form clusters surrounded by a minimal amount of connective tissue. By these changes, the follicle is transformed into a more or less spherical **corpus luteum**. In the corpus luteum of the human ovary, two kinds of lutein cells are distinguishable. Those arising from the granulosa cells are called **granulosa lutein cells,** whereas smaller, more deeply staining cells, arising from cells of the theca interna are **theca lutein cells.** Both types of lutein cells have an abundance of smooth endoplasmic reticulum, mitochondria with tubular cristae, and lipid droplets in their cytoplasm—characteristics typical of steroid-secreting cells (Fig. 23-8). Despite their similar ultrastructure, they have different functions. The principal steroid secreted by the granulosa lutein cells is **progesterone**, whereas the theca lutein cells secrete mainly **estradiol** and **estrone**.

In a cycle in which the ovum was not fertilized, the corpus luteum regresses in about 9 days. Its lutein cells undergo apoptosis, and invading macrophages phagocytize and digest their residues. A pale-staining fibrous scar, called a **corpus albicans** persists at the site for several months (Fig. 23-9 [see Plate 31]). In a cycle in which the ovum was fertilized and successfully implanted in the uterus, the corpus luteum persists and grows further under the influence of **gonadotrophic hormones** secreted by the developing placenta. For the first 2 months of pregnancy, the hypertrophied corpus luteum is the major source of the steroids needed to maintain pregnancy.

Histophysiology

The cyclic activity of the ovary is dependent on two gonadotrophic hormones of the hypophysis: **follicle-stimulating hormone (FSH)** and **luteinizing hormone (LH)**. Although formation of primary follicles appears to be independent of hormones, their further development to antral follicles, and beyond, requires FSH which stimulates proliferation of granulosa cells and activates an enzyme that is essential for steroid synthesis. Cells of the theca interna secrete androgenic steroid precursors that diffuse into the follicle, where the granulosa cells convert them to estradiol. Proliferation of granulosa cells and their synthesis of an increasing amount of estradiol, raises the concentration of this hormone in the blood. These increased levels, in turn, act back upon the hypothalamus and hypophysis, stimulating a midcycle surge of LH that induces ovulation. Thereafter, the granulosa cells reduce their production of estradiol and secrete increasing amounts of progesterone,

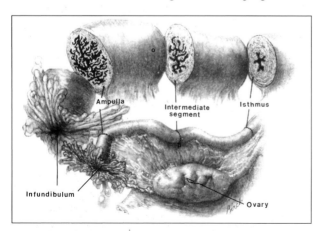

Fig. 23-10 Drawing illustrating the mucosal pattern of the several segments of the oviduct. Location of the cross sections is indicated on the intact oviduct below. (From M.J. Eastman and L.M. Hellman, eds., *Williams Obstetrics*, 13th ed., Appleton, Century, Crofts, New York, 1961; labeling added.)

the hormone that prepares the uterine mucosa for reception of the ovum. The elevated level of LH triggering ovulation is also responsible for the transformation of the postovulatory follicle into a corpus luteum.

THE OVIDUCTS

The oviducts are two tubes, about 12 cm in length, extending laterally from the fundus of the uterus, in the free upper border of the broad ligament (Fig. 21-1, Fig. 23-10). The oviduct receives the ovum, provides an appropriate environment for its fertilization, and transports it to the uterus. Four regions are distinguished. The portion traversing the wall of the uterus is its **interstitial segment.** The slender medial third is the **isthmus.** Lateral to this, it expands slightly to form the **ampulla**, and this is continuous with the funnel-shaped **infundibulum,** which opens into the peritoneal cavity near the lateral pole of the ovary. Radiating from the ostium (opening) of the infundibulum are numerous slender tapering processes, called the **fimbriae** of the oviduct (Fig. 23-10).

The wall of the oviduct consists of a moderately thick layer of smooth muscle covered by a thin serosa of peritoneum. In its interior, the mucosa forms longitudinal folds projecting into its lumen. These vary in their length and degree of branching in the four segments of the oviduct. In the interstitial segment and isthmus, they are simply low ridges. Farther laterally, they increase in length and number and become elaborately branched thin folia (leaflike structures) in the ampulla. In cross sections at this level, the lumen is a labyrinthine system of narrow spaces between the numerous ramifying folia (Fig. 23-11).

The oviduct is lined by a simple columnar epithelium. Its cells are tall in the infundibulum and ampulla but gradually decrease in height toward the uterus. They are of two types: ciliated and nonciliated (Fig. 23-12 [see Plate 31]). Their relative numbers and activity are influenced by the level of circulating estrogens. Early in the **follicular phase** of the cycle, the cells become taller and begin to form cilia. In the **preovulatory phase,** the mean percentage of ciliated cells on the fimbriae is 48%, but it declines to about 4% in the late **luteal phase.** Cyclic changes are also evident in the nonciliated cells, which show evidence of increased synthetic activity, which reaches a peak at midcycle and declines thereafter.

The beating of cilia on the fimbriae creates currents in the overlying film of fluid that move the fertilized ovum into the tubal infundibulum, and those of the ampulla and isthmus contribute to its transport to the uterus. The function of the nonciliated cells is less well understood. Although the nature of their secretion is not known, it probably creates an intralumenal environment that sustains the motility of the spermatozoa and enables them to undergo **capacitation,** the series of biochemical changes that enables them to fertilize an ovum. The environment must also enable the fertilized

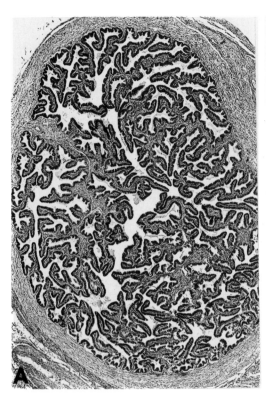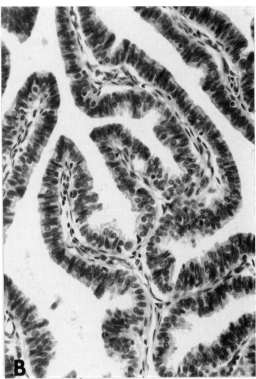

Fig. 23-11 Photomicrographs of the ampulla of the oviduct of a 23-year-old woman. (A) Low magnification to show the elaborately branching folia of the mucosa reducing the lumen to a labyrinthine system of narrow clefts. (B) Higher magnification of one of the folds of mucosa showing the columnar epithelium.

ovum to develop to the multicellular blastocyst stage during its passage down the oviduct.

The muscularis of the oviducts does not have distinct layers. The innermost bundles of smooth muscle are mainly circular, but toward the periphery, longitudinal bundles appear in increasing number, and near the surface, bundles with this orientation predominate. Bundles of smooth muscle extend into the fimbriae, and their contraction, as well as that of the muscularis of the infundibulum, brings the ostium of the oviduct into close contact with the ovary at midcycle, favoring entry of the fertilized ovum. Rhythmic contractions then sweep along the oviduct toward the isthmus, contributing to ovum transport.

UTERUS

The human uterus is a pear-shaped organ with a thick muscular wall. It is about 7 cm long, 4 cm wide at its upper end, and 2.5 cm in depth. It is slightly flattened anteroposteriorly and is normally tipped forward. Its rounded upper portion is referred to as the **fundus,** and its wide upper two thirds is the body, or **corpus.** A narrower portion below this is the **isthmus,** and a cylindrical lower segment is the **cervix** (Fig. 23-1). The lower end of the cervix that projects into the vagina is its **portio vaginalis.** The flattened uterine cavity is triangular in outline and is continuous with the lumen of the

interstitial segment of the oviducts on either side of the fundus. At its narrow lower end, the lumen is continuous with the **cervical canal,** which opens into the vagina.

Myometrium

The myometrium is 1.25 cm thick and is made up of interlacing bundles of smooth muscle separated by connective tissue. Four ill-defined layers can be distinguished. In the two innermost layers, the orientation of the smooth muscle is mainly longitudinal. The next layer is less compact and contains numerous blood vessels. Peripheral to this is a layer in which circularly oriented fibers predominate, and in the thin outermost layer, they are again longitudinal. The two outermost layers are continuous with the muscularis of the oviducts. Smooth muscle decreases and connective tissue increases in the isthmus of the uterus, and the cervix consists almost exclusively of dense connective tissue containing many elastic fibers. During pregnancy, considerable enlargement of the uterus is required to accommodate the growing fetus. This is accomplished by hypertrophy of the existing smooth-muscle cells and addition of new cells. There is also an increase in the collagen content of the uterine wall. After pregnancy, these changes are reversed by a decrease in the size and number of smooth muscle cells.

Leiomyoma (fibroid tumor) is the most common tumor of women (1 in 4). It is a benign tumor derived from smooth-muscle cells of the myometrium. The cells proliferate slowly in a concentric pattern and the tumor may attain a diameter of several centimeters. They are usually asymptomatic but may cause excessive menstrual bleeding.

The **cervix** surrounds a cervical canal about 3 cm in length that is continuous above with the uterine lumen through a constriction called the **internal os.** It is continuous below with the vagina through the **external os.** The canal is lined by tall columnar epithelial cells with nuclei displaced to the base by mucous droplets that occupy much of the cytoplasm. Highly branched **cervical glands,** extending into the submucosa, are lined by a similar epithelium. The mucus secreted by these glands contains the enzyme lysozyme. It cleaves the proteoglycans of bacterial cell walls and is believed to be important in the defenses against the bacterial flora of the lower reproductive tract. Near the external os, there is an abrupt transition from simple columnar epithelium to stratified squamous epithelium covering the portion of the cervix that projects into the vagina. The wall of the cervix contains few smooth-muscle cells and is composed mainly of dense connective tissue. Late in pregnancy, changes in the fibrous and amorphous components make the cervix softer and more pliable, facilitating its dilatation by the advancing head of the fetus.

Endometrium

Endometrium is the term applied to the mucosa lining the uterine cavity. It consists of a simple columnar epithelium from which tubular glands extend downward into a very thick lamina propria, commonly referred to as the **endometrial stroma.** From puberty until menopause, the endometrium undergoes monthly cyclic changes in its thickness and histological appearance in response to fluctuating levels of ovarian hormones. At the end of a cycle in which no ovum is fertilized, the greater part of its thickness sloughs off, accompanied by extravasation of blood from the vessels of its stroma. The products of these degenerative changes appear as a bloody vaginal discharge, the **menstrual flow,** that continues for 3–5 days.

Two zones of the endometrium are distinguished. The upper half to two-thirds, which will be sloughed off at the next menstrual flow, is called the **functionalis,** whereas the deeper portion which persists and regenerates the functionalis in the next cycle is called the **basalis.** To understand the changes occurring in menstruation, some knowledge of the blood supply is needed. The uterine arteries course longitudinally in the **broad ligament** along the sides of the uterus. Branches penetrate to the

vascular layer of the myometrium. Their branches, called **arcuate arteries,** take a circumferential course to the midline where they anastomose with arcuate arteries from the other side. Penetrating branches of the arcuate arteries, called **straight arteries**, give off lateral branches that supply the basalis of the endometrium and continue as **coiled** or **spiral arteries** that supply the functionalis. Late in the menstrual cycle, there is a vasoconstriction of the coiled arteries that leads to the necrotic changes in the endometrium culminating in menstruation.

Cyclic Changes

For descriptive purposes the menstrual cycle is divided into **proliferative, secretory,** and **menstrual phases.** The proliferative phase coincides with the secretion of estrogens by the developing follicles, the secretory phase is correlated with the secretion of progesterone by the functional corpus luteum, and the menstrual phase is associated with a rapid decline in hormonal stimulation.

Proliferative Phase: Beginning at the end of the menstrual flow, on about the 5th day of the cycle, and extending to day 14, proliferation of cells in the epithelium of the basalis results in restoration of the surface epithelium and a progressive lengthening of the **endometrial glands.** This is accompanied by active proliferation of the stromal cells. These regenerative changes in the first 2 weeks of an ideal 28-day cycle, result in growth of the endometrium from a postmenstrual thickness of 0.5 mm to 2–3 mm. The glands are initially relatively straight and lined by a columnar epithelium (Fig. 23-13A,B). Later, they become more sinuous (Figs. 23-13D and 23-13E) and their columnar epithelial cells accumulate glycogen, displacing the nucleus toward the apex. Concurrent with these changes, the coiled portions of the branches of the arcuate arteries, that were lost during menses, regenerate and take on a spiral course as they lengthen. By the 14th day of the cycle, the endometrium has completed its regeneration and is prepared for receipt of an implanting blastocyst (Fig. 23-13B).

Secretory Phase: In this phase, extending from the 15th to the 28th day of the cycle, the glands of the functionalis become more tortuous and acquire lateral sacculations that result in a larger lumen, irregular in outline (Figs. 23-13C). The glycogen content of the cells diminishes and the lumen contains a glycoprotein secretion. The glands in the basalis remain more slender and their walls are relatively straight. Elongation and convolution of the coiled arteries continues and the stroma becomes edematous.

Menstrual Phase: In a cycle in which an ovum is not fertilized, marked vascular changes begin in the endometrium about 2 weeks after ovulation. The endometrium is blanched for hours at a time, owing to constriction of the coiled arteries. The glands cease to secrete and the stroma is invaded by large numbers of leukocytes. After about 2 days of intermittent interruption of blood flow, the vasoconstriction of the coiled arteries becomes continuous,

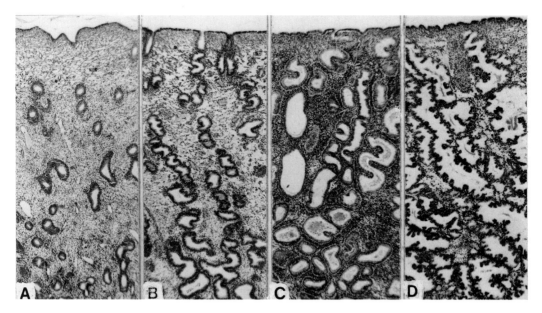

Fig. 23-13 Photomicrographs of the human endometrium in different phases of its differention: (A) proliferative phase, 9th day of cycle. (B) early secretory phase, 15th day; (C) later secretory phase, 19th day; (D) gestational hyperplasia, 12th day of pregnancy. (Courtesy of A. Hertig.)

depriving the functionalis of oxygenated blood, while blood flow to the basalis is uninterrupted. The ischemic (blood deficient) functionalis begins to degenerate. Several hours later, the constricted arteries reopen, but the walls of their distal portions, now damaged by ischemia, rupture and blood escapes into the stroma and breaks out into the uterine lumen. This is followed by exfoliation (shedding) of clumps of necrotic endometrium, and by the third or fourth day of menses, the entire functionalis of the endometrium has sloughed off. Blood loss is normally about 35 ml, but larger amounts are common. The basalis remains intact and soon begins to regenerate a new functionalis.

Endometriosis is a condition in which endometrial tissue exists outside of the uterine cavity, on the ovaries, on the broad ligament of the uterus, or on the pelvic floor. Opinion is divided as to whether it is caused by regurgitation of bits of endometrium through the oviducts during menstruation, or abnormal differentiation from peritoneum. Patients complain of abdominal pain and dymenorrhea (painful menstruation).

Histophysiology

The changes in the endometrium described above are dictated by hormones produced by the ovary. The corpus luteum that formed after ovulation degenerates toward the end of an anovulatory cycle and the consequent rapid decline in circulating progesterone and estradiol results in cessation of secretion and early regressive changes in the functionalis of the endometrium. The falling level of these hormones also triggers the vascular changes in the endometrium that culminate in menstruation. On the other hand, if fertilization and implantation have occurred, **chorionic gonadotrophins** secreted by the developing placenta result in the maintenance of the corpus luteum, now called the **corpus luteum of pregnancy,** and it continues to secret **estrogen** and **progesterone,** which stimulate further endometrial development and secretion (Fig. 23-13D).

FERTILIZATION

While ovulation is in progress, the fimbria of the oviduct are sweeping over the surface of the ovary. Beating of cilia on their epithelium creates currents in the film of fluid on that surface, drawing the ovum into the oviduct, where spermatozoa await its arrival. The granulosa cells adhering to the ovum's **zona pellucida** are quickly dispersed exposing its surface. The zona is composed of three glycoproteins that have been designated **ZP1, ZP2,** and **ZP3.** In its formation in the developing ovarian follicle, molecules of ZP2 and ZP3 copolymerized to form microfilaments that are cross-linked by molecules of ZP1 to form a firm meshwork in the zona. Certain oligosaccharides of ZP3 serve as sperm receptors. A specific protein in the plasmalemma of the sperm head binds to the receptors on the zona and this binding triggers the **acrosome reaction** of the spermatozoon (Fig. 23-14). This involves fusion of the acrosomal membrane with the overlying plasmalemma at multiple sites, creating openings through which enzymes of the acrosome are released. These digest a channel through the zona pellucida, through which the

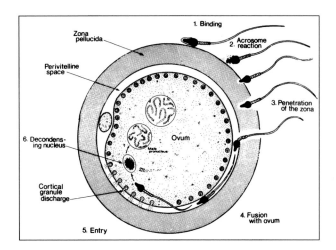

Fig. 23-14 Diagram of the various steps in fertilization of an ovum. (1) Sperm head binds to zona; (2) acrosome reaction is induced; (3) zona is penetrated; (4) sperm head binds to oolemma and the membranes fuse; (5) sperm head sinks into ooplasm and its nucleus decondenses in preparation for its conjugation with the oocyte nucleus.

vigorously motile spermatozoon enters the perivitelline space between the zona and the oolemma. The membrane on the postacrosomal region of the sperm head then fuses with the oolemma and the sperm nucleus enters the cytoplasm of the ovum, where its chromatin begins to decondense. Fusion of the membranes triggers the **cortical reaction** of the ovum. Thousands of **cortical granules** in its peripheral cytoplasm undergo exocytosis, releasing enzymes into the perivitelline space. These destroy the sperm-receptors of the zona pellucida, thus preventing the

binding and entry of other spermatozoa.

Entry of the spermatozoon into the ovum initiates completion of the second meiotic division, which production of a second polar body. This is followed by completion of fertilization by fusion of the decondensed sperm nucleus with the nucleus of the ovum, restoring the diploid chromosome number.

IMPLANTATION

As the fertilized ovum passes down the oviduct, it divides repeatedly, forming a small spherical mass of cells, called the **morula.** Upon reaching the lumen of the uterus on about the fourth day, it consists of many more cells, and these have become arranged in a fluid-filled hollow sphere called the **blastocyst.** After a day or two in the lumen of the uterus, this attaches to the surface of the secretory endometrium (Figs. 23-15, and 23-16A). At this stage, there is a cluster of cells at one pole of the blastocyst, called the **inner cell mass,** that is destined to form the embryo proper. The remainder of the sphere consists of **trophoblast cells** that actively invade the endometrium (Figs. 23-16A and 23-16B). Rapid proliferation of the trophoblast gives rise to an inner layer of **cytotrophoblast,** made up of separate cells, and an outer layer of **syncytiotrophoblast,** which is a multinucleate layer of protoplasm in which no cell boundaries are discernible. The cytotrophoblast is mitotically active and the new cells formed fuse with and are incorporated into the surrounding syncytial trophoblast.

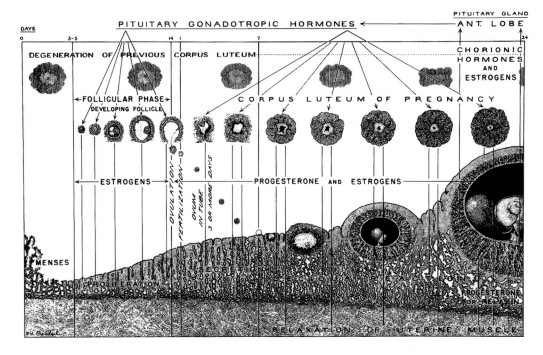

Fig. 23-15 Diagrammatic representation of the histological changes in the endometrium and correlated changes in the follicle and corpusluteum in the ovary. The hormones controlling these events are also shown. (From N.J. Eastman, ed., William's Obstetrics, 11th ed., Appleton, Century, Crofts, New York, 1956.)

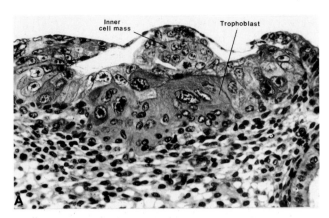

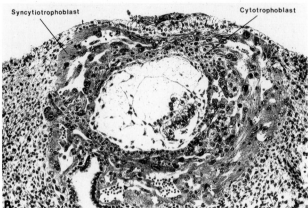

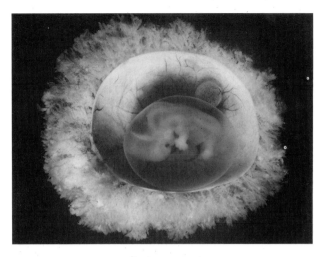

Fig. 23-17 Photograph of a 40-day human embryo (Carnegie No. 8537) showing the myriad placental villi projecting from the entire surface of the chorion frondosum. (From D.G. McKay and M.V. Richardson, American Journal of Obstetrics and Gynecology 69:735, 1955; courtesy of Carnegie Institution of Washington).

Fig. 23-16 Photomicrographs of early human implantation sites. (A) At 7 days, the embryo is a small sphere of cells called the inner cell mass. On one side, the the trophobast is invading the endometrium. (B) At 9 days, the embryo is a bilaminar disk. The differentiation of inner cytotrophoblast and outer syncytiotrophoblast is now evident, and lacunae are appearing in the syncytiotrophoblast. (From A. Hertig and J. Rock, Carnegie Contributions to Embryology. No 125, 1941. Courtesy of Carnegie Institution of Washington.)

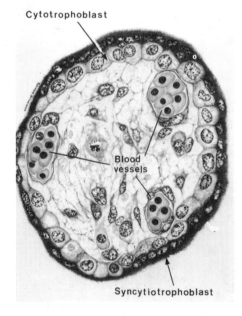

Fig. 23-18 Drawing of a placental villus from a human embryo. Cytotrophoblast on the inside and syncytial trophoblast on the outside. Vessels in the mesenchyme of the core contain nucleated primitive erythroblasts.

Erosion of the the endometrium by the trophoblast enables the embryo and its investments to sink deeper into it. By the 9th to 11th day, it is entirely within the endometrium, surrounded by a thin layer of cytotrophoblast and a thicker layer of syncytial trophoblast (Fig. 23-16B). As this outer layer continues to invade the endometrium, it becomes permeated by a labyrinthine system of intercommunicating lacunae, filled with blood liberated from endometrial blood vessels eroded by the syncytial trophoblast. At 11 days after ovulation, the embryo proper is a bilaminar disk consisting of a plate of columnar epithelial cells, the **ectoderm**, and a thinner layer of cuboidal cells, the **endoderm**. At its margins, the ectodermal plate is continuous with a thin layer of squamous cells that enclose a small **amniotic cavity** (Fig. 23-16B). The endoderm is continuous at its margins with a sheet of squamous cells that enclose the **yolk sac**. Between these structures and the trophoblast, there is a space, called the **exocoelem**, which is traversed by thin strands of **extraembryonic mesenchyme** (Fig. 23-16B). The broad peripheral zone of trophoblast is henceforth referred to as the **chorion**.

From the 15th day onward, cords of trophoblast grow outward into the endometrium forming the **primary chorionic villi.** These are soon invaded at their base by mesenchyme that advances in their interior to their tips, converting the primary villi into **secondary chorionic villi** (Fig. 23-17). These consist of an outer layer of syncytiotrophoblast and an inner layer of cytotrophoblast around a core of mesenchyme (Fig. 23-18). The villi are bathed by blood flowing sluggishly through a system of lacunae that collectively form the **intervillous space**. From the ends of the secondary chorionic villi, columns of syncytial trophoblast grow across this intervillous space, and upon reaching the other side, they spread along it, coalescing with similar outgrowths of neighboring villi to form a continuous **trophoblastic shell**, interrupted only at sites of communication of maternal blood vessels with the intervillous space. Throughout the remainder of pregnancy, the intervillous space is lined by trophoblast and traversed by villi that are fixed to the maternal tissue by their continuity with the trophoblastic shell or **basal plate** (Fig. 23-19). The villi absorb nutrients from the maternal blood and excrete wastes into it.

Meanwhile, endothelial-lined spaces have developed in the mesenchyme within the cores of the villi and these coalesce to form blood vessels that communicate with vessels that are developing in the **body stalk** (later to become the umbilical cord). By the 22st day, the embryo has developed a heart, and fetal blood then begins to circulate through the vessels of the placental villi. Thereafter, these are referred to as **tertiary villi.** Later in pregnancy, the villi begin to branch and their branching continues in the weeks that follow increasing their total surface area.

The endometrium responds to invasion by the trophoblast with changes in its stroma. The fusiform stromal cells enlarge and take on a polygonal epithelioid form and are henceforth called **decidual cells** (Fig. 23-20 [see Plate 32]). The endometrium so modified is referred to as the **decidua.** The portion of the decidua beneath the developing embryo is termed the **decidua basalis;** the portion extending over its adlumenal surface is called the **decidua capsularis.** That lining the rest of the uterus, away from the products of conception, is the **decidua vera.** The contact of the fetal trophoblast with the maternal decidua is a confrontation between cells of different genotypes. Why fetal cells bearing antigens inherited from the father are not subject to immunological rejection is still not understood.

During the first 8 weeks of pregnancy, villi are equally numerous around the entire circumference of the chorion (Fig. 23-17), but thereafter the villi penetrating the decidua basalis rapidly increase in number and length, whereas those penetrating the decidua capsularis degenerate. By the third month, the adlumenal portion of the chorion, now devoid of villi, is smooth and relatively avascular and is called the **chorion laeve.** The portion invading the decidua basalis is now called the **chorion frondosum.** This discoid basal area of long trophoblastic villi will go on to form the fetal portion of the definitive **placenta.** By that time, the branching of the villi has continued until their total surface area is about 10 m². The additional surface area achieved by the microvilli of the syncytial trophoblast would probably bring the total surface to nearly 90 m².

By four and half months of gestation, the uterine lumen is largely obliterated by the growing fetus and its membranes. The decidua capsularis has degenerated and the chorion laeve has fused with the decidua vera on the opposite side of the uterine lumen. The subsequent develop-

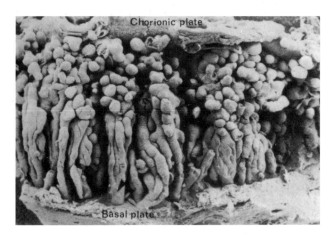

Fig. 23-19 *Scanning electron micrograph of a portion of the placental disk of a macaque at 31 days of gestation. Near the chorionic plate, the villi are developing numerous side branches. (From B. King, Anatomy and Embryology 165:361, 1982.)*

ment of the placenta involves a great increase in the number and length of the villi of the chorion frondosum and expansion of the blood-filled intervillous spaces.

In the fetal portion of the developing placenta, the cytotrophoblast cells cease to divide and progressively decrease in number. By the fifth month, those remaining no longer form a continuous layer. These remanents ultimately fuse with and are incorporated into the syncytial trophoblast. The syncytial trophoblast is not of uniform thickness. Thick areas containing clusters of nuclei alternate with thin areas devoid of nuclei. Dilated fetal capillaries, in the core of the villi, are closely applied to the thin areas, so the barrier between the fetal and maternal blood is little more than 2 μm in thickness, facilitating gas exchange between them.

Histophysiology of the Placenta

Blood, poor in oxygen, is carried from the fetus to the placenta in the **umbilical arteries** and circulates in the capillaries of the placental villi. Venous blood returning from the villi is carried via the **umbilical veins** to their junction with the inferior vena cava near the heart. On the maternal side of the circulation, blood from the arcuate arteries of the uterus passes through coiled arteries of the decidua into the intervillous space, where it flows over the surface of the placental villi and through communications between the intervillous space and veins of the decidua basalis. Oxygen, carbon dioxide, fatty acids and electrolytes can pass through the syncytiotrophoblast by diffusion. Amino acids cross the barrier by active transport. Immunoglobulins and other macromolecules are taken up by receptor-mediated endocytosis and moved across the barrier in transport vesicles.

The placenta is a major endocrine organ producing hormones essential for maintenance of pregnancy. **Chorionic** gonadotrophin, one of the hormones secreted by the trophoblast, is detectable very early in pregnancy and increases rapidly up to the fifth month. It is similar to luteinizing hormone of the hypophysis and serves to maintain the corpus luteum in the maternal ovary and to stimulate its secretion of progesterone. The placenta also secretes **progesterone** that acts locally on the endometrium, stimulating proliferation of cells of the decidua. It also acts on the myometrium, inhibiting uterine contraction during pregnancy. In many mammals, the placenta also secretes **placental lactogen,** a hormone that stimulates development of the mammary gland of the mother, in anticipation of parturition. No such action has been verified for the human.

FEMALE GENITALIA

The genitalia of the female include the **vagina,** the **clitoris,** the **labia majora,** and the **labia minora.** The vagina is a fibromuscular tube 8–9 cm in length extending from the uterine cervix to the vestibule of the external genitalia. In the virgin, its opening is partially closed by a crescentic fold, or fenestrated membrane, called the **hymen.** The vaginal mucosa consists of stratified squamous epithelium, 150–200 µm thick, with a lamina propria rich in elastic fibers. As in the epidermis, antigen-presenting Langerhans cells are present in the lower layers of the epithelium. The superficial cells of the epithelium undergo little keratinization. Their cytoplasm is filled with glycogen in the middle of the menstrual cycle, but this diminishes later in the cycle. Cells are constantly exfoliating from the epithelium of the cervix and vagina, and leukocytes, which abound in the lamina propria, migrate through the epithelium into the lumen. Examination of these cells in **vaginal smears** is a common clinical procedure for detection of cells exfoliated from early cancer of the cervix uteri. The vaginal epithelium has no associated glands and the film of fluid that lubricates its surface is evidently contributed, in large measure, by the glands in the cervix. The relatively thin muscularis of the vagina is composed of interlacing bundles of smooth muscle oriented both longitudinally and circumferentially, with longitudinal bundles greatly predominating in the outer half of the muscular coat.

The **labia majora** are two rounded longitudinal folds that extend from the mons pubis anteriorly to the perineum posteriorly. On their lateral surface, the skin bears coarse hairs. On their inner surface, the skin is smooth, hairless, and contains multiple sebaceous glands. The interior of the folds consists mainly of adipose tissue.

The **labia minora,** medial to the labia majora, are thin flexible folds covered with stratified squamous epithelium that has a very thin keratinized layer. It is devoid of hairs but contains numerous sebaceous glands. The labia minora have a core of spongy connective tissue containing networks of elastic fibers. Unlike the labia majora, they contain no adipose tissue. The space between the two labia

minora is called the **vestibule.** It contains the orifices of the urethra, anteriorly, and of the vagina, posteriorly. The labia converge anteriorly and form a thin fold over the dorsum of the **clitoris,** the homolog of the penis. This fold is comparable to the prepuce on the penis in the male. The clitoris is made up of two very small cylinders of erectile tissue that end in a small **glans clitoridis,** corresponding to the glans penis of the male.

Two **glands of Bartholin,** about 1 cm in diameter, open onto the medial surface of the labia minora. They are tubuloalveolar glands corresponding to the bulbourethral glands of the male. They secrete a lubricating mucus. Several smaller mucus-secreting **vestibular glands** around the opening of the urethra correspond to the glands of Littré in the male.

MAMMARY GLANDS

Although not strictly a part of the reproductive tract, the mammary glands are important accessory glands that have evolved in mammals to nourish their offspring. In the human female, they reach their greatest development at about age 20. Atrophic changes begin at 40 and become marked after the menopause. In addition to these long-term changes related to age, the breasts undergo slight changes in size in each menstrual cycle, and striking changes in size and functional activity during pregnancy and lactation.

The mammary gland is a compound tubuloalveolar gland consisting of 15–20 lobes drained by an equal number of **lactiferous ducts** that open at the tip of the **mammary papilla** (nipple). The lobes are separated by connective tissue and varying amounts of adipose tissue. Unlike other major glands, which have a single large duct, the mammary gland is an assemblage of independent units, each having its own excurrent duct. Within the nipple, each lactiferous duct is slightly dilated to form a **lactiferous sinus.**

Inactive Gland

At birth, the gland consists only of short branching lactiferous ducts with no associated alveoli. As puberty approaches, the ducts elongate and branch under the influence of ovarian hormones, and small spherical masses of epithelial cells appear at the ends of the smallest branches of the duct system. These do not have a lumen but are capable of developing into functional acini later, in response to appropriate hormonal stimulation. Between the epithelial cells and the basal lamina, are stellate **myoepithelial cells** which have several long radiating processes. These form a wide-meshed network around each spherical mass of epithelial cells. In the adult female, cyclic changes in the glandular tissue are minimal. The slight increase in breast size and sense of fullness experienced by some

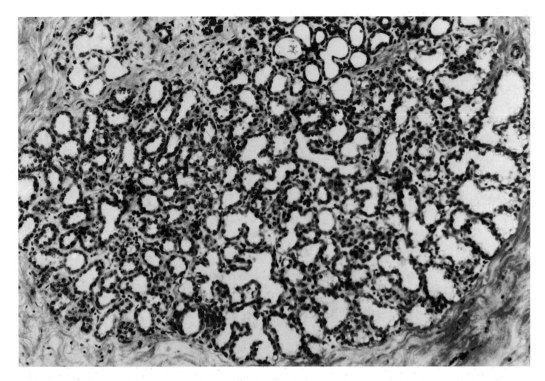

Fig. 23-21 Photomicrograph of a small area of human mammary gland at 8 months of pregnancy. The gland is prepared for lactation but is not yet secreting.

women around midcycle are probably due to increased blood flow and some edema of the connective tissue of the breast.

> *Carcinoma of the breast is a common malignant tumor of older women. It is relatively slow growing, and with frequent physical examinations, it can often be detected early enough for a successful surgical cure.*

Active Gland

The elevated levels of estrogens and progesterone, during pregnancy bring about major changes in the mammary glands. There is rapid growth in length and branching of the duct system, expansion of the pre-existing spheres of cells at the ends of the ducts, and a proliferation of additional true acini (Fig. 23-21). These changes are accompanied by increasing infiltration of the stroma by lymphocytes, plasma cells, and eosinophils. The histological appearance of different regions of the active gland varies considerably, suggesting that not all areas are in the same functional state at the same time. In some areas, the walls of dilated acinar ducts and acini are thin and the lumen is filled with milk. In other areas, the lumen is narrow and the epithelium taller. Thus, the epithelial cells vary from columnar to low cuboidal. They are generally acidophilic but may have some basophilia

near the base. Droplets of lipid accumulate in the cytoplasm and in the lumen (Fig. 23-22).

In electron micrographs, there are parallel arrays of cisternae of the rough endoplasmic reticulum in the basal

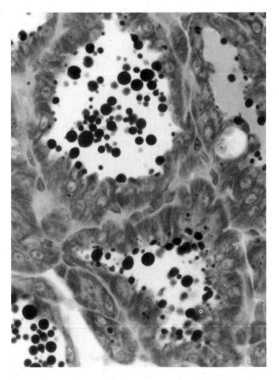

Fig. 23-22 Photomicrograph of lactating mammary gland of a mouse, fixed in osmium tetroxide to preserve lipid. There are many lipid droplets in the lumen. (Courtesy of N. Feder.)

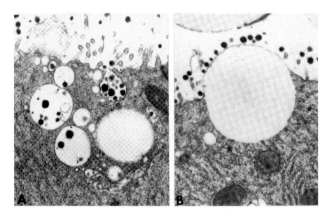

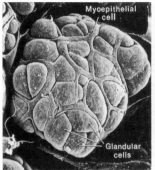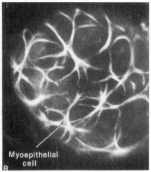

Fig. 23-23 Electron micrographs of mammary gland secretion. (A) Exocytosis of vesicles containing multiple, small granules of milk protein; (B) lipid droplet protruding into the lumen covered by a portion of the apical plasma membrane. It would later be extruded, enveloped in a detached portion of the cell membrane. (Courtesy of A. Ichikawa.)

Fig. 23-24 (A) Scanning micrograph of an acinus of the mammary gland showing myoepithelial cells occupying grooves between the bases of the secretory cells. (Courtesy of T. Nagato, Cell Tissue Research 209:1, 1980.) (B) Acinus of a mammary gland stained with a fluorescent probe for actin. (Courtesy of J. Emerman and W. Vogl, Anatomy Record 216:405, 1986.

cytoplasm, and a large supranuclear Golgi complex. Two distinct types of secretory product are identifiable: (1) vesicles containing multiple, small, dense granules and (2) large droplets of lipid. The mode of secretion of these two products differs. The protein-containing vesicles arise in the Golgi complex and fuse with the apical plasmalemma, discharging their content, as in other glandular cells (Fig. 23-23A). The synthesis of the lipid component of milk does not appear to involve the endoplasmic reticulum or the Golgi complex. Small lipid droplets arise throughout the cytoplasm and fuse to form progressively larger lipid drops. These project into the lumen of the acinus covered only by the plasmalemma and they are then pinched off, enclosed in a detached portion of the cell membrane (Fig. 22-23B).

At the base of the epithelium, processes of the myoepithelial cells occupy recesses in the base of the epithelial cells (Fig. 22-24A). They are filled with actin filaments. In whole mounts, these can be stained with a fluorescent specific probe for actin (Fig. 22-24B). Lymphocytes are occasionally found between the bases of the epithelial cells, and plasma cells are common in the surrounding connective tissue.

Histophysiology

The growth and differentiation of the ducts and acini of the gland, initiated by increased estrogens and progesterone in the early weeks of pregnancy, continues after the placenta becomes the dominant source of these hormones. Actual secretion of milk is suppressed until birth of the baby. After delivery of the placenta there is a precipitous

drop in the hormones that had inhibited secretion by the prepared gland. In the absence of this inhibition, **prolactin,** secreted by the pars distalis of the hypophysis, is a powerful lactogenic stimulus, and full lactation is established within a few days.

Once lactation is initiated, the cells secrete continuously, but release of milk is episodic. Between breast feedings, milk is stored in the acini and small ducts. At feeding time, psychic and sensory stimuli associated with handling the baby are relayed to the hypophysis, resulting in the release of a surge of **prolactin** from its anterior lobe and **oxytocin** from its posterior lobe. Prolactin causes increased secretion into the acini, and oxytocin causes contraction of the myoepithelial cells around the alveoli, resulting in expulsion of the accumulated milk. When these complex mechanisms proceed smoothly, the average milk production of a mother feeding one baby is in excess of 1100 ml/day, and a mother of twins may produce over 2100 ml/day. Milk contains water and electrolytes (88%), protein (1.3%), and carbohydrate (3.3%) plus immunoglobulins (IgE and IgA) produced by plasma cells in the connective tissue of the gland. The principal protein component is **casein** and the principal carbohydrate is **lactose.**

After weaning of the baby, interruption of the neurohormonal stimuli and distension of the gland result in cessation of secretion, a collapse of the acini, a sloughing and autolysis of cells, and elimination of their residues by macrophages. Despite the widespread autolytic activity, some viable epithelial cells remain, forming acini without a lumen, and the myoepithelial cells persist. In a subsequent pregnancy, growth and differentiation of a functioning gland is repeated. In old age, the gland undergoes gradual atrophy of the acini and terminal portions of the duct system, reverting to the prepubertal condition.

QUESTIONS*

1. Concerning corpora albicantia which one, if any, of the following statements is correct?

   A. appear in the fetal ovary
   B. may be seen in postmenopausal ovaries
   C. develop from growing follicles
   D. secrete gonadotropins
   E. none of the above

2. Concerning spiral arteries, which one, if any, of the following statements is correct?

   A. supply the maturing ovarian follicles
   B. supply the corpus luteum
   C. supply the endometrial basalis
   D. supply the endometrial functionalis
   E. none of the above

3. Concerning the vagina, which one, if any, of the following statements is correct?

   A. contains mucous glands
   B. contains serous glands
   C. is aglandular
   D. is avascular
   E. none of the above

4. Progesterone is produced by

   A. theca interna cells
   B. the corpus albicans
   C. theca folliculi cells
   D. granulosa lutein cells
   E. the zona pellucida

5. Concerning the mammary gland, all the the following statements are correct except one. Which is the false statement?

   A. It is a compund tubuloalveolar gland.
   B. It secretes colostrum.
   C. It reaches its greatest development at about 20 years of age.
   D. It contains myoepithelial cells.
   E. It is under the direct control of FSH.

6. During the menstrual cycle, all of the following undergo more or less obvious changes **except**

   A. vagina
   B. ovary
   C. endometrium
   D. oviduct
   E. myometrium

7. Milk ejection is caused by which one of the following hormones?

   A. vasopressin
   B. estrogen
   C. oxytocin
   D. somatomammotropin
   E. progesterone

8. The glassy membrane

   A. surrounds the corpus albicans
   B. surrounds the granulosa of the ovarian follicle
   C. surrounds the theca interna of the ovarian follicle
   D. surrounds the theca externa of the ovarian follicle
   E. none of the above

9. The zona pellucida

   A. is typical of primordial follicles
   B. is produced by the theca externa
   C. supports the theca interna
   D. supports the theca externa
   E. none of the above

10. The placental barrier consists of all of the following **except**

    A. syncytial trophoblast
    B. cytotrophoblast
    C. endometrium
    D. capillary endothelium
    E. connective tissue

11. Which one, if any, of the following does **not** have secretory cells?

    A. vagina
    B. cervix
    C. endometrium
    D. ampulla of the oviduct
    E. none of the above

12. The ovarian cycle is under control of

    A. oxytocin
    B. FSH
    C. estrogen
    D. estradiol
    E. progesterone

*Answers on page 307.

24

EYE

CHAPTER OUTLINE

KEY WORDS

Accommodation
Anterior Chamber
Aqueous Humor
Bowman's Membrane
Bruch's Membrane
Choriocapillaris
Choroid
Ciliary Body
Ciliary Muscle
Cone
Conjunctiva
Cornea
Corneoscleral Coat
Crystallin
    Membrane
Dilator Pupillae
Fovea
Glands of Moll
Glands of Zeis
Iris
Larimal Duct
Lacrimal Puncta
Lacrimal Sac
Lens
Levator Palpebral
    Superioris

Limbus
Melanin
Muscle
Meibomian Gland
Nasolacrimal Duct
Optic Papilla
Ora Serrata
Orbicularis Oculi
    Muscle
Orbit
Pedicle
Posterior Chamber
Retina
Retinene
Rhodopsin
Rod
Schlemm's Canal
Sclera
Sphincter Pupillae
Superior Tarsus
Tenon's Capsule
Uvea
Vitreous Body
Vitreous Cavity

The acquisition of stereoscopic vision, evolution of a large brain, and freeing of the hands from a locomotor function enabled our hominid ancestors to develop manipulative skills that contributed to the ascendency of humans. In this chapter, we consider the eyes, the complex photoreceptor organs that enable us to sense the form, color, and movement of objects in our field of vision. Each eye occupies an **orbit,** a hemispherical cavity in the front of the skull that protects it and permits a range of eye movements. The wall of the eyeball is made up of three layers: (1) a thick, fibrous, outer layer, the **corneoscleral coat;** (2) a vascular middle layer, the **uvea;** and (3) a photosensitive inner layer, the **retina** (Fig. 24-1). The corneoscleral layer has a transparent anterior portion, the **cornea,** and an opaque posterior region, the **sclera,** that encapsulate the greater part of the eyeball and protect the delicate structures within the organ. The transparency of the cornea permits light to enter the eye and reach the retina at the back of the eye. The fibrous sclera and intraocular fluid pressure maintain the spherical shape of the eye. The uvea carries its blood supply. Its anterior margin includes the **ciliary body,** a beltlike regional specialization, containing smooth muscle that can change the shape of the lens to bring light from different distances to focus on the retina. Thus, the ciliary body is the agent of visual **accommodation,** corresponding to the focusing device on a camera. The **iris,** a thin continuation of the ciliary body anterior to the lens, is able to constrict or dilate to vary the diameter of the pupil and thus control the amount of light entering the eye. It is, therefore, an adjustable optical diaphragm, corresponding the aperture-setting device on a camera. The multilayered retina lining the posterior two-thirds of the eye contains the **rods** and **cones,** the receptors for light. It also contains complex neural networks that encode visual information and send it through the optic nerve to the **visual cortex** of the brain.

The interior of the eye has three chambers: (1) the **anterior chamber** between the cornea and the iris, (2) the **posterior chamber** between the iris and lens, anteriorly, and the vitreous body, posteriorly, and (3) the **vitreous cavity,** the large spherical space between the lens and the retina (Fig. 24-1). The transparent media in the path of the light are, in sequence, the **cornea,** the **aqueous humor** (the fluid content of the anterior chamber), the **lens,** and the **vitreous body,** a gelatinous translucent substance that fills the posterior chamber.

SCLERA

The sclera is a thick, fibrous layer, ranging in thickness from 0.6 mm near the corneoscleral junction to 1.0 mm at the porterior pole of the eye. It consists of flat bundles of collagen fibers, networks of elastic fibers, and occasional flattened fibroblasts between the fiber bundles. It is connected by loose strands of thin collagen fibers to **Tenon's capsule,** a thin sheet of connective tissue separating the

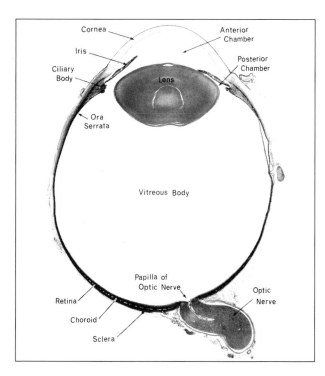

Fig. 24-1 Photomicrograph of a meridional section of the eye of a rhesus monkey. (Courtesy of H. Mizoguti.)

eyeball from the adipose tissue that fills much of the bony orbit behind the eyeball. A narrow **episcleral space** between the sclera and Tenon's capsule permits the eyeball to rotate. Movements of the eyeball depend on extraocular muscles with origins on the wall of the orbit and insertions onto the sclera.

CORNEA

The cornea is slightly thicker than the sclera, measuring 1.1 mm in the center and 0.6mm at its periphery. Within it, five layers are identifiable in histological sections: (1) the **corneal epithelium,** (2) **Bowman's membrane,** (3) the **corneal stroma** (substantia propria), (4) **Descemet's membrane,** and (5) the **endothelium** (Fig. 24-3). The epithelium consists of about five layers of unkeratinized cells. It has a very rich supply of sensory nerve endings and has a remarkable capacity for regeneration. Minor injuries are repaired by a gliding movement of neighboring cells to fill the defect, followed by an increased rate of mitosis in the basal layer. **Bowman's membrane,** beneath the epithelium, is not a membrane in the usual sense of the word, but is a lamina 10–12 μm thick, consisting of a feltwork of randomly oriented thin fibrils of collagen. It ends abruptly at the margin of the cornea. The **stroma** or **substantia propria,** making up 90% of the thickness of the cornea (Fig. 24-3), is a connective tissue with a highly ordered arrangement of its bundles of collagen fibers. They form thin lamellae arranged in many layers. Within each lamella, the fibers are parallel, but those of successive

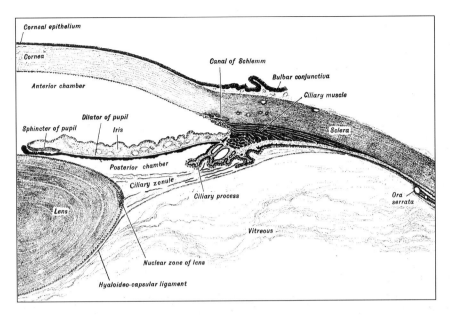

Fig. 24-2 Drawing of the sclerocorneal junction, iris, lens, and ciliary body as seen in a meridional section of the eye.

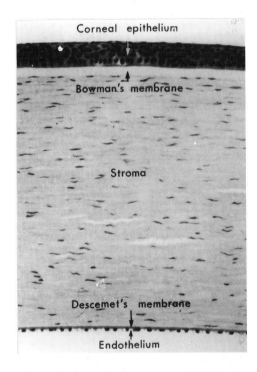

Fig. 24-3 Photomicrograph of a section of the human cornea. (From T. Kuwabara, in R.O. Greep, ed., Histology, 2nd ed., McGraw-Hill Book Co., New York, 1966.)

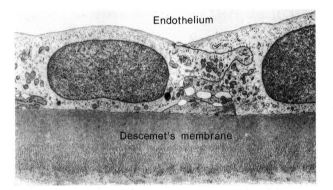

Fig. 24-4 Electron micrograph of the endothelium and underlying Descemet's membrane. (Courtesy of T. Kuwabara.)

simple squamous **endothelium** on the inner surface of the cornea (Fig. 24-4).

The cornea is avascular and depends on diffusion of oxygen from the atmosphere or from the aqueous humor in the anterior chamber. Its transparency is attributable, at least in part, to the uniform diameter and changing orientation of the collagen fibers in its successive layers. With this arrangement, scattered rays of light cancel each other by destructive interference. When corneal edema occurs, the increase in the amount of interfibrillar fluid results in cloudiness of the cornea.

SCLEROCORNEAL JUNCTION

The transition from the highly ordered, transparent cornea to the opaque connective tissue of the sclera is called the **sclerocorneal junction,** or the **limbus.** On its inner surface, there is a shallow depression occupied by a

lamellae change direction so that they are nearly at a right angle to those of the neighboring lamellae. The cells are thin flattened fibroblasts lodged in narrow clefts between successive lamellae. Cells and fibers are embedded in a ground substance, rich in chondroitin sulfate and keratan sulfate. **Descemet's membrane** is simply a very thick basal lamina (7–10 μm) consisting of an hexagonal array of very thin, atypical collagen fibrils. It is a product of the trabecular meshwork made up of strands of connective tissue covered by an endothelium that is continuous with that on the posterior surface of the cornea (Fig. 24-6). Aqueous humor, percolating through the maze of endothelium-lined spaces of the meshwork, finds its way into **Schlemm's canal,** a tubular space that encircles the periphery of the cornea. Twenty-five to 50 slender channels, radiating from the outer wall of the canal, communicate with deep veins of the limbus, which drain into the episcleral veins. Thus, aqueous humor, following this path, drains into the circulatory system.

> *In older individuals, decreased outflow of fluid through the trabecular meshwork and Schlemm's canal leads to* **glaucoma.** *The resulting elevation in intraocular pressure results in a progressive loss of peripheral vision. This is a major cause of blindness. Medications may slow the progress of the disorder. If this fails, laser surgery on the trabecular meshwork may improve drainage.*

The corneal epithelium is continuous, at the limbus, with the epithelium of the **conjunctiva,** the mucous membrane that covers the anterior surface of the eyeball around the cornea. At its periphery, the conjunctiva is reflected from the eyeball onto the inner surface of the eyelids. At the margin of the cornea, Bowman's membrane terminates and is replaced by connective tissue underlying the epithelium of the conjunctiva. Radially arranged loops of blood capillaries in this layer extend a few millimeters into the cornea. Metabolites diffusing from these vessels contribute to the nutrition of the avascular central portion of the cornea.

THE UVEA

The **uvea** is the middle layer of the wall of the eyeball. It has three regions: the **choroid,** the **ciliary body,** and the **iris.** The choroid is the highly vascular portion of the uvea that underlies the retina and provides it with oxygen and other metabolites. The **ciliary body** is a specialized anterior region of the uvea that extends from the anterior margin of the retina, the **ora serrata,** to the sclerocorneal junction Figs. 24-5 [see Plate 32] and 24-6). The **iris** is a thin diaphragm that continues from the ciliary body over the anterior surface of the lens. Its inner edge outlines the **pupil** of the eye.

Choroid

The choroid is a thin, highly vascular layer immediately beneath the sclera. It contains many blood vessels surrounded by loose connective tissue rich in fibroblasts, macrophages, lymphocytes, and plasma cells. Melanocytes, present in limited numbers, give this layer a brown color. The inner portion of this layer, the **choriocapillaris,** contains a dense network of capillaries essential for the nutrition of the retina. These are lined by endothelium that is fenestrated on the side toward the retina. The choroid is separated from the retina by **Bruch's membrane,** a refractile layer 1–4 μm in thickness. The choroid ends anteriorly at the ora serrata, the irregularly scalloped anterior margin of the retina.

Ciliary Body

The ciliary body is a circumferential thickening of the uvea between the ora serrata and the lens. It is involved in suspension of the lens and in **accommodation** (the changes in the shape and position of the lens that bring light rays to focus on the retina). In a meridional section of the eyeball, its shape is that of a slender inverted triangle with its base toward the anterior chamber (Figs. 24-2 and 24-5 [see Plate 32]). About 70 radially oriented ridges, the **ciliary processes,** project from its base toward the lens. These are covered by a bilaminar epithelium and have a core of loose connective tissue. Slender **zonula fibers** originating in the basal lamina of the ciliary epithelium pass between its cells and insert into the capsule of the lens, holding it in place (Fig. 24-2).

The bilaminar **ciliary epithelium** is an anterior continuation of the retina. Due to its origin from the two layers of the invaginated embryonic optic cup, the ciliary epithelium is exceptional in that the apices of the cuboidal cells of its outer layer are apposed to the apices of the cells in the lower layer, and there is a basal lamina on both surfaces of the epithelium. The cell apices in the two layers are joined by desmosomes, but there are small intercellar spaces between them. The cells of the layer adjacent to the core of the ciliary processes are filled with melanin pigment granules (Fig. 24-6). Those of the unpigmented outer layer contain many mitochondria and cisternae of rough endoplasmic reticulum. The plasmalemma adjacent to the basal lamina is elaborately infolded as in other epithelia transporting water and ions. The ciliary epithelium produces the **aqueous humor,** a clear fluid containing most of the soluble constituents of the blood but very little protein. This fluid moves from the posterior chamber through the pupil into the anterior chamber, from where it is drained through the trabecular meshwork and canal of Schlemm. Maintenance of the optimal intraocular pressure depends on an accurate balance between the rate of its production by the ciliary epithelium and the rate of its outflow to the episcleral veins. When this balance is disturbed, intraocular pressure is increased, resulting in serious damage to the optic nerve and retina.

The bulk of the ciliary body consists of the **ciliary muscle,** the muscle of accommodation. It is made up of bundles of smooth muscle of differing orientation. One group close to the sclera is oriented anteroposteriorly and stretches the sclera. Others radiate medially toward the

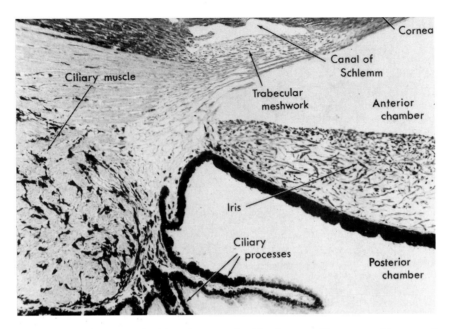

Fig. 24-6 Photomicrograph of the sclerocorneal angle of a normal human eye. (Courtesy of T. Kuwabara.)

vitreous, and still others, at the base of the ciliary processes, are oriented circularly. Contraction of the circular fibers eases tension on the zonula fibers, permitting the lens to become more convex, thus changing its refractive power. Connective tissue of the ciliary body and blood vessels from highly vascular choroid form the core of the ciliary processes.

Iris

The iris arises from the ciliary body and projects toward the anteroposterior axis of the eye, anterior to the lens. It separates the anterior from the posterior chamber and consists of highly vascular loose connective tissue, covered on its posterior surface by a continuation of the ciliary epithelium. The layer of this epithelium, which is not pigmented on the ciliary body, becomes heavily pigmented on the iris. The other layer becomes less pigmented on the iris and its cells are transformed into myoepithelial cells with long radiating processes filled with myofilaments. Collectively, the myoepithelial cells of the iris constitute the **dilator pupillae** that increases the diameter of the pupil. In the stroma of the iris near the pupil, there is a thin flat ring of circumferentially oriented smooth-muscle cells, forming the **sphincter pupillae** (Fig. 24-7). Its contraction reduces the diameter of the pupil. The ability to change the diameter of the pupil permits vision over a wide range of light intensities. Moreover, when the pupil constricts in bright light, the depth of focus is increased and aberrations (imperfections in the refraction of a lens) are minimized. The anterior surface of the iris is not covered by epithelium but is made up of a discontinuous layer of fibroblasts and melanocytes. The stroma of the iris consists of loose connective tissue containing many blood vessels. These

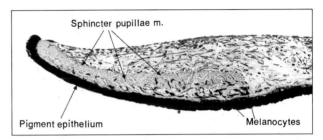

Fig. 24-7 Photomicrograph of a section through the human iris. (Courtesy of T. Kuwabara.)

are atypical, in that they lack smooth muscle in their wall, regardless of their size. The color of the iris depends on the number of melanocytes in its stroma. If they are few, the light reflected from the pigmented epithelium on its posterior surface will appear blue. If they are abundant, the iris will appear brown.

REFRACTIVE MEDIA OF THE EYE

The refractive media of the eye are the **cornea,** the **lens,** and the **vitreous body.** The structure of the cornea has been described above. Its refractive power, which is a function of its index of refraction (1.376) and its radius of curvature (7.8 mm), is twice as high as that of the lens. The biconvex lens is quite elastic and therefore capable of slight changes in shape. It is about 10 mm in diameter and 3.7–4 mm in thickness, but its thickness can increase to 4.5 mm in accommodation (the bringing of near subjects into focus upon the retina). The lens is covered by a homogeneous, highly refractile lens capsule rich in type IV collagen and proteoglycans. Beneath the capsule, on the anterior surface of the lens, is a layer of cuboidal epithelial

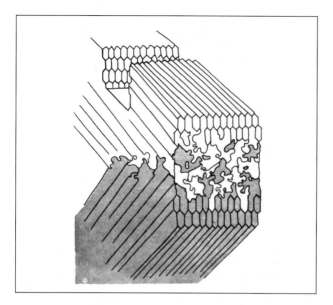

Fig. 24-8 Schematic drawing of the arrangement of the lens fibers. They have an hexagonal cross section except in the suture area, where there may be considerable interdigitation of fibers converging from opposite sides of the lens. (From T. Wanko and M. Green, Structure of the Eye, Academic Press, New York, 1961.)

cells, the **subcapsular epithelium**. Toward the equator of the lens, these cells become columnar. Further differentiation and elongation of cells, in this equatorial region, results in long **lens fibers** that make up the bulk of the lens. The term lens fiber is unfortunate, for each of these is a

modified epithelial cell, shaped like a six-sided prism 7–10 mm long, 8–12 μm wide, and only 2 μm thick (Fig. 24-8). They number about 2000 in the human lens. They have a curved course from the anterior toward the posterior surface of the lens. The outer fibers are nucleated, whereas the deeper fibers have lost their nuclei. They are arranged in precise rows in multiple layers. In some regions, their surfaces are elaborately interdigitated (Fig. 24-8). Elsewhere, they have only a few short, rounded processes that fit into depressions of conforming shape in the adjacent fiber (Fig. 24-9B). The cytoplasm of the lens fibers contains few organelle but has many intermediate filaments and a large amount of a family of proteins called **crystallins.**

> *Inflammatory ocular disease, metabolic disorders, or aging may result in **cataracts**, an opacification of the lens that causes blurred vision. This can be corrected by removing the lens from its capsule and its replacement with a plastic lens.*

The **vitreous body,** between the lens and the retina, is a colorless, transparent, gelatinous mass. It is 99% water, with a liquid phase and a solid phase. The liquid phase contains highly hydrated long molecules of hyaluronic acid, and the solid phase consists of a network of very thin collagen fibers, 6–15 nm in diameter. Near its periphery, it contains a few cells called **hyalocytes** that probably synthesize the collagen and much of the hyaluronic acid of the vitreous body.

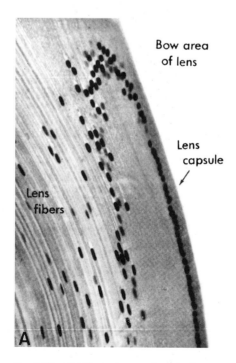

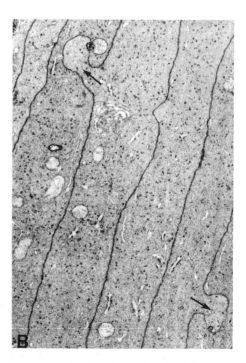

Fig. 24-9 (A) Photomicrograph of the bow area of the human lens, where the epithelial cells become greatly elongated to form the lens fibers. (B) Electron micrograph of cortical fibers of the human lens. The cytoplasm is homogeneous and contains few organelles. Short processes extend from one fiber into a depression of corresponding shape in the neighboring fiber (at arrows). (Micrographs courtesy of T. Kuwabara.)

THE RETINA

The retina contains the photoreceptors essential for vision. Its photosensitive portion extends from the papilla of the optic nerve at the back of the eye to the posterior margin of the ciliary body. Its outmost layer, the **pigment epithelium,** is separated from the choroid by **Bruch's membrane,** a thin layer on the inner surface of the choroid. The supranuclear cytoplasm of the pigment epithelial cells is filled with melanin granules, and these extend into long apical processes that occupy spaces between the outer segments of the rods and cones of the retina. The melanin granules absorb light that has passed through the photoreceptor layer of the retina, preventing its reflection from the outer tunics of the eyeball. The basal cytoplasm of the pigment epithelial cells contains abundant smooth endoplasmic reticulum that is thought to be the site of storage of vitamin A utilized by the rods and cones. The plasmalemma at the cell base is infolded and interdigitated with basal processes of neighboring cells.

With aging, extracellular material may accumulate in the pigment epithelium and there may be large breaks in Bruch's membrane and an associated proliferation of subretinal blood vessels. These changes lead to **macular degeneration** *with slowly progressive loss of vision.*

Photoreceptor Cells

The photoreceptor cells are the **rods** and **cones.** Both are long slender cells oriented parallel to one another and perpendicular to the layers of the retina (Fig. 24-10 [see Plate 32]). Rods greatly outnumber the cones. In the human, their number is estimated to be about 120 million. The smaller number of cones are distributed among them, a uniform distance apart (Fig. 24-11). The photosensitive portion of the rod is its cylindrical **outer segment,** which is made up of a very large number of closely spaced, membranous disks oriented transverse to the long axis of the cell (Fig. 24-12). Each of these is a membrane-limited saccule flattened into a disk about 2 μm in diameter and 14 nm thick (Fig. 24-13A). The outer segment of the rod is continuously renewed. Disks at its tip are exfoliated and ingested by the cells of the underlying pigment epithelium, and new disks are formed, at the same rate, at the base of the outer segment. The outer segment is totally renewed in 10–14 days. The outer segment is connected to the **inner segment** by a slender stalk, containing a short cilium that emerges from a centriole in the distal end of the inner segment (Fig. 24-13A). The outer portion of the inner segment is filled with long mitochondria (Fig. 24-12). Its inner portion expands into an ovoid cell body containing the nucleus, a small Golgi complex, occasional tubules of endoplas-

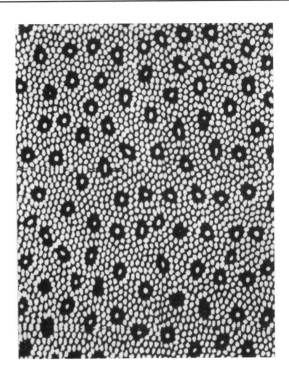

Fig. 24-11 Photomicrograph of a section through the outer segments of the photoreceptors of monkey retina, showing their uniform distribution, and the relative numbers of rods and cones. Micrograph is printed as a negative. White dots surrounded by a black ring are the cones. (Courtesy of E. Raviola.)

mic reticulum, and longitudinally oriented microtubules. Toward the vitreous cavity, the cell body tapers down to a thin cell process called the **inner fiber.** This ends in a terminal expansion, the **spherule,** which synapses with the second of a series of neurons that conduct the visual stimulus to the brain (Fig. 24-12, 24-14). The spherule is invaginated into a cuplike form around postsynaptic elements that are dendrites of the **bipolar cells** of the retina. The cytoplasm of the spherule contains a dense **synaptic rod,** or ribbon, immediately surrounded by a halo of synaptic vesicles (Fig. 24-14).

The membrane of the disks in the outer segment of the rod contains **rhodopsin (visual purple),** which consists of a pigment, **retinene,** bound to a large protein molecule. When exposed to light, retinene dissociates from the protein, a process called **"bleaching."** In the dark, the complex is reconstituted. Bleaching of rhodopsin by light initiates the visual stimulus. Rhodopsin is synthesized in the inner segment of the rod, transported through the stalk to the outer segment, and incorporated in the new disks being formed there.

The cones number 6–7 million. Like the rods, they consist of an outer segment connected to an inner segment by a slender stalk. However, the shape of the outer segment is conical instead of cylindrical (Figs. 24-10 and 24-12.). Near its base, the two membranes of the disks are occasionally continuous with the plasmalemma along one side, suggesting that they may form by invagination of this membrane (Fig. 24-13B). Tracer studies provide no

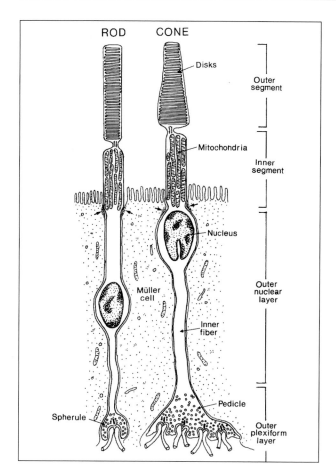

Fig. 24-12 Drawing of a rod and a cone, and the intervening Müller cell. Note the greater size of the cone inner fiber and its expanded pedicle.

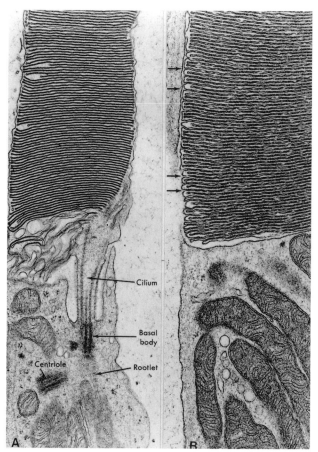

Fig. 24-13 (A) Electron micrograph of portions of the outer and inner segment of a rod. Note the cilium in the stalk conntecting the two. (B) Corresponding region of a cone. Note that some of the disks are open to the intracellular space (arrows). (Courtesy of T. Kuwabara.)

evidence of movement of the disks from base to tip, and there appears to be no exfoliation of disks and their ingestion by the cells of the pigment epithelium. Cones contain no rhodopsin. There are at least three functional types of cones, but they cannot be distinguished morphologically. Each of the cell types contains a photopigment, **iodopsin,** which absorbs photons in one of three regions of the light spectrum; 419 nm (blue), 531 nm (green), and 558 nm (red). As in the rods, the outer portion of the inner segment is rich in mitochondria (Fig. 24-15). The expanded portion containing the nucleus is relatively short. The inner fiber of the cone is thicker than that of the rod and, as it approaches the next layer of the retina, it expands into a broader ending, called the **pedicle,** which contains multiple invaginated synapses with the bipolar and horizontal cells (Fig. 24-12).

Layers of the Retina

In histological sections, seven layers are recognizable above the pigment epithelium: **photoreceptor layer, outer nuclear layer, outer plexiform layer, inner nuclear layer, inner plexiform layer, ganglion cell layer,** and the **nerve fiber layer** (Figs. 24-16 and 24-17). The photore-

ceptor layer consists of the outer segments of the rods and cones. The densely staining, outer nuclear layer includes the myriad nuclei of the rods and cones and the base of their inner fibers. The lightly staining, outer plexiform layer is largely devoid of nuclei and contains the spherules of the rods, the pedicles of the cones, and their synapses. The inner nuclear layer contains the cell bodies and nuclei of three cell types: the **bipolar cells,** the **horizontal cells,** and the **amacrine cells.** One type of bipolar cell, oriented perpendicular to the layers of the retina, connects the photoreceptor cells with large neurons in the ganglion cell layer. Its dendrites are in synaptic contact with the spherules of two or three rods, and its axon contacts up to four ganglion cells. A second type of bipolar cell (monosynaptic bipolar cell) connects a single rod cell to a smaller type of **ganglion cell.** A third type connects several cone pedicles to both large and small ganglion cells. The horizontal cells, oriented parallel to the layers of the retina, have very long processes that branch into groups of shorter processes in the plexiform layer (Fig. 24-17). Some horizontal cells contact 10 or more rod spherules. Others make contact with six or seven cone pedicles. The function of the horizontal cells is poorly

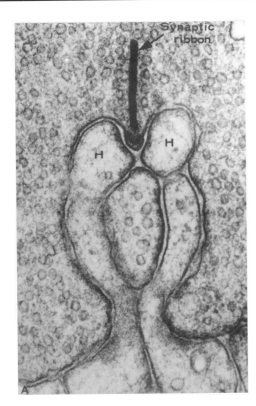

Fig. 24-14 Electron micrograph of the invaginated synapse of a rod spherule in the rabbit retina. Two deeply inserted processes (H) probably arise from a horizontal cell. (Courtesy of E. Raviola.)

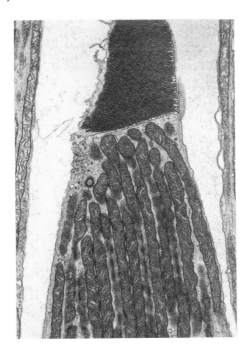

Fig. 24-15 Electron micrograph of the inner segment of a cone, showing the high concentration of mitochondria in the ellipsoid.

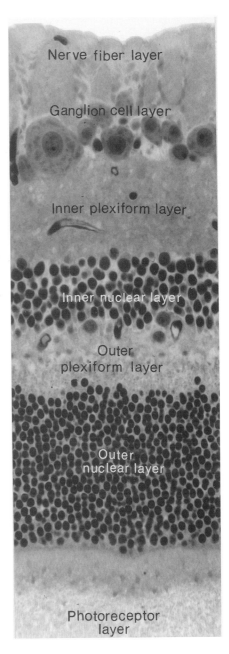

Fig. 24-16 Photomicrograph of the retina of a cat. The innermost layer is at the top. (Courtesy of A.J. Ladman.)

understood. They do not appear to have an axon and may simply serve to integrate the stimuli of groups of photoreceptors. The function of the several kinds of amacrine cells is equally obscure. They are situated in the inner portion of the inner nuclear layer and have numerous dendrites but no recognizable axon. Their processes contact the axonal endings of bipolar cells, and dendrites of multiple ganglion cells (Fig. 24-17).

The ganglion cell layer contains the cell bodies of large neurons that have been called ganglion cells only because of their resemblance to cells in the peripheral ganglia of the nervous system. They are the terminal link in the chain of neurons between the photoreceptor cells and the brain. They receive input from the bipolar cells, and their long axon becomes one of the many fibers of the optic nerve running from the retina to the visual cortex of the brain. There are at least two categories of ganglion cells in the primate retina, differing greatly in size. Their axons, in the nerve fiber layer at the inner surface of the retina, converge

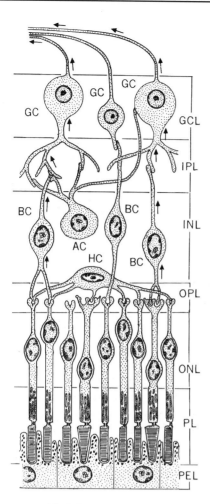

Fig. 24-17 A simplified drawing of the principal cell types of the retina. P. E.—pigment epithelium. H. C.—horizontal cell; B. C.—bipolar cell; A. C.—amacrine cells; G. C.—ganglion cell. GCL—ganglion cell layer; IPL—inner plexiform layer; INL—inner nuclear layer; OPL—outer plexiform layer; PL—photoreceptor layer; PEL—pigment epithelial layer.

upon the papilla of the optic nerve (**optic papilla**). This small round area, devoid of photoreceptors, is the so-called **"blind spot"** of the retina.

As a specialized portion of the central nervous system, the retina contains supporting elements comparable to the neuroglia of the brain. Among these are the radially oriented **Müller cells,** which are supporting cells unique to the retina. The cell body is a long slender pillar of varying width, crossing the layers of the retina and extending throughout the greater part of its thickness. At the inner and outer plexiform layers, it gives off many lateral branches that occupy the spaces between the neuronal processes in those layers. In electron micrographs, there is a conspicuous row of zonulae adherentes between the outer ends of the Müller cells and the cell bodies of the photoreceptor cells. Early histologists, using the light microscope, erroneously described this dark line as an "outer limiting membrane." The term is no longer used.

The Fovea

Slightly lateral to the optic papilla there is a shallow depression in the inner surface of the retina, about 1.5 mm in diameter, called the **fovea.** Beneath it, the bipolar and ganglion cells are displaced laterally, making the retina here thinner. (Fig. 24-18). A central area of the fovea, 500 μm in diameter, contains up to 30,000 cones and no rods. The cones are narrower and more closely packed than elsewhere. The fovea is in the visual axis of the eye and the rays of light pass directly to the outer segments of the cones without passing through inner nuclear and ganglion cell layers. This is therefore the area of greatest visual acuity in the retina.

HISTOPHYSIOLOGY OF VISION

In brief, the eye functions in the following way. The rays of light emanating from an illuminated object are refracted by the cornea onto the lens and are further bent by it to come to focus on the photosensitive retina. There, a greatly reduced inverted image of the object is formed and the quanta of incident light are transduced by the rods and cones, into nerve signals. These are processed by the network of retinal neurons and translated into nerve impulses that are conducted to the brain over the fibers of the optic nerve.

The rods and cones differ in their light sensitivity. Rods are active in dim illumination (**scotopic vision**), whereas cones are active in daylight conditions (**photopic vision**). The retinal rod is extremely sensitive to light. It is capable of responding to a single photon (the smallest unit of light energy). It requires many more photons to activate a cone cell, and signal transduction is by a different mechanism. In the rod cell, there are several thousand ion channels in its membrane. In darkness, these are held open by binding of cyclic guanosine monophosphate (cGMP), and there is free flow of ions into and out of the cell. Thus, the rods are depolarized in darkness and are releasing transmitter. When light is absorbed by rhodopsin in the disks of the outer segment, a change in its molecular configuration results in a lowering of the concentration of cGMP. This closes the ion channels, interrupting the steady inflow of Na^+ and Ca^{2+}

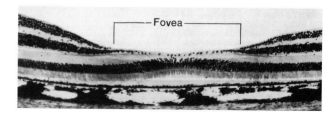

Fig. 24-18 Photomicrograph of the fovea of a macaque retina showing the marked reduction in thickness in this area of maximal acuity. (Courtesy of H. Mizoguti.)

and causing hyperpolarization of the membrane. The electrical signal created spreads to a bipolar cell, and then to the ganglion cells. These generate action potentials that are conducted to the visual cortex of the brain. In the recovery phase of the process, the visual pigment is regenerated in the disks, and calcium is pumped back into the rods. These events require energy generated by the mitochondria in the outer part of the inner segment.

ACCESSORY STRUCTURES

Eyelids

The eyelids are formed during embryonic development as folds of skin that advance over the front of the eye. The skin on their outer surface is thinner than that elsewhere on the face and its stratified squamous epithelium has few papillae. There are a few sebaceous glands and fine hairs, visible only with magnification. Deep to the subcutaneous loose connective tissue, there are transversely oriented bundles of striated muscle that constitute the palpebral portion of the **orbicularis oculi muscle,** which closes the eyelids. The upper lid is raised by the **levator palpebral superioris muscle.** Its origin is in the roof of the orbit and it terminates in a thin fascia that inserts onto the **superior tarsus,** which is a convex, hemispherical plate of dense connective tissue that stiffens the lid and makes it conform to the curvature of the underlying eyeball (Fig. 24-19).

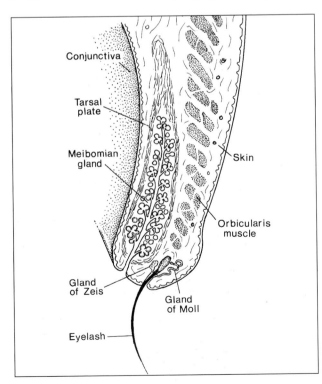

Fig. 24-19 Drawing of a section of an eyelid, showing its principal components.

Embedded within the tarsus are 20 or more parallel **Meibomian glands** that are drained by individual ducts opening in a single row along the free edge of the lid. A much smaller **inferior tarsus,** containing about 20 Meibomian glands, is found in the lower lid. The secretion of these modified sebaceous glands forms a thin lipid layer over the tear film. This retards its evaporation.

The **eyelashes** are coarse hairs set obliquely in three or four rows along the edge of the lids. They are replaced at intervals of 100–150 days. Associated with their follicles are modified sweat glands, called the **glands of Moll,** and modified sebaceous glands, the **glands of Zeis** (Fig. 24-19). The secretion of both is delivered into the infundibulum of the follicles of the eyelashes.

Conjunctiva

At the lid margins, the skin on their outer surface is continuous with the **palpebral conjunctiva** on their inner surface. This thin, transparent, mucous membrane lines the inner surface of the lids, and at their base, continues onto the front of the eyeball as the **bulbar conjunctiva** which terminates at the margin of the cornea. The conjunctival epithelium is stratified with two or three layers of cells. The basal layer is columnar and those at the surface are low cuboidal or squamous. There are a few goblet cells in this epithelium and their secretion contributes to the tear film. The potential space between the eyelids and the eyeball is called the **conjunctival sac.**

Lacrimal Glands

An almond-shaped lacrimal gland is situated above the temporal quadrant of each eyeball. It consists of several lobules drained by 6–12 ducts that open into the conjunctival sac. It is a tubuloalveolar gland in which the alveoli are somewhat distended and lined by serous columnar cells, containing pale, secretory granules. Intercellular secretory canaliculi can be found between the cells. Between the epithelium and its basal lamina are branching myoepithelial cells that contribute to expulsion of the secretion from the acini. The secretion of the lacrimal gland forms a tear film over the bulbar conjunctiva and the cornea. This fluid is drained into two tiny orifices, the **lacrimal puncta,** one on the edge of each lid at its medial end. These are the openings of two short **lacrimal ducts** about 1 mm in diameter and 8 mm long, lined by stratified squamous epithelium. These join to form a single very short duct opening into the **lacrimal sac.** This is the expanded upper end of a **nasolacrimal duct** that courses downward to open into the inferior meatus of the nasal cavity. The lacrimal sac and nasolacrimal duct are lined by ciliated, pseudostratified, columnar epithelium containing some goblet cells.

QUESTIONS*

1. In the eye, the zonule is composed of suspensory ligaments which connect the

   A. iris and ciliary body
   B. ciliary body and ciliary muscles
   C. cornea and sclera
   D. anterior and posterior chambers
   E. lens and ciliary body

2. Which of the following is the most highly vascular tissue of the eye?

   A. choroid
   B. sclera
   C. cornea
   D. lens capsule
   E. tunica fibrosa

3. The thickest layer of the cornea is the

   A. substantia propria
   B. Bowman's membrane
   C. Descemet's membrane
   D. epithelium
   E. endothelium

4. Which of the following properties shows the **least** difference between the cornea and the sclera?

   A. the degree of vascularity
   B. the degree of transparency
   C. the structure of Bowman's membrane
   D. the structure of the overlying epithelium
   E. the abundance of collagen fibers

5. The blind spot of the eye corresponds to the location of the

   A. fovea
   B. macula lutea
   C. ora serrata
   D. optic nerve head
   E. limbus

6. The flow of aqueous humor out of the eye is via the

   A. uveal tract
   B. Tenon's space
   C. lacrimal duct
   D. canal of Schlemm
   E. choriocapillaris

7. The lens of the eye is held in place by suspensory ligaments which insert into the

   A. iris
   B. ciliary body
   C. ora serrata
   D. cornea
   E. uvea

8. The fovea is a region of high visual acuity principally due to the high density of

   A. cones
   B. rods
   C. ganglion cells
   D. synapses
   E. rhodopsin

9. The corneal–scleral junction is also known as the

   A. ora serrata
   B. zonule of Zinn
   C. limbus
   D. stroma
   E. orbital septum

10. Aqueous humor is secreted by the

    A. ciliary processes
    B. suprachoroidal lamina
    C. conjunctiva
    D. iris
    E. zonule

*Answers on page 307.

25

EAR

KEY WORDS

Acoustic Meatus	Otoconium
Ampula	Otolith
Auditory Canal	Otolithic Membrane
Auditory Ossicle	Oval Window
Auricle	Perilymph
Basilar Membrane	Pinna
Cerumen	Reissner's Membrane
Cerumenous Gland	Round Window
Cochlear Duct	Scala Media
Crista Ampullaris	Scala Tympani
Cupula	Scale Vestibuli
Endolymph	Schrapnell's
Eustachian Tube	Membrane
Helicotrema	Stapedius Muscle
Incus	Stapes
Kinocilium	Stereocilium
Macula Sacculi	Stria Vascularis
Macula Utriculi	Tectorial Membrane
Malleus	Temporal Bone
Mastoid Process	Tensor Tympani
Modiolus	Tip-Link
Organ of Corti	Tympanic Membrane
Osseous Labyrinth	Vestibule

The ear is the organ of hearing, a sensitive sensory organ that has two major functions: (1) It receives sound of frequencies between 16 and 20,000 cycles per second and translates this into nerve impulses that are interpreted in the auditory center of the brain. (2) It senses linear and rotational acceleration of the head and generates nerve impulses that induce the corrective body movements necessary to restore a state of equilibrium. The organ has three regions: the **external ear,** the **middle ear,** and the **internal ear.**

THE EXTERNAL EAR

The **auricle** (**pinna**) is an irregularly shaped plate of elastic cartilage with a perichondrium rich in elastic fibers. It is covered by skin that is closely adherent to the perichondrium, except on the posterior surface of the ear where there is a small amount of subcutaneous connective tissue. The skin bears a few fine hairs and their associated sebaceous glands. Sweat glands are few or absent.

The **external auditory meatus (acoustic meatus)** is a canal about 2.5 cm in length, extending inward from the auricle (Fig. 25-1). Coarse hairs project into the outer third of the canal, and the sebaceous glands associated with their follicles are exceptionally large. The skin lining the canal also contains **cerumenous glands.** These coiled tubular glands are modified sweat glands. They secrete **cerumen,** a brownish waxy material. The ducts of the glands open

either onto the surface of the skin or into the necks of the hair follicles. At its inner end, the **auditory canal** is closed by the ovoid, translucent, **tympanic membrane** or eardrum (Fig. 25-1). This is covered on its outer surface by a thin layer of epidermis, and on its inner surface by the squamous epithelium that lines the **tympanic cavity.** Between these two epithelia, there is a tough layer of connective tissue containing both collagen and elastic fibers. In its anterior upper quadrant, the tympanic membrane is thinner and this region is referred to as **Schrapnell's membrane.** Vibration of the tense tympanic membrane by the sound waves initiates the hearing process.

THE MIDDLE EAR

The middle ear, or **tympanic cavity,** is an irregular space within the **temporal bone,** bounded laterally by the tympanic membrane. It communicates posteriorly with the air-filled spaces within the **mastoid process** of the temporal bone, and anteriorly with the **eustachian tube** that courses downward from the middle ear to the nasopharynx. The cavity is lined by squamous epithelium. A thin lamina propria intervenes between the epithelium and the periosteum of the surrounding bone. Near the opening of the eustachian tube, there is a transition from squamous epithelium to the ciliated pseudostratified epithelium that lines the tube. The act of swallowing or yawning briefly opens the eustachian tube, allowing the

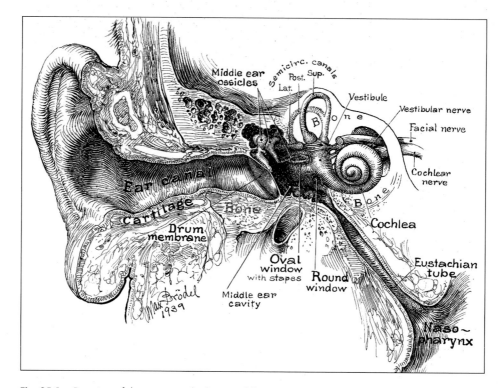

Fig. 25-1   Drawing of the anatomical relations of the various components of the human ear. From M. Brodel in J. Malone, M. Guild, and B. Crowe, eds., Three Unpublished Drawings of the Human Ear, W.B. Saunders Co., Philadelphia, 1946.)

pressure in the tympanic cavity to equalize with that of the atmosphere. The contents of the tympanic cavity include the **auditory ossicles,** and the **tensor tympani,** and **stapedius muscles.**

The auditory ossicles are a chain of three minute bones, the **incus, malleus,** and **stapes,** which extend across the tympanic cavity from the tympanic membrane to the **oval window,** an opening in the bony wall between the middle ear and the inner ear (Fig. 25-1). The three bones articulate at diarthrodial joints and are covered by the squamous epithelium lining the cavity. Their pistonlike action transforms the energy of the sound waves vibrating the tympanic membrane into more forceful oscillations of pressure in the fluid of the inner ear.

> *A bacterial infection of the middle ear (**otitis media**) is a common complication of upper-respiratory-tract infections. There is fever and severe earache as the lining of the cavity thickens and inflammatory cells (pus) accumulate in the cavity. This process may lead to perforation of the tympanic membrane and drainage into the auditory canal. Treatment is by antibiotics. The infection sometimes spreads into the air spaces of the mastoid process (**mastoiditis**). If persistent, mastoidectomy may be required.*

INNER EAR

The several components of the inner ear occupy a series of communicating cavities in the petrous portion of the temporal bone that collectively comprise the **osseous labyrinth.** It is occupied by the **membranous labyrinth,** consisting of two small sacs, the **utricle** and **saccule,** three **semicircular ducts** (anterior, posterior and lateral), emanating from the utricle, and the **cochlear duct** occupying the spiral bony canal of the osseous labyrinth (Fig. 25-2).

All portions of the membranous labyrinth contain a fluid called the **endolymph.**

The wall of the membranous labyrinth is separated from the wall of the osseous labyrinth by a **perlymphatic space** that contains a fluid of different composition called the **perilymph.** The central portion of the osseous labyrinth, called the **vestibule,** contains the utricle and saccule and these are often referred to as the **vestibular organs.**

The function of the vestibular organs is to maintain the normal position of the body. They respond to acceleration of the head by generating nerve impulses to the brain, which initiate reflexes that restore normal body position.

Utricle and Saccule

The **utricle** and the **saccule** are two small sacs occupying slightly expanded areas in the wall of the central portion of the vestibule (Fig. 25-2). Their wall consists of an outer fibrous layer, a more delicate intermediate layer of highly vascular connective tissue, and an inner layer of low-cuboidal epithelium. In certain specialized receptor regions, however, the epithelium is more complex. There is an area, 2–3 mm in diameter, in the floor of the utricle called the **macula utriculi** which consists of columnar **hair cells** and **supporting cells** (Fig. 25-3). On the free surface of each hair cell, there is a bundle of 40–80 unusually long and thick stereocilia (the "hairs") and a single cilium (Fig. 25-4). The interior of the stereocilia is filled with microfilaments of actin that extend downward into a thick terminal web. Within the bundle, the stereocilia are aligned in rows, with those in the successive rows increasing in length from 1 μm on one side to 100 μm on the side adjacent to the cilium. The cilium has the usual "9+2" arrangement of internal microtubules, but the central pair may be absent in its distal portion. Because its internal structure is typical of motile cilia elsewhere in the body, it has been regarded as a kinocilium, but it is questionable whether it is motile.

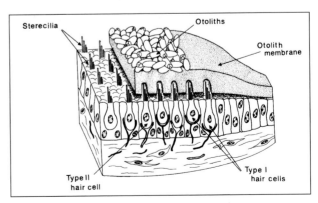

Fig. 25-3 Drawing of the macula utriculi showing the relation of the otolithic membrane to the hair cells. The drawing is cut away, at the left, to show the stereocilia on the rows of hair cells. (Redrawn from D.E. Parker, Scientific American 243:125, 1980.)

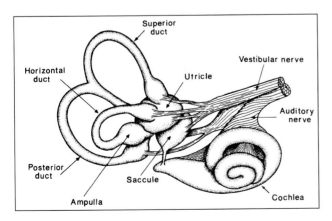

Fig. 25-2 Drawing of the membranous labyrinth of the human ear. (Redrawn from D.E. Parker, Scientific American 243:120, 1980.)

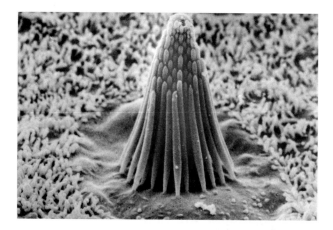

Fig. 25-4 Scanning micrograph of the bundle of stereocilia on a hair cell of the bullfrog. The bundle on vestibular hair cells of the human is very similar. (Courtesy of David Corey.)

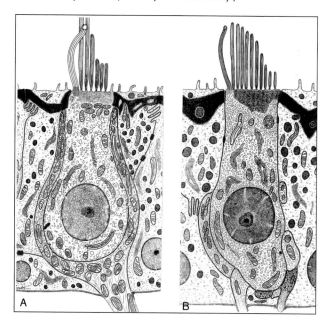

Fig. 25-5 (A) Drawing of the ultrastructural features of the type I vestibular hair cell. (B) A comparable depiction of the type II hair cell which lacks a nerve calyx.

Two kinds of hair cells are distinguishable (Figs. 25-5A and 25-5B). **Type I** has a rounded base and a narrower neck, and much of its length is surrounded by a deep, chalice-shaped afferent nerve ending, called the **calyx. Type II** is longer, more columnar, and it is not enclosed in a calyceal nerve ending. Instead, there are multiple, small afferent nerve endings in contact with its base. Synaptic ribbons are found in the peripheral cytoplasm adjacent to each afferent nerve ending. Between the hair cells, there are columnar **supporting cells** that bear numerous short microvilli on their free surface, but they are otherwise unspecialized.

The stereocilia and kinocilium of the hair cells project into the under side of a moderately thick gelatinous layer of glycoprotein that is probably secreted by the supporting cells. Traditionally, this layer has been has been called the

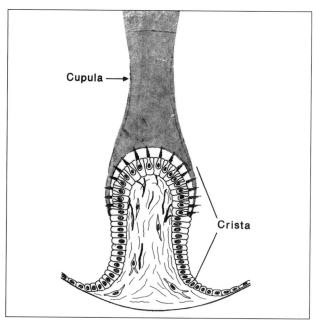

Fig. 25-7 Drawing of the crista ampullaris. (Redrawn from D.E. Parker, Scientific American 243:120, 1980.)

otolithic membrane, but "membrane" is clearly inappropriate. Embedded in the upper surface of this layer of glycoprotein are a multitude of crystalline bodies 3–5 μm in diameter, called **otoliths** or **otoconia** (Fig. 25-3). These consist of calcium carbonate and protein and are thought to provide the layer with additional inertia, resisting its displacement. Thus, when linear acceleration is applied to the head, this gelatinous layer and its otoliths tend to remain stationary, whereas the hair cells beneath tend to move slightly, bending the stereocilia (hairs) and triggering nerve impulses to the brain.

The **saccule** is lined by an epithelium similar to that of the utricle, and on its anterior wall, there is a **macula sacculi** that has a structure similar to that of the macula utriculi. However, because the macula is in the vertical anterior wall of the saccule and that of the utricle is in its horizontal floor, their hair cells respond to head movements in different directions (see below).

SEMICIRCULAR DUCTS

The **semicircular ducts,** occupying the bony semicircular canals, emerge from the utricle and return to it. The three ducts are lined by cuboidal epithelium and contain the fluid called **endolymph.** Each has a small dilatation near the utricle, called the **ampulla.** In the floor of each ampulla, there is a transverse ridge, called the **crista ampullaris** (Figs. 25-6 [see Plate 32] and 25-7). As in other sensory areas of the inner ear, the epithelium over the top of the crista consists of hair cells and supporting cells. Here, the hair cells do not extend down to the basal lamina but occupy rounded recesses between neighboring sup-

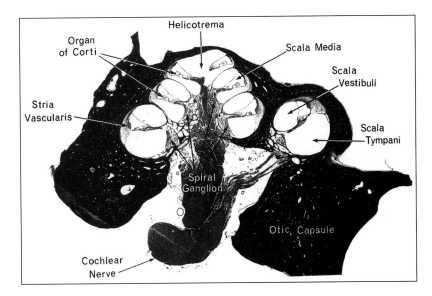

Fig. 25-8 Photomicrograph of a section through the axis of the cochlea, showing the scala vestibuli, scala tympani and the organ of Corti on the basilar membrane in the scala media. (Courtesy of H. Mizoguti.)

porting cells. On their free surface, they have a tuft of stereocilia and a single kinocilium. The ends of these extend upward into the base of a conical, gelatinous structure, called the **cupula,** which projects into the lumen of the ampulla.

The endolymph in the semicircular ducts has considerable inertia and, when the head is quickly rotated, it tends to remain stationary as the wall of the duct moves. This results in a slight movement of the crista ampullaris relative to the endolymph, in a direction opposite to the direction of head rotation. The slight movement of the cupula bends the stereocilia embedded in its base, activating the receptors. Thus, the hair cells act as minute strain gauges, responding to movement of their stereocilia toward the kinocilium.

Cochlea

The **cochlea** is anterior to the vestibule and is conical in form, 5 mm in height and 9 mm in breadth across its base. It consists of a spiral bony canal about 35 mm in length that makes two and three-quarters turns around a central pillar of spongy bone, called the **modiolus** (Figs. 25-1 and 25-8). At its base, the **cochlear canal** communicates with the tympanic cavity through two openings in its lateral wall: the **oval window** (fenestra vestibuli) and the **round window.** The oval window is closed by the foot-plate of the stapes, the third of three auditory ossicles in the tympanic cavity. The round window is closed by a membrane.

A narrow ridge projects from the modiolus of the cochlea into the spiral cochlear canal. From its edge, the **basilar membrane** extends across the canal to join a thickening of the endosteum on the opposite side. From this latter area, a second membrane, the **vestibular mem-**

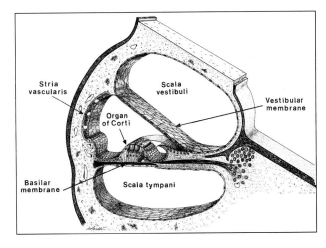

Fig. 25-9 Schematic representation of a section through one of the turns of the cochlea, showing the organ of Corti on the basilar membrane.

brane (Reissner's membrane), extends obliquely across the canal at an angle to the basilar membrane (Fig. 25-9). The lumen of the canal is thus divided into three spiral chambers: the **scala vestibuli** above the vestibular membrane, the **scala media,** between the vestibular membrane and the basilar membrane, and the **scala tympani** below. The scala media, also called the **cochlear duct,** contains **endolymph** and ends blindly at the tip of the spiral. The scala vestbuli and scala tympani contain **perilymph** and they communicate at the apex of the cochlea through a small opening, the **helicotrema.**

The vestibular membrane consists of two layers of squamous epithelium and their intervening basal lamina. The epithelium on the side toward the scala vestibuli is extremely thin. That on the side toward the scala media is slightly thicker and its cells have short clavate microvilli on their free surface. In both epithelia, the cells are joined by tight

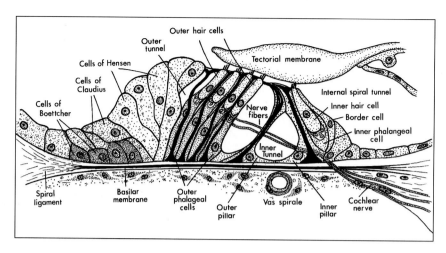

Fig. 25-10 Drawing of a section of the organ of Corti from the upper part of the first coil of the human cochlea. (Redrawn and slightly modified from J. Held, Untersuchungen uber der feineren Bau des Ohrlabyrinthes der Wiebetiere, Vols. I and II, Teubner, Leipzig, 1908.)

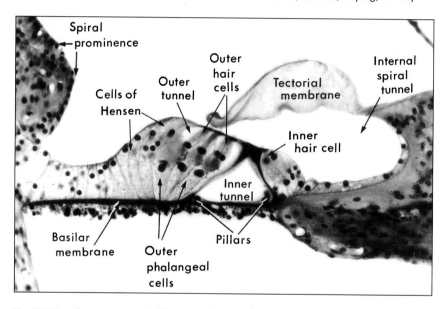

Fig. 25-11 Photomicrograph of the organ of Corti of a cat. The tectorial membrane has been lifted off of the hair cells during specimen preparation. (Courtesy of H. Engstrom.)

junctions, their lateral surfaces are interdigitated, and the cell base is elaborately infolded. These features suggest that they are involved in water and electrolyte transport. The epithelium on the side toward the scala media is continuous, at the lateral wall of the canal, with a thicker stratified epithelium, the **stria vascularis,** which contains an intraepithelial plexus of capillaries. The cells of the superficial layer of the stria have many microvilli, and their base is infolded to form a labyrinthine system of narrow cell processes filled with mitochondria. The cells of the basal layer contain fewer mitochondria and have processes that interdigitate with cells of the upper layer and surround the capillaries. The specialized epithelium of the stria vascularis is involved in water transport and maintenance of the electrolyte composition of the endolymph in the scala media.

On the basilar membrane, the epithelium is columnar and is highly specialized to constitute the receptor for auditory stimuli, the **organ of Corti,** (Figs. 25-10 and 25-11). This consists of hair cells and several types of supporting cells. One of the latter, the **phalangeal cells,** have a columnar base with a cup-shaped upper end that is occupied by the rounded base of a hair cell. A slender lateral process of the cell extends upward to the surface of the epithelium and expands into a platelike structure joined to the apex of the hair cell and to surrounding supporting cells by junctional complexes (Fig. 25-12). The cell body contains conspicuous bundles of filaments and microtubules that converge on the lateral process and continue in it to the surface of the epithelium. The well-developed cytoskeleton of these supporting phalangeal cells gives them the stiffness necessary to maintain the position of the hair cells. Two rows of a second type of supporting cell, the **outer** and **inner pillar cells,** are separated at their base by a wide intercellular space called the **inner tunnel** (Figs.

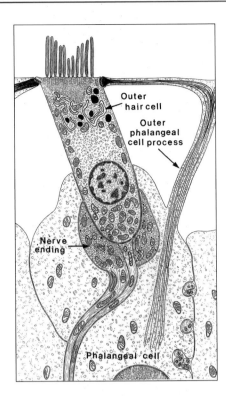

Fig. 25-12 Schematic representation of the relationship between an outer hair cell and the head of the process of its supporting phalangeal cell.

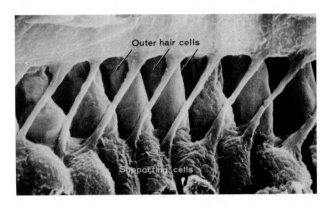

Fig. 25-13 Scanning micrograph of the outer hair cells and the slender processes of their supporting phalangeal cells. (Courtesy of H. Engstrom.)

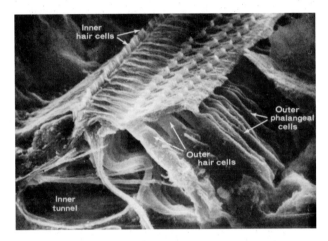

Fig. 25-14 Scanning micrograph of a guinea pig organ of Corti cut transversely, at the lower left, and and viewed longitudinally. Note the rows of hair cells (top) and the outer phalangeal cells at the right. (Courtesy of H. Engstrom.)

25-10, and 25-14). Their apices, however, are in contact with each other and with the hair cells in the rather stiff **reticular lamina,** which is a mosaic of the apical ends of the hair cells and the platelike heads of the their supporting phalangeal cells. The pillar cells on either side of the tunnel are tall cells with an unusual shape. They have a broad base containing the nucleus, but they narrow to a slender cylindrical body that is not in contact with neighboring cells. This then widens, at the apex, into a thin plate attached by junctional complexes to other cells of the reticular lamina (Figs. 25-13 and 25-14). Microtubules arising in the basal cytoplasm converge into a dense bundle that completely fills the slender body or pillar of the cell. Interspersed among the microtubules are 6-nm microfilaments. In the apical plate, the microtubules diverge and many of them end in the junctional complexes with adjacent cells. These bundles of microtubules give the pillars the stiffness to buttress the reticular plate containing the upper ends of the hair cells.

The hair cells of the organ of Corti are arranged in parallel ranks. The **inner hair cells** form a single row along the entire length of the organ (Figs. 25-14 and 25-15). On the apical surface of each is a U-shaped bundle of 50–60 hairs. A kinocilium is lacking. Some distance lateral to the inner hair cells there are three rows of taller **outer hair cells,** with their stereocilia distributed in a W-shaped pattern (Fig. 25-15). The stereocilia are stiffened by a dense bundle of actin filaments in their interior. They vary in length in a stepwise manner, so that the bundle has a short side and a long side. A thin fiber called a **tip-link** runs

diagonally from the tip of each stereocilium to the tip of the next stereocilium in the row (Fig. 25-16). The tips of the stereocilia are embedded in the **tectorial membrane**. Again, this is not a true membrane but a gelatinous sheet of glycoprotein stiffened by integral 4-nm filaments of a protein related to keratin (Figs. 25-10 and 25-11). The rounded base of each hair cell is set in a chalice-shaped depression in the body of the supporting phalangeal cell, with afferent and efferent nerves interposed between the supporting cell and the hair cell.

HISTOPHYSIOLOGY OF THE INNER EAR

Vestibular Function

The vestibular apparatus, consisting of the utricle, saccule, and semicircular ducts, responds to acceleration of the head during any disturbance of equilibrium, by sending nerve impulses to the brain that initiate reflexes which restore the body to its normal position. The receptor for

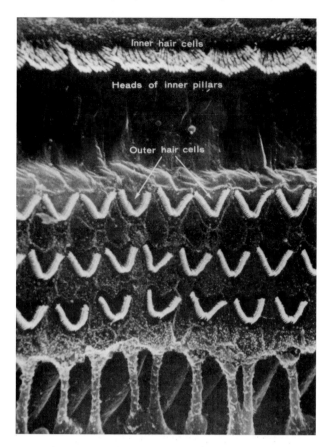

Fig. 25-15 Scanning electron micrograph of guinea pig organ of Corti as seen from above. The W-shape of the bundles of stereocilia on the outer hair cells is less clear than in the human. (Courtesy of H. Engstrom.)

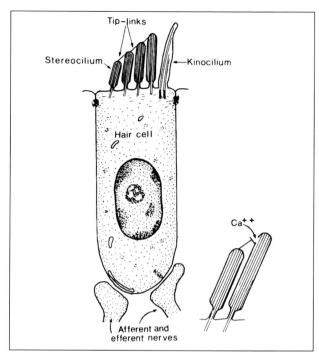

Fig. 25-16 Drawing of a vestibular hair cell showing the stereocilia and the tip-links connecting them. Deflection of the stereocilia causes the tip-links to open ion channels, permitting influx of Ca+ ions. (Redrawn from J.T. Corwin and M.E. Warchol, *Annual Reviews in Neuroscience* 14:301, 1991.)

Auditory Function

Sound waves produce vibrations of the tympanic membrane that are transmitted, via the malleus, incus, and the stapes, to the fluid in the cochlear canal. The auditory ossicles have an amplifying effect, transforming a very low pressure on the eardrum to a 20-fold greater pressure on the fluid in the cochlea. The foot-plate of the stapes acts like a piston, alternately compressing and easing the pressure on the fluid. This results in a vibration of the basilar membrane that causes a rocking motion of the organ of Corti and produces shearing forces that move the stereocilia with respect to the overlying tectorial membrane. When the bundle is deflected toward the tall side of the bundle, the tip-links between successive rows of stereocilia are stretched, resulting in opening of **transduction channels** near the tips of the stereocilia. This permits entry of Ca2+ ions, creating an inward current that depolarizes the hair cell membrane. This triggers an increase in the release of neurotransmitters at the basolateral surface of the hair cells, activating the sensory nerve endings. The tip-links thus serve as gating springs opening the ion channels. Deflection of the bundle toward its short side tends to close the channels, decreasing the rate of neurotransmitter release.

Thus, unlike other types of sensory cells, hair cells do not depend on a cascade of chemical reactions to generate a signal. Such a process would be too slow for detection of sound. To process sound in the high frequencies of human

linear acceleration of the head is the horizontally oriented **macula utriculi.** When the head undergoes linear acceleration, the otolith membrane remains relatively stationary, whereas the hair cells beneath it move slightly with the wall of the utricle, causing a deflection of the stereocilia in the direction opposite to that of the head movement. The information relayed to the brain initiates the corrective movements. The orientation of the **macula sacculi,** on the other hand, is nearly vertical and it responds to sudden movements of the head at a right angle to those that activate the macula of the utricle.

The receptors that detect angular acceleration of the head are situated in the ampullae of the three semicircular canals. The anterior (or superior) semicircular duct and the posterior semicircular duct are oriented approximately vertically, at an angle to one another, and the lateral duct is nearly horizontal. Angular acceleration of the head causes motion of the wall of one of the canals relative to the endolymph in the lumen. As the cupula is displaced, the stereocilia of the underlying hair cells are flexed in the opposite direction, resulting in depolarizing of the cells and an increase in frequency of their impulses to the brain. The brain responds by activating muscles influencing the position of the eyes and other groups that tend to correct any disturbance of equilibrium.

hearing, it is estimated that the hair cells would have to turn current on and off more than 10,000 times a second. The mechanism that makes this possible depends on the tip-links and the fact that the inner resting potential of the hair cells is negative, whereas that of the surrounding endolymph is positive, making the transmembrane potential across the apices of the hair cells higher than that of any other cell type. This increases their sensitivity to slight movement of their hairs. A deflection of only 3 nm is the threshold for hearing. This is comparable to deflection of the top of the Eiffel tower by a thumb's breadth. A deflection of 50–120 nm results in a near maximal response.

The perception of sound intensity (loudness) is called **amplitude discrimination.** This sense is dependent on the degree of displacement of the basilar membrane at any given frequency. The ability of the ear to distinguish the **frequency** (pitch) of a sound has long been attributed to differences in width of the basilar membrane along its length and to differences in length of the stereocilia on the hair cells. Each tone was believed to produce maximal amplitude of vibration in a different region of the membrane, with the sound of high frequency having the greatest effect on the membrane near the base of the cochlea, and the sound of low frequency producing maximal vibration near the helicotrema. Nerve fibers from each level along the membrane are thought to conduct impulses to an area of the brain where there are neurons that are activated by specific frequencies. This passive mechanism, based on the differing width of the basilar membrane along its length, still holds, but there is recent experimental evidence for an active fine-tuning of frequency selectivity by motor activity of the hair cells. The outer hair cells normally vary in length, from 20–50 μm near the base of the cochlea to 75–90 μm near its apex. Isolated hair cells, in the absence of a basilar membrane, have been found to respond to mechanical or electrical stimulation by a slight change in their length. Long cells respond best to low frequencies, and short cells to high frequencies. The best frequency for inducing a motor response, in a given cell, is correlated with the length of the cell and its original position in the cochlea.

There are only about 16,000 hair cells in the human cochlea and they have little or no capacity for regeneration. Millions of people suffer from impaired hearing due to loss of, or damage to, their hair cells. We live in an environment in which loud sounds are common, and about 40% of our hair cells are lost by the age of 65. In experimental animals, a 2-h exposure to a loud noise, such as a loud rock band, is enough to seriously damage the bundles of sterocilia in the inner ear.

QUESTIONS*

1. What is the most probably source of the endolymph?

   A. Reissner's membrane
   B. stria vascularis
   C. tympanic membrane
   D. helicotrema
   E. endolymphatic sac

2. The bony petrous portion of which bone is filled with perilymph?

   A. stapes
   B. parietal
   C. occipital
   D. temporal
   E. none of the above

3. What structure connects the middle ear with the oral cavity or nasopharynx

   A. oval window
   B. malleus
   C. cochlea
   D. auditory (eustachian) tube
   E. none of the above

4. Human otoconia are mostly composed of which of the following?

   A. calcium carbonate
   B. sodium carbonate
   C. sodium chloride
   D. potassium phosphate
   E. none of the above

5. Which of the following is **not** found on the basilar membrane?

   A. inner hair cells
   B. outer hair cells
   C. pillar cells
   D. phalangeal cells
   E. the stria vascularis

6. Sensory hair cells in the cristae ampullaries contact which of the following?

   A. gelatinous cupola
   B. gelatinous otolithic membrane
   C. tectorial membrane
   D. Reisner's membrane
   E. Hensen's cells

7. With which part of the ear do you associate hairs, sebaceous and ceruminous glands?

   A. tympanic cavity
   B. auditory tube
   C. external auditory meatus
   D. all of the above
   E. none of the above

8. The perception of different frequencies of sound is principally due to properties of the

   A. basilar membrane
   B. tympanic membrane
   C. round window
   D. Reissner's membrane
   E. tectorial membrane

9. The tensor tympani and stapedius are mainly composed of

   A. bone
   B. dense connective tissue
   C. striated muscle
   D. low-cuboidal epithelium
   E. elastic cartilage

10. Within the inner ear, the scala vestibuli and scala tympani communicate with each other through the

    A. ductus reuniens
    B. oval window
    C. round window
    D. helicotrema
    E. cochlear window

*Answers on page 307.

ANSWER KEY

Chapter 1

1e, 2c, 3d, 4c, 5c, 6c, 7c, 8b, 9e, 10e, 11b

Chapter 2

1e, 2d, 3d, 4d, 5c, 6a, 7b, 8e, 9e, 10b

Chapter 3

1a, 2d, 3d, 4c, 5d, 6d, 7c, 8b, 9a, 10d

Chapter 4

1c, 2d, 3c, 4c, 5c, 6c, 7e, 8b, 9e, 10d

Chapter 5

1b, 2b, 3d, 4c, 5e, 6b, 7a, 8e

Chapter 6

1e, 2d, 3c, 4d, 5a, 6b, 7b, 8d

Chapter 7

1c, 2c, 3c, 4a, 5d, 6b, 7b, 8e, 9b, 10c

Chapter 8

1a, 2a, 3c, 4d, 5b, 6e, 7c, 8a, 9a, 10d

Chapter 9

1a, 2c, 3e, 4a, 5d, 6c, 7c, 8d, 9c, 10d

Chapter 10

1d, 2c, 3e, 4a, 5b, 6c, 7c, 8d, 9a, 10b, 11a, 12e

Chapter 11

1a, 2b, 3c, 4c, 5b, 6a, 7a, 8e, 9e, 10c

Chapter 12

1b, 2e, 3d, 4c, 5b, 6e, 7a, 8d, 9e, 10d

Chapter 13

1a, 2a, 3e, 4b, 5c, 6c, 7b, 8e, 9d, 10c, 11c, 12a, 13c, 14d

Chapter 14

1e, 2a, 3b, 4c, 5c, 6b, 7d, 8e, 9b, 10a, 11c, 12e

Chapter 15

1e, 2b, 3e, 4e, 5c, 6d, 7b, 8c, 9b, 10a

Chapter 16

1e, 2b, 3d, 4e, 5a, 6b, 7d, 8c, 9b, 10d

Chapter 17

1b, 2e, 3b, 4d, 5d, 6c, 7d, 8c, 9c, 10e, 11b, 12d

Chapter 18

1e, 2d, 3d, 4a, 5a, 6c, 7c, 8c, 9b, 10e, 11d, 12e

Chapter 19

1a, 2e, 3e, 4c, 5c, 6e, 7e, 8c, 9b, 10e

Chapter 20

1d, 2e, 3d, 4b, 5c, 6e, 7d, 8c, 9e, 10e, 11b, 12a

Chapter 21

1d, 2e, 3d, 4e, 5c, 6c, 7c, 8d, 9b, 10d, 11b, 12b

Chapter 22

1c, 2d, 3d, 4d, 5e, 6c, 7c, 8d, 9c, 10b

Chapter 23

1b, 2d, 3c, 4d, 5e, 6e, 7c, 8b, 9e, 10c, 11a, 12b

Chapter 24

1e, 2a, 3a, 4e, 5d, 6d, 7b, 8a, 9c, 10a

Chapter 25

1b, 2d, 3d, 4a, 5e, 6a, 7c, 8a, 9c, 10d

INDEX

Lymph nodes, 144–146
Lymph nodules, of intestines, 205
Lymphokines, 40
Lymphopoiesis, 89–90
Lysosomes, 9
Lysozyme, 204

M
M-band, of skeletal muscle, 99
M-cells, of GI mucosa, 205
Macrophage, 39, 49–50
Macula adherens (desmosome), 24
Macula sacculi, 300
Macula utriculi, 299
Macula densa, of kidney, 247
Major histocompatability complex, 138
Malignant melanoma, 173
Malleus, 299
Malpighian bodies, 147
Mammary Gland, 281–283
Mammotropes, of hypophysis, 153
Manchette, 259
Mast cells, 51–52
Medullary cavity, bone, 70
Megakaryocytoblast, 89
Megakaryocytes, 89
Meibomian glands, 295
Meiosis, 15, 258
Meissner's corpuscles, 178
Meissner's plexus, 194
Melanin, 111, 172
Melanocyte stimulating hormone, 155
Melanocytes, 173–173
Melanosomes, 172
Melatonin, 164
Membrane coating granules, 172
Meninges, 121
Menopause, 272
Merkel cells, 174
Merkel endings, 179
Mesangium, 244
Metaphase, of mitosis, 15, 258
Microfilaments, 11–12
Microglia, 120
Microtubules, 12–13
Mitochondrion, 8–9
Mitosis, 14
Moll's glands, 295
Monocyte, of blood, 38–39
Mononuclear phagocyte system, 39
Monocytopoiesis, 89
Motor end plate, 102
Motor unit, skeletal muscle, 102
Mucocutaneous junctions, 174
Mucous neck cells, stomach, 196–197
Muller cells, of retina, 294
Multiple sclerosis, 116
Mumps, 189
Muscle, 93–106
    cardiac, 103–106
    skeletal, 96–113
    smooth, 94–96
Muscular dystrophy, 97
Myasthenia gravis, 103
Myelin sheath, 114–116
Myeloblasts, 87
Myelocyte, basophilic, 87–88
    eosinophilic, 88
    neutrophilic, 88
Myocardium, 126
Myoendocrine cells, 105
Myoepithelial cells, 177, 271
Myoid cell, of testis, 256
Myometrium, 275

Myoneural junction, 102
Myosin, 12

N
Nails, 177
Nephrons, 243–249
Nephrolithiasis, 244
Nerve impulse, 113
Nervous system, 109–122
Neurofibrils, 111
Neurofilaments, 12
Neuroglia, 119–120
Neurohypophysis, 155–156
Neurokeratin, 114
Neuron, 110–113
    axon of, 112–113
    dendrites of, 112
    perikaryon of, 110
Neurophysins, 155
Neurotransmitters, 113
Neutrophils, 35–37
Nexus, 24
Nissl bodies, 110
Node of Ranvier, 114
Norepinephrine, 113
Normoblast, 86
Nose, 230
Nuclear envelope, 3
    fibrous lamina of, 4
    perinuclear cisterna of, 3
Nuclear pore complex, 3
Nucleosomes, 4
Nucleolus, 4–5
    pars fibrosa, 4
    pars granulosa, 4
Nucleus, 3–5
Nucleus pulposus, 67

O
Odontoblast, 184
Olfactory epithelium, 230
Oligodendrocyte, 112, 115, 120
Oocytes, 270
Oral cavity, 181–190
Organ of Corti, 301
Organelles, cytoplasmic, 2, 5–10
Ossification, endochondral, 65, 75–77
Ossification intramembranous, 74
Osteoblast, 65, 71
Osteoclast, 72–73
Osteocytes, 72
Osteogenesis imperfecta, 46
Osteon, 74
Osteoprogenitor cells, 70–71
Otoliths, 300
Ovary, 270–274
Oviducts, 274–275
Ovulation, 273
Ovum (oocyte), 273
    fertilization of, 277
    implantation of, 278–279
Oxyntic cells (parietal cells), 198
Oxyphil cells, parathyroid, 159
Oxytocin, 155, 283

P
Pacinian corpuscles, 179
Pancreas, 221–226
Pancreatitis, 224
Paneth cells, 204
Papillae, circumvallate, 182
    dermal, 175
    filiform, of tongue, 182
    foliate, of tongue, 182

fungiform, of tongue, 182
Parathyroid glands, 159–160
Parathyroid hormone, 78
Parietal cells, 197
Parotid glands, 188–189
Pemphigus, 17
Penis, 266
Perforin, 140
Perichondrium, 64
Perimysium, 97   *Pericytes, 131*
Perinuclear cisterna, 3
Perineurium, 116
Periosteal collar, 75
Periosteum, 70
Peritoneum, 207
Peroxisomes, 9
Peyer's patches, 205
Phagocytosis, 16
Phalangeal cells, 301
Pia arachnoid, 121
Pia mater, 121
Pigment epithelium, eye, 291
Pillar cells, 301
Pinealocytes, 164
Pineal gland, 164–165
Pinocytosis, 15–16
Placenta, 280
Plasma cell, 50
Plasmalemma (cell membrane), 2
Platelet demarcation channels, 86
Platelets, of blood, 32–35
Pleura, 237
Pneumonocyte (alveolar cell), 235
Podocyte, of nephron, 243
Polychromatophilic erythroblast, 86
Polymorphonuclear neutrophil, 35–37, 88
Pompe's disease, 11
Pores of Kohn, 235
Portal lobule, liver, 212
Proerythroblast, 86
Progesterone, 274
Prolactin, 152–153, 283
Promyelocytes, 87
Prostate gland, 265
Prostatic hyperplasia, 265
Proximal convoluted tubule, 245
Pseudopodia, 16
Pulmonary alveoli, 234–236
Pulmonary surfactant, 236
Purkinje cell, 118
Purkinje fibers, 106
Pyloric glands, 198–199

R
Regional enteritis, 207
Renal corpuscle, 243
Reproductive system, female, 270–283
Reproductive system, male, 256–266
Respiratory bronchioles, 234
Respiratory system, 230–238
Reticular cells, 144
Reticular fibers, 46
Reticulocyte, 32, 87
Reticulum, endoplasmic, 6–7
    rough (RER), 6
    smooth (SER), 6
    sarcoplasmic, muscle
Retina, 291
Rhodopsin, 291
Ribonucleoprotein (RNA), 4
Ribonucleic acid, 5
    messenger (mRNA), 5–7
    ribosomal (rRNA), 5–7
    transfer (tRNA), 6–7